A Text Book Of

PHARMACEUTICS - I

As Per PCI Regulations

FIRST YEAR B. PHARM.
Semester I

Dr. Ashok A. Hajare
M. Pharm. Ph.D.
Professor and Head,
Department of Pharmaceutical Technology,
Bharati Vidyapeeth
College of Pharmacy, Kolhapur, Maharashtra, India

Dr. Durgacharan A. Bhagwat
M. Pharm. Ph.D.
Assistant Professor,
Department of Pharmaceutics,
Bharati Vidyapeeth
College of Pharmacy, Kolhapur, Maharashtra, India

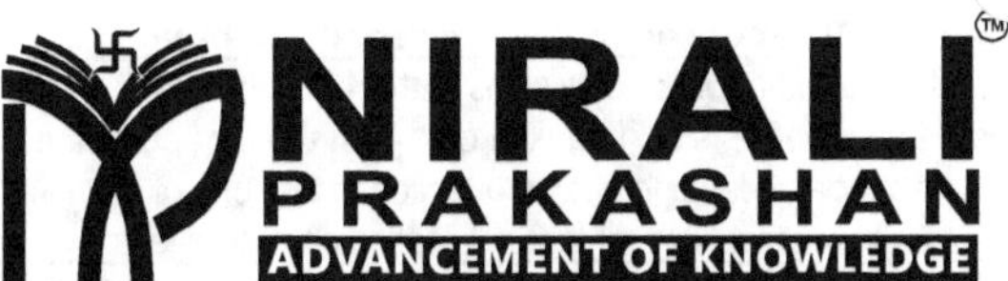

N3923

PHARMACEUTICS - I   **ISBN 978-93-86700-51-3**

Fifth Edition   :   **February 2020**

©   :   **Authors**

Published By :

NIRALI PRAKASHAN

Abhyudaya Pragati, 1312, Shivaji Nagar
Off J.M. Road, PUNE – 411005
Tel - (020) 25512336/37/39, Fax - (020) 25511379
Email : niralipune@pragationline.com

➤ **DISTRIBUTION CENTRES**

PUNE

Nirali Prakashan   :   119, Budhwar Peth, Jogeshwari Mandir Lane, Pune 411002, Maharashtra
(For orders within Pune)   Tel : (020) 2445 2044; Mobile : 9657703145
                               Email : niralilocal@pragationline.com

Nirali Prakashan   :   S. No. 28/27, Dhayari, Near Asian College Pune 411041
(For orders outside Pune)   Tel : (020) 24690204; Mobile : 9657703143
                               Email : bookorder@pragationline.com

MUMBAI

Nirali Prakashan   :   385, S.V.P. Road, Rasdhara Co-op. Hsg. Society Ltd.,
                               Girgaum, Mumbai 400004, Maharashtra; Mobile : 9320129587
                               Tel : (022) 2385 6339 / 2386 9976
                               Email : niralimumbai@pragationline.com

➤ **DISTRIBUTION BRANCHES**

JALGAON

Nirali Prakashan   :   34, V. V. Golani Market, Navi Peth, Jalgaon 425001, Maharashtra,
                               Tel : (0257) 222 0395, Mob : 94234 91860; Email : niralijalgaon@pragationline.com

KOLHAPUR

Nirali Prakashan   :   New Mahadvar Road, Kedar Plaza, 1st Floor Opp. IDBI Bank, Kolhapur 416 012
                               Maharashtra. Mob : 9850046155; Email : niralikolhapur@pragationline.com

NAGPUR

Nirali Prakashan   :   Above Maratha Mandir, Shop No. 3, First Floor,
                               Rani Jhanshi Square, Sitabuldi, Nagpur 440012, Maharashtra
                               Tel : (0712) 254 7129; Email : niralinagpur@pragationline.com

DELHI

Nirali Prakashan   :   4593/15, Basement, Agarwal Lane, Ansari Road, Daryaganj
                               Near Times of India Building, New Delhi 110002 Mob : 08505972553
                               Email : niralidelhi@pragationline.com

BENGALURU

Nirali Prakashan   :   Maitri Ground Floor, Jaya Apartments, No. 99, 6th Cross, 6th Main,
                               Malleswaram, Bengaluru 560003, Karnataka; Mob : 9449043034
                               Email: niralibangalore@pragationline.com

Other Branches : Hyderabad, Chennai

niralipune@pragationline.com | www.pragationline.com

Also find us on www.facebook.com/niralibooks

Preface

It is indeed a matter of great pride for us that, the *Pharmacy Council of India (PCI), New Delhi has framed Bachelor of Pharmacy (B. Pharm.)* course regulations 2014. The Pharmaceutics-I is a very important subject at First year of the course. It gives us a great pleasure to present this book in the hand of readers. The book is strictly written as per syllabus framed by PCI under Section 6, 7 & 8 of Regulation 2014 and we had made an attempt to make it simple and understandable to the readers. The sequence of syllabus content is designed unit wise imparting better understanding of subject matter. In this book wherever needed full forms and abbreviations, pictorial diagrams, tabular data, examples of formulation including marketed products and manufacturers are given. Model questions are given at the end of every subunit to exercise on contents studied.

We owe a great debt of gratitude to Hon. Dr. Patangraoji Kadam, Founder, Bharati Vidyapeeth Pune, for their encouragement. We are indeed very grateful to Prof. Dr. Shivajirao Kadam, Pro-Chancellor, Bharati Vidyapeeth University, Pune for his consistent and cheerful support and Dr. Vishwajit Kadam, Secretary Bharati Vidyapeeth, Pune for encouragement and motivation. We honestly extend our gratitude to Dr. H. N. More, Principal, Bharati Vidyapeeth College of Pharmacy, Kolhapur for freedom to work and timely help. We are thankful to Mrs. Snehal Patil Librarian for her co-operation during literature work.

We thank Mrs. Suvarna and Mrs. Shital, Digvijay and Aarush and our parents from bottom of heart for sustained support, encouragement and for their forbearance.

We are thankful to Mr. Jignesh Furia, Akbar Shaikh, Anagha Kaware, Chaitali Takle of Nirali Prakashan, Pune and Staff of Nirali Prakashan for bringing out nicely printed book.

Dr. A. A. Hajare
Dr. D. A. Bhagwat

∎∎∎

Syllabus

Unit I [10 Hours]
- **Historical Background and Development of Profession of Pharmacy:** History of Profession of Pharmacy in India in relation to Pharmacy Education, Industry and Organization, Pharmacy as a Career, Pharmacopoeias: Introduction to IP, BP, USP and Extra Pharmacopoeia.
- **Dosage Forms:** Introduction to Dosage Forms, Classification and Definitions.
- **Prescription:** Definition, Parts of Prescription, Handling of Prescription and Errors in Prescription.
- **Posology:** Definition, Factors Affecting Posology. Pediatric Dose Calculations based on Age, Body Weight and Body Surface Area.

Unit II [10 Hours]
- **Pharmaceutical Calculations:** Weights and Measures – Imperial and Metric System, Calculations involving Percentage Solutions, Alligation, Proof spirit and Isotonic solutions based on Freezing Point and Molecular Weight.
- **Powders:** Definition, Classification, Advantages and Disadvantages, Simple and Compound Powders – Official Preparations, Dusting Powders, Effervescent, Efflorescent and Hygroscopic Powders, Eutectic Mixtures, Geometric Dilutions.
- **Liquid dosage forms:** Advantages and Disadvantages of Liquid Dosage Forms. Excipients used in Formulation of Liquid Dosage Forms. Solubility enhancement techniques.

Unit III [08 Hours]
- **Monophasic liquids:** Definitions and Preparations of Gargles, Mouthwashes, Throat Paint, Eardrops, Nasal Drops, Enemas, Syrups, Elixirs, Liniments and Lotions.
- **Biphasic liquids:**
  - ➤ **Suspensions:** Definition, Advantages and Disadvantages, Classifications, Preparation of Suspensions; Flocculated and Deflocculated Suspension and Stability Problems and Methods to Overcome.
  - ➤ **Emulsions:** Definition, Classification, Emulsifying Agent, Test for the Identification of Type of Emulsion, Methods of preparation and Stability Problems and Methods to Overcome.

Unit IV [08 Hours]
- **Suppositories:** Definition, Types, Advantages and Disadvantages, Types of Bases, Methods of Preparations, Displacement Value and its Calculations, Evaluation of Suppositories.
- **Pharmaceutical Incompatibilities:** Definition, Classification, Physical, Chemical and Therapeutic Incompatibilities with Examples.

Unit V [07 Hours]
- **Semisolid Dosage Forms:** Definitions, Classification, Mechanisms and Factors Influencing Dermal Penetration of Drugs, Preparation of Ointments, Pastes, Creams and Gels, Excipients used in Semi Solid Dosage Forms, Evaluation of Semi Solid Dosages Forms

■■■

Contents

∎∎∎

UNIT I

Chapter 1 ...

Historical Background and Development of Profession of Pharmacy

LEARNING OBJECTIVES

Pharmaceutics course is not only introductory for the Pharmaceutical Sciences but it is helpful to the students to explore the historical evolution, the potential and the perspectives of their scientific field.

The objectives of this chapter include:

- Recall the history of pharmacy, pharmaceutical practice, development of pharmacy profession and pharmaceutical industry in India.
- To acquaint the young pharmacy students with the official pharmaceutical literature, its importance and scope.
- To inform students about historical development of pharmacy education in India.
- To improve pharmacists participation in the organizational activities at various levels.
- To spread awareness among the students about career opportunities in the pharmaceutical field.
- To create awareness of latest advances and discoveries in the dosage forms.
- To know the history of profession of pharmacy

1.1 HISTORY OF PHARMACY PROFESSION

The history of pharmacy profession can be traced back to third millennium BC in Samaria. Samarian people developed a cuneiform writing style on clay tablets which included lists of drugs of animal, vegetable and mineral origin that were used in the management of diseases, and prescriptions with details of the ingredients used in their compounding. Greeks were one of the first patrons of pharmacy profession. This profession can be traced back to the Sumerian population, living in modern day Iraq. Knowledge of preparation and application of natural products for healing is as old as man himself. Earliest known records of preparation of medicines are Babylonian 2600 BC. They called for combination of pharmaceutical, medical and religious measures. The *Ebers Papyrus* document dating back to 1550 BC describes prescriptions and modes of administration of drugs including gargles, inhalations, suppositories, ointments and lotions.

The Ancient Egyptians preparing specific medicine were known as *Pastophor*. Egyptians commonly used mortar and pestles, hand mills, sieves, balances for their compounding of suppositories, gargles, pills, inhalations, troches, lotions, ointments, plasters and enemas.

(1.1)

Pharmacy was viewed as a high status branch of medicine, and again, like the Sumerians, these pharmacists were also priests who worked and practiced in the temples. The papyrus 'The Ebers Papyrus' a continuous scroll some 60 feet long and foot wide written during 1500 B.C. includes 800 prescriptions (formulas) and 700 drugs. The drugs are chiefly botanical such as acacia, castor bean, fennel etc. The vehicles were beer, wine, milk and honey. Many of the pharmaceutical formulas employed about two dozen or more medicinal agents, a type of preparation are called 'Polypharmacal'. Literature indicates that the Egyptians were involved in making and using infusions, ointments, lozenges, suppositories, lotions, enemas, and pills.

In China, a comprehensive theory for diagnosis and treatment was developed. The text *Huangdi Neijing* listed the basic principles of pharmaceutical drug use in the third century BC. In India Ayurvedic medicine was first described around 800 BC. Documents list the use of drugs together with charms for expelling demons and make reference to the god of medicine, *'Dhanvantari'*. The *'Charaka Samhita'* includes reference to drugs of animal, plant and mineral origin used until the first century AD. Hippocrates (460 BC) is considered to be the 'Father of Medicine'. He is associated with a number of documents known collectively as the *Hippocratic Corpus* dating to 420–370 BC, which list 200–400 drugs of vegetable origin and describe the method of preparation of gargles, ointment and pessaries. Hippocrates a Greek physician is credited with the introduction of scientific pharmacy and medicine, oath of ethical behaviour for the healing profession and honored by being called the 'Father of Western Medicine'.

King of Pontus (presently Turkey), Mithridates (134–63 BC) experimented with poisons and antidotes, tried them on himself and prisoners of war. Arabian Christian twin brothers Damian and Cosmas practiced pharmacy and medicine together until their martyred in 304 AD. Dioscorides (40-90 AD) a Greek physician and botanist, is known for his work which deals with botany as an applied science of pharmacy. Dioscorides prepared the document *De Materia Medica* around AD 60–78. Galen was physician around AD 160. He compiled medical knowledge of the time drawing on the documents by Hippocrates and Dioscorides. He described the use of formulations made-up of numerous plants which were referred to as 'galenicals'. In ancient Japan pharmacists were highly respected. In the Imperial household, the pharmacist was even ranked above the two personal physicians of the Emperor.

The Arabic period, stretching from the 7th to the 12th century is regarded as the period of transmission of the cultural and scientific heritage of Antiquity and of the East to the West. Monks, trained as apothecaries, preserved an advanced knowledge during the Middle Ages (5th to 12th centuries); raised medicinal herbs in cloister gardens, for the treatment of ill and injured in their care. Profession of pharmacy started acquiring shape during 9th century in the civilized world around Baghdad. It slowly spread to Europe as alchemy and finally developed into chemistry. The first known chemical process was carried out by the artisans of Mesopotamia, Egypt, and China.

Pharmacy always existed, but not so for pharmacists. Since initially medicine and pharmacy were not independent from one another. A person uses to made diagnosis also provides medicines. The physician was a man of authority without formal education. When the physician could no longer cope with his work, he hired assistants to collect herbs for him and make preparations under his supervision. These assistants were called pharmacopolae but they were not pharmacists. Arabs with their clear insight and mathematical approach realized that this situation could not persist. The simultaneous exercises of medicine and pharmacy were incompatible. The people dealing with the health of patients supposed to acquire professional and ethical education. The mutual control between physician and pharmacist provided a much higher degree of safety in a domain where people care most for their health and life. The Arabs were of thought that those who prepare medicines could do so in an independent profession. Ultimately this thought separated medicine and pharmacy. The first pharmacy shop was opened in Bagdad in 770 under Caliph Al-Mansoer. Pharmacists that time had much experience with medicines but did not possess the required education. This situation was changed by Caliph Al Mamoen, who ruled Bagdad from 813 to 833 and pharmacists started acquiring professional education.

Frederic II in 1231 made constitution with legal norms in relation to medicine which had been established by the Arabs. He divided medicine into dogmatic medicine which makes diagnoses; manual medicine, which performs surgical interventions; and pharmaceutical medicine, which collects mixes and conserves medicines. The profession of pharmacy was honorable form initial days. Pharmacists were often called Sayadilah in Arabic works and Sandaliin Latin. Arabs who founded pharmacy also expanded the pharmaceutical armamentarium. Arabs and the Mohammedans met each other on their pilgrimage to Mecca, provided for the exchange of ideas as well as of goods between people from India, China and Spain that introduced many new drugs in the field of medicine. Arabs developed number of new drug delivery forms such as syrups, pellets, preserves, confections, marmalades.

The earliest recorded shop dealing with sales of medicines in London was opened in 1345. In England, Chaucer in his treatise *'The Knight's Tale'* (written around 1386) used the word 'pharmacy' to describe a medical preparation of plants "Farmacies of Herbs". Between the 1500s and 1700s, the distinctions between alchemy and medicinal chemistry were somewhat blurred. Chemist and druggist was a term first used to describe both chemical and drug merchants and practitioners of the emerging profession of pharmacy from the late 1700s.

The term apothecary, often used between the 1600s and 1800s, for individuals living in London who had passed the examinations of the Worshipful Society of Apothecaries of London, founded in 1617. The role of the apothecary developed out of the role of the spicer who involved in trading crude drugs and preparing medicines. Apothecaries were strongly involved in dispensing but they were supposed to do all work including handling of drugs and chemicals, examining and treating patients. Apothecaries did not charge for these services but only for the medicines supplied. Following a ruling in the Rose Case (1701-1703/4), apothecaries became legally ratified members of the medical profession to prescribe and dispense medicines.

Unable to attract apothecaries or physicians to the new world, John Winthrop, Governor of Massachusetts colony (1630 – 1649), sought advice by correspondence and performed apothecaries service in his own house for citizen of colony. As apothecaries moved into a more advisory role, chemists and druggists developed themselves in the area of preparation and supply of medicines. It resulted into competition between them with the apothecaries. The apothecaries tried to control the chemists and druggist's activities in 1748 with a proposed new law to control the supply of medicines. But this didn't progress. In America first hospital pharmacy began operations in 1752; one year after Pennsylvania hospital was established in Philadelphia house. John Morgan, first as hospital pharmacist, later as physician, championed independent practice of two professions. In the early 1800s, an Association was formed to put together a proposal to Parliament to set-up a body that examined and regulated apothecaries, surgeon-apothecaries, midwives and dispensing chemists. The chemists and druggists were of the opinion that they were best to set their own standards being more experienced in handling prescriptions and making medicines than the apothecaries. To resolve the issue between chemist and druggists and apothecaries 'Apothecaries Act' was passed in 1815 which stated that apothecaries will not have control over making medicines. Under this Act, apothecaries who passed specified course of Worshipful Society of Apothecaries were licensed to conduct practice as general practitioners and called as licentiate. Licentiates practiced in London and the provinces. The establishment of the General Medical Council in 1858 and growth in University training courses for medical students in the later 1800s limited the significance of the Society of Apothecaries in the training of general practitioners. Non-professional trained dispensers were employed by doctors and health institutions such as hospitals. They were trained assistants who compounded prescriptions under supervision. From 1815 onwards, the 'Society of Apothecaries' started assistants' examination and qualifying candidates were to compound and dispense drugs under the supervision of an apothecary, pharmacist or doctor. Apothecary's failure was due to impotent or inappropriate use, under dosage, over dosage and poisoning of drugs. Whereas apothecary's success was attributed to experience, mere coincidence of appropriate drug selection, natural healing, and in consequential effect of the drug or placebo effects.

At this time, it often referred to scientists who promoted the use of chemical-based therapeutics. The word 'pharmacist' was first used in a publication in England in 1834. By the time the new Pharmaceutical Society adopted the term in the 1840s. Legislation in 1852 stated that the term 'pharmaceutical chemist' should only be used by people who had passed the Society's 'major' examination, or by certain unexamined members of the Pharmaceutical Society who owned their own businesses. A 'Register of Pharmaceutical Chemists' was compiled, but not published, from 1852 onwards. The term Pharmaceutical Chemist was retained after 1868, when registration became compulsory. Under the 'Pharmacy Act 1868' in England the term Chemist and Druggist was used by the Pharmaceutical Society to denote those who had passed its minor examination, and so met the minimum requirement to register as a pharmacist. After 1868, the use of the title chemist and druggist became legally restricted to registered pharmacists only. However, it was certainly in use from the 18th century. At the beginning of the 19th century most people those who were involved in compounding and dispensing have called themselves chemists and/or druggists. The terms pharmacist and pharmaceutical chemist came later in the 1800s and shortened to chemist. By the mid of 19th century 'pure' scientific chemists had their own Chemical Society, formed in 1841.

In the 19th century pharmacy completely sprouted out from medicine and started developing as a separate profession. This century witnessed various milestones being set in the field of pharmacy. In 1821, first 'School of Pharmacy' was established in United States at Philadelphia. The first U. S. Pharmacopoeia was published in 1820. 'American Pharmacist Association' was founded in 1852. The first 'National Formulary' was published in 1888.

1.2 HISTORY OF PHARMACY PROFESSION IN INDIA

Pharmacy is the health profession that links the health sciences with the chemical sciences that work to ensure safe and effective use of pharmaceutical drugs. Pharmacy practice includes traditional practice of compounding and dispensing of medications. History of pharmacy profession in India can be divided in to three parts as ancient history, pre-independence and post-independence.

Ancient Pharmacy Profession

A little is known about history of ancient Indian pharmacy. In ancient India the sources of drugs were of vegetable, animal and mineral origin. They were prepared empirically by few experienced persons. Knowledge of that medical system was usually kept secret within a family. There were no scientific methods of standardization of drugs. In mythological literature it is reported that Lord Brahma was the first teacher of Universe who wrote "Ayurveda" in 5000 BC. Sushruta, the son of Vishwamitra, did his work in the field of surgery. The Ayurveda work on internal medicine whereas Sushruta-Samhita deals mainly with surgical medicine. Charaka and Sushruta were physicians as well as pharmacists who studied more than 1000 herbs. The Ayurveda had been used by his devotees for medical purposes. It eventually spread over Asia with the advanced evolution of Buddhism.

Archaeological evidence suggests the Indus people lived a settled life approximately in 2500 BC. The people in cities were enjoying the cleanest and hygienic daily life with elaborate civic sanitation systems. The whole conception shows a remarkable concern for health. The term Ayurveda (i.e., science of life) is found in Ramayana and Mahabharata and in the Atharva-Veda. The Aryans invaded India about 1500 BC and the Vedic age started. Vedic literature indicates that Lord Dhanvantari was worshiped as "God of Health". The reference of use of various herbs in treating diseases is mentioned in 'Rig-Veda". The Rig-Veda texts contain the hymns for Soma and those for herbs. The concept of hospital was developed and practiced during rein of king "Ashoka The Great" in 226 BC.

In Tamil Nadu during 900 AD discovered organized practice of hospital activity for the treatment of patients with diseases. India, being rich in flora and fauna, wide variety of herb was mainly used to treat disease like piles, jaundice, dropsy, hemorrhage etc. During period of 15th century European practitioners were greatly influenced by Indian drugs and herbs. In 1563 Portuguese practitioner Garcia de Orta reported use of Indian herbs in his treatise "Cologuiousdos stroples a drogus da indica". British traders brought the practice of allopathic system to India in 15th century.

The first general hospital was setup at Madras in 1664. The first college in India was established at Madras in the name of Madras Medical College in 1835 where professional training was given to students for treating patients with drugs. Next year in 1836, Calcutta Medical College was started at Calcutta. The Indian system of medicine declined during the Muslim rule while the Arabic or the Unani-Tibbi system flourished. The Allopathic system came into India with the British traders who later become the rulers. Under British Rule Allopathic system got state patronage and become popular by the close of 19th Century. Allopathic system during last decades of British rule explored to the greatest level that it overruled traditional Indian system of medicine.

Pre-independence Pharmacy Profession

The beginning of pharmacy profession can be traced back to 19th century when first chemist shop was opened by Scotch Bathgate at Calcutta in 1811. In India during independence various activities related to pharmacy practice were performed according to 'London Pharmacopoeia". This situation forced back traditional practice in India and compelled to import drugs from European countries.

In 1840 Goa Medical College was started at Panjim. 'Bengal Dispensatory and Pharmacopoeia' was published in 1841 at Bishop's College Press Calcutta by order of Government. In 1868 'Pharmacopoeia of India' was published under editorship of Waring. The compilation of vernacular names of Indian medicinal plants and herbs was carried by Mohideen Sheriff in 1869. The inception of pharmacy profession in India was marked by the first class of the chemist and druggist conducted at the Madras Medical College in 1870s to train students to gain skills in pharmacy practice. The first of its kind two-year professional course 'Chemist and Druggist Diploma' was started in Madras Medical College in 1874. Pharmacy education pattern was based on the instructions provided by the Pharmaceutical Society of Great Britain.

In 1878, 'Opium Act' was implemented that dealt with cultivation of poppy and the manufacture, transport, export, import and sale of opium. A formal training of the compounders was started in 1881 in Bengal. The pharmacy profession entered India almost simultaneously. In 1889 'Indian Merchandise Act' was implemented to avoid misbranding of goods in general. In 1894 'Indian Tariff Act' passed for levy of customs duty on goods including foods, drinks, drugs, chemicals and medicines imported into India or exported there from. 'Sea Customs Act' in 1894 was enforced to prevent import of goods with false trade descriptions. In 1901 'City of Bombay District Municipal Act' that was concerned with food was passed.

Health Scenario in India during 1901-1930 was not good. The people were well under the poverty line and were undernourished. The systems of treatment for the prevalent diseases and ailment were the Ayurvedic and Unani systems of medicine and the Allopathic system. The British government established small centers for production of small pox vaccine and for plague at Haffkine Institute Mumbai and King's Institute Madras. Pasteur institutions were set-up to manufacture Anti-rabbis vaccines. In India first pharmaceutical company 'Bengal Chemical and Pharmaceutical Works' started in 1901 at Calcutta by Acharya Prafulla Chandra Ray. In 1903 a small pharmaceutical unit at Parel (Mumbai) was started by Prof. T. K. Thakkar. Following the experience of setting-up an industry he started second unit 'Alembic Chemical Works' at Baroda in 1907. Some of the British who owned pharmacies during independence include Spencer and Company at Madras, Madon and Co. Bombay and Whitehall Pharmacy at Calcutta and Kemp and Co. Bombay.

In 1909 'Bengal Excise Act' was implemented. In 1912 'United Provinces (now Uttar Pradesh) Prevention of Adulteration Act' was passed that refers to adulteration of foods and drugs. In 1914 'Punjab Excise Act' was enforced. In 1916 'United Provinces Municipalities Act' for inspection of shops and seizure of adulterated substances was implemented. In 1919 'Bihar and Orissa Prevention of Adulteration Act' and 'Madras Prevention of Adulteration Act' was implemented. In the same year 'Poisons Act' was implemented to regulate the import, possession and sale of poisons. In 1920 'The Calcutta Chemist and Druggist Association' was formed which in 1926 changed their name as 'Bengal Chemists and Druggist Association'. The 'Pharmacist Association' was formed by chemist and druggist of Madras in 1923 which was changed in 1925 as 'Pharmaceutical Society of India'. Qualified pharmacist in Madras practiced pharmacy profession till India become independent. In 1925 'Bombay Prevention of Adulteration Act' was enforced.

Drugs in India were mostly exported in crude form and imported in finished form. During World War-I (1914 – 1920) the imports of drugs was slowed down but after war it was resumed to regular. There were no any restrictions on the quality of drugs imported, thus manufacturers abroad took advantage of the situation. They dumped inferior quality medicines and adulterated drugs. Markets were full of all sorts of useless and deleterious drugs and were sold by unqualified men. In absence of any control over quality of drugs, adulteration of drugs was rampant in the country. In response to this situation and to control pharmacy practice in 1930 'Dangerous Drug Act' was passed. Government of India on 11[th]August 1930, appointed a 'Drug Enquiry Committee' (DEC) under the chairmanship of Late Col. R. N. Chopra to see into the problems of Pharmacy in India and recommend the measures to be taken to avoid unethical practices. The committee report was published in 1931.

Qualified professionals from Banaras Hindu University (BHU) 'BHU Pharmaceutical Society' in 1935. In December 1935 'United Provinces Pharmaceutical Association' (UPPA) was registered which in 1936 became Indian Pharmaceutical Association (IPA). In 1937 Government of India brought 'Import of Drugs Bill' that was withdrawn in later. In 1940 'Allied Manufacturers and Distributors Association Ltd.' was formed in Mumbai.

In the same year British government bought 'Drug Bill' to regulate the import, manufacture, sale and distribution of drugs in British India. This Bill was finally adopted as 'Drugs Act of 1940'. This Act covered recommendations given by DEC headed by Chopra. Up to 1940 all the allopathic drugs were imported from Europe but in later years some of these drugs were begun to be produced in India.

In 1941 the first 'Drugs Technical Advisory Board' (DTAB) under this act was constituted. The first pharmacist post was created and filled at KEM hospital Mumbai. First 'All India Pharmaceutical Conference' (AIPC) was held at Banaras in January 1941 organized by IPA. Central Drugs Laboratory in Calcutta was established under Directorship of Col. Chopra on 1st February 1947 with four scientific divisions.

1.3 PHARMACEUTICAL EDUCATION

India was deprived of pharmacy education till start of 19th century. There was no recognized specialized education and only traditionally experienced professionals were involved in practice. Just after the publication of the report Pt. Madan Mohan Malaviya introduced 'Pharmaceutical Chemistry' subject in the three years' bachelor's degree course in science (B. Sc.). Mahadeo Lal Shroff 'The Father of Pharmacy Education in India' in 1937 started first B. Pharm. course at BHU. 'Indian Journal of Pharmacy' (IJP), first journal in India, was published 1939 as a quarterly journal devoted to the science and practice of pharmacy in all its branches. The first post-graduation course in pharmacy, M. Pharm., was introduced in 1940 at BHU.

In 1943, Indian Government appointed a committee under the chairmanship of Sir Joseph Bhore to make a survey of existing position in respect to the health care delivery organization in India and to make recommendation for future developments. This committee recommended three-tier system for education in pharmacy. In 1944, graduate course in pharmacy was started at the Punjab University, Lahore (currently in Pakistan). The B. Pharm. course at BHU was industry oriented while that at Punjab University was oriented towards Pharmacy practice. Though the profession was oriented towards pharmacy practice at the introductory stage but as it grew it became more industry oriented. In 1945 'Doctor of Philosophy' (Ph.D.) course was introduced at BHU. In the same year 'Drugs Rule' under the 'Drugs Act 1940' was established. In 1945, Government of India brought the Pharmacy Bill to standardize the Pharmacy Education in India. The 'Pharmacopoeial List' was published in 1946 under the chairmanship of Col. R. N. Chopra. Pharmacopoeial List contained lists of drugs in use in India at those times which were not included in British Pharmacopoeia. To regulate, control and standardize pharmacy education in India 'Pharmacy Bill' was passed by the Legislature in 1947.

Post-independence Pharmacy Profession

In 1948 Indian Pharmaceutical Congress Association (IPCA) was formed at Calcutta. IPCA is a federation of five national pharmaceutical associations, *viz*. The Indian Pharmaceutical Association (IPA), The Indian Pharmacy Graduates' Association (IPGA), The Indian Hospitals Pharmacist Association (IHPA), The Association of Pharmaceutical Teachers of India (APTI) and The All India Drugs Control Officers Confederation (AIDCOC) as its constituents. IPCA is the apex body representing the Indian Pharmacists working in various capacities in India. Currently, IPCA has more than 20,000 pharmacists as its members. The first Indian Pharmaceutical Congress (IPC) was organized at Calcutta in December 1948 with Prof. M. L. Shroff as its President. In 1948 'Indian Pharmacopoeial Committee' was constituted under the chairmanship of late Dr. B. N. Ghosh.

The "Pharmacy Act' was came in force in 1948 which provided statutory regulations for pharmacy institutions in India. Under this Act the 'Pharmacy Council of India' (PCI) was established in 1949. First D. Pharm. course was started in 1949 at Institute of Pharmacy Jalpaiguri in West Bengal. With the enactment of 'Pharmacy Act 1948' Pharmacy Council of India through the State Pharmacy Councils took measures to bring within its fold, a large number of Pharmacists who otherwise have been deprived of being classified as Registered Pharmacists. The first 'Education Regulation' (ER) was framed in 1953 and has come in force in some states in 1954 but other states lagged behind. Now it is mandatory to all states to follow ER. The ER's then amended in 1972, 1981, 1991 and in 2014. In 1953 PCI made D. Pharm. as a compulsory minimum qualification to work as a pharmacist in India.

The IPA and IPCA held joint conferences in Dec. 1952 and Dec. 1953. For the IPA, these were the Thirteenth and Fourteenth Conferences and for the IPCA, the Fifth and the Sixth. Government of India in 1953 appointed 'Pharmacy Enquiry Committee' under chairmanship of Major General S. L. Bhatia to make comprehensive enquiry in to the working of pharmaceutical industry and to recommend what steps the Government should take to establish it on sound lines in the interest of the country's health care delivery and economy. The committee recommended pay scales for pharmacists. In 1954, IPCA and IPA jointly decided that IPCA will organize annual conference where as IPA will carry out all other professional activities. The Pharmaceutical Conference held its sessions at different places to publicize Pharmacy as a whole. In 1954 'Drugs and Magic Remedies Act' was passed to stop misleading advertisement. In 1955 'Medicinal and Toilet Preparation Act' was passed to enforce uniform duty for all states of India for alcohol products.

First edition of Indian Pharmacopoeia was published in 1955. In 1960, All India Council for Technical Education (AICTE) drafted syllabus for M. Pharm. course. Indian Drug Manufacturers Association (IDMA) was founded in 1961 at Mumbai. 'Mudaliar Committee', in 1962, was constituted for the development of the health services infrastructure and the health care at the primary level. In 1963 'Indian Hospital Pharmacist Association' (IHPA) was formed at Delhi. In 1964 first issue of 'Indian Journal of Hospital Pharmacist" (IJHP) was published under the able leadership of Dr. B. D. Miglani. The journal was published from Delhi since last 5 decades and recently overall responsibility of publication of this journal is transferred to Manipal University, Karnataka. 'Organization of Pharmaceutical Producers of India' (OPPI) a premier association of research and innovation driven pharmaceutical companies in India and was also a scientific and professional body, established in 1965 at Mumbai. It caters to the needs of research based pharmaceutical industry to achieve the healthcare objectives of the nation.

Second edition of Indian Pharmacopoeia was published in 1966. India joined 'Commonwealth Pharmaceutical Association' (CPA) in 1970. CPA is made-up of six geographical regions across the commonwealth: Eastern and Southern Africa; West Africa; Americas; Pacific; Central Asia and Europe with its head quarter at London. In 1978, Dr. Yelavarthy Nayudamma Committee recommended to held Graduate Aptitude Test in Engineering (GATE) to pharmacy students to study M. Pharm. course with scholarships. In 1979 the name of IJP was expanded to the 'Indian Journal of Pharmaceutical Sciences' (IJPS). In 1979, all pharmacy associations merged to form 'All India Organization of Chemist and Druggist' (AIOCD) and Mr. V. L. Tyagrajan was the first President. This organization with its head quarter at Mumbai is now recognized as the only true representative body of the Pharmaceutical Trade in India.

'Indian Pharmacy Graduates Association' was established In 1973 at New Delhi. Indian Government under the chairmanship of Jaysukhlal Hathi in 1975 constituted 'Hathi Committee' to take comprehensive look into the drug industry and to enquiry in to the various facets of drugs in India. The process of appointing Pharmacy Inspector was initiated in for different parts of the India. In 1984 'Pharmacy Act' was amended to restrict the practice of pharmacy to qualified registered pharmacist only. The Drugs Act 1940 has been modified from time-to-time and presently the provisions of the Act cover cosmetics and ayurvedic, Unani and homeopathic medicines in some respects.

The third edition of Indian Pharmacopoeia was published in 1985. In order to provide protection to society from danger of addictive substances 'Narcotic and Psychotropic Substances Act' was introduced in 1985. The 'Drug Price Control Order' was passed in 1996. The Government of India controls the price of drugs in India by amending DPCO from time to time. The fourth edition of Indian Pharmacopoeia was published in 1996. In 55th IPC at Chennai charter 'Pharma Vision 2020' was released at the hands of The President of India Dr. A. P. J. Abdul Kalam. The 'Pharmacy Roadmap' a document that proposed activities that may help in shaping the future of pharmacy profession and a pharmaceutical service in India by 2020 was released in 58th IPC held at Mumbai. The fifth edition of Indian Pharmacopoeia was published in 2007. In 2010 sixth edition of Indian Pharmacopoeia was published. In 2010 PCI framed regulations for staring Pharm. D. course under 'Pharmacy Act 1948'.

Currently there are over 5 million pharmacists involved in practice of pharmacy profession. Approximately 55% of them are in community practice, 20% are in hospital pharmacist, 10% are in industries and regulatory. Every year nearly 20000 D. Pharm., 30,000 B. Pharm., 6000 M. Pharm., 700 Pharm. D. and more than 100 Ph. D. students entering in to the field of pharmacy profession. Diploma pharmacy people largely handle the pharmacy profession. State Pharmacy Councils in the states organize 'Refresher Training Programmes for Retail/Hospital Pharmacists' at various places in the states. Significant developments are underway to improve consumer awareness among the pharmacist to provide direct patient care. Since last three decades PCI, IPA and leaders in pharmacy profession has collectively undertaken initiatives to improve activities of pharmacy profession.

International organizations are entering India in community practice and health insurance. Currently foreign direct investment (FDI) in health industry in India is increasing. Awareness is developing rapidly for quality pharmaceutical care only by pharmacist trained in direct patient care. Now-a-day in India pharmacy profession is becoming very popular due to its wide scope. Equal to other highly demanded professions like doctors and engineering people are attracted to pharmacy profession too. It has resulted into numerous specialty educations in the field of pharmacy.

Pharmaceutical field in India is largely concentrated at city places. There are number of organizations and association in India working for welfare of every individual within the preview. Indian Pharmaceutical Association (IPA) Mumbai, Indian Drug Manufacturers Association Mumbai (IDMA), Indian Drug Manufacturers Association Hyderabad, Indian Drug Manufacturers Association Delhi and Confederation of Indian Industry, Delhi, Indian Pharma Machinery Manufacturers Association (IPMMA), New Delhi, Association of Pharmacy Teachers of India (APTI), Bengluru, Indian Hospital Pharmacists' Association (IHPA), Pillani and Chemist and Druggist Association (CDA) at Taluka, District and State level are some of them. As per Pharmacy Act 1948 every person completing diploma, degree, post-graduation or doctoral education in Pharmacy has to register his/her name at State Pharmacy Council office.

Changeover of pharmacy profession from pharmacy practice at introductory stage to industry oriented in later led to development of modern Indian pharmaceutical industry, which is now the 4th in terms of volume and 14th in terms of value. As mentioned in charter 'Pharma Vision 2020' the future prediction for the Indian pharma industries is expected to become the super power by the year 2020. The profession is going to face newer challenges in this century and the PCI and state councils must be prepared to face them and provide right solutions for overcoming them. The Pharmacists is not going to be only a seller or dispenser of drugs, but, is going to play a vital role in health services of the country by patient counseling and community services to the society at large. But in real sense the future of a pharmacy is in pharmacy practice and it is now observed that pharmacy in India is going back to from where it started.

Bachelor of Pharmacy (Practice) Regulations, 2014

The Pharmacy Council of India has started a two year bridge program for uplifting the diploma holders into bachelors' level through notification of Bachelor of Pharmacy (Practice) Regulations, 2014 on 18th December, 2014. Students completing diploma in pharmacy (D. Pharm.) will be required to undergo a two years 'bridge course' in pharmacy before being allowed to register with the State Pharmacy Councils from 2017. With this, all the new pharmacists will have to hold a degree-level qualification to enter the profession after two years. The aim is to increase the professional skills of the pharmacists and to upgrade their qualification and standard into a common degree level all over the country. Patient-counselling, hospital pharmacy management, community pharmacy management, pharmacovigilance and drug information dispensation are the major subjects selected for this course.

The Bachelor of Pharmacy (B. Pham.) and Master of Pharmacy (M. Pharm.) Course Regulations, 2014

Pharmacy Council of India, with the approval of the Central Government made 'The Bachelor of Pharmacy (B.Pham.) and Master of Pharmacy (M. Pharm.) Course Regulations, 2014' on 10th December, 2014. This new regulations include duration of course, minimum qualification required to obtain admission to this course, syllabus for B. Pharm. and M. Pharm. course, mode and pattern of examinations. In this regulation Choice based credit system (CBCS) is adopted by PCI for pharmacy courses. As per the philosophy of Credit Based semester system, certain quantum of academic work *viz*. theory classes, tutorial hours, practical classes, etc. are measured in terms of credits. On satisfactory completion of the courses, a candidate earns credits.

Pharmacy Practice Regulations, 2015

In exercise of the powers conferred by Section 10 and 18 of the Pharmacy Act, 1948 (8 of 1948), the Pharmacy Council of India, with the approval of the Central Government makes Pharmacy Practice Regulations, 2015 on 15 tn January, 2015. As per the rules Dispensing of Drugs should be carried by the Qualified Registered Pharmacists only. Renting of Registration Certificates to Pharmacy owners are strictly prohibited. The Pharmacists who rented their Registration Certificates without attending dispensing services considered as misconduct and subjected for Cancellation of their Registration Certificates permanently. The Pharmacists during working times should wear a white clean apron, black badge plate consists of Name and Registration Number of Pharmacists. The Registration Certificates should be displayed visible to the public. Along with dispensing services pharmacists should provide their professional services like patients counselling, adverse drug reactions reporting, primary care to all uncomplicated simple illnesses. For this purpose a separate cell should be arranged within the Pharmacy. Pharmacists may charge consultation fees for their professional services.

1.4 INDIAN PHARMACEUTICAL INDUSTRY

Indigenous medicines were in use prior to the British rule in India. 'Western medicines' scientifically termed as allopathic came to be known only during the British Era. The pioneering efforts of some few indigenous people led to the steady start of the modern pharmaceutical industry. British Government did set-up some medical institutions for education in modern pharmaceutical research. The Bengal Chemical and Pharmaceutical Works (BCPW) was established in 1892. Subsequent efforts in this direction by others have also been recorded. Drug production meeting around 13% of Indian drug product requirement was produced by several other indigenous firms during and after the World War II. Around 1930's efforts were also made in producing synthetic bulk drugs.

Prior to therapeutic revolution there was not much difference between the activities of indigenous and foreign companies in India as they were essentially involved in manufacturing and not in inventing. Indigenous sector dominated the pharmaceutical industry in India until 1950. The therapeutic revolution led to the change in equations between Indian pharmaceutical industry and global multinationals. During 1940's and 1950's new medicines were marketed by multinational corporations (MNC's) in India but indigenous industry remained unaffected. The focus was exclusively on manufacturing and not on research. This in a way strengthened the skills in developing new manufacturing technologies. A collaborative effort between Council of Scientific and Industrial Research (CSIR) and private manufacturing industry led to development, application and advancement of substantial skills in the pharmaceutical industry in India. However, post 1950 MNC's gained the ground with new medicines being introduced in the Indian markets. A strong product patent system under the 'British Patents and Designs Act 1911' led to increasing influence of MNCs in the Indian pharmaceutical markets. Initially Government was not much concerned about creating national champions during that period. A faulty system of industrial licensing aggravated the problem, as it inclined in favor of easy entry for MNCs prior to 1970s. Another reason was that MNCs carried certain special type of processing of formulations, which was not carried out by Indian companies during that period. India was one of the unique countries which provided for special and national treatment to MNCs. Thus by 1970s, the share of indigenous companies was reduced from 62% (1950) to 32% in 1970. The share of MNCs stood at 68% in 1970s, which increased from 32% held in 1952.

However, it must be noted that during 1950's, the government established the Indian Drugs and Pharmaceuticals Limited (IDPL) and Hindustan Antibiotics Limited (HAL) with both indigenous and foreign technology collaboration. This provided the necessary impulsion to the private industry players and put in some confidence during the later stages of pharmaceutical industry development. The contribution of the CSIR laboratories is also well recognized for the private sector having developed substantial reverse engineering skills post 1970. During late 1960s and in 1970s, there was an intentional attempt to give preference to national industry. The socialist policy advocated by the government and comprehensive review of legislations and policies having a potential to restrain domestic participation made the way for growth of the domestic generic industry in India. Ayyangar report examining the legislation came to a conclusion that foreign patent holders dominated the industry through large number of patent filing and grants. It was observed that the patents law in force failed to work in national interest. Thus Patents Act, 1970 came in which restricted patents only to process in case of pharmaceuticals and agricultural chemicals. The term of patents was reduced to 7 years. Apart from this, the Foreign Exchange Regulation Act, 1973 and the National Drug Policy, 1978 provided essential momentum to the growth of the Indian generic industry. Thus post 1970 reversed the foreign domination of the pharmaceutical industry in India. Large scale bulk drug production was possible and this led to the change the scene of industry.

In late 1980 and early 1990, the Indian generic industry steadily increased the exports and came to be recognized as an important player in global generic industry. Substantial price controls in 1979 through the 'Drug Price Control Order' (DPCO) based on National Drug Policy 1978 were major efforts in the direction of ensuring equitable access to health. This led to entry of large number of firms thus contributing to the fundamentals of the present top generic companies in India. The technical skills expanded by the generic industry in reverse engineering pharmaceutical products developed elsewhere are also remarkable. After 1990s, export led growth and increase in domestic consumption led to a dominating share of Indian firms in the market. In 1998, the domestic companies held 68% of the market share which grew to 77% in 2003. Even in the new economic context of liberalization, privatization and globalization, the foreign companies faced substantial barrier in penetrating into the Indian markets. However, post 2005; the industry witnessed new trends with rapid developments. The large and the medium industry attempted to make strategies themselves for the developments. The generic industry had different bargain contributed by increased technical collaborations, merging and acquisitions.

The Indian pharma industry has grown from ₹ 237 crores (1980) to about ₹ 1040 billion (2009-10). The country now ranked third in terms of volume of production and fourteenth largest by value. The share of export of drugs, pharmaceuticals and fine chemicals was more than ₹ 4755 billion. The domestic pharma industry has recently achieved some historic milestones through world class cost effective generic drugs manufacturer of AIDS medicines. Many Indian companies are part of an agreement where major AIDS drugs are supplied to people living with AIDS in Africa. Many Indian manufacturers supplies anti-retroviral drugs to USA. Indian healthcare sector has grown from 4% average household income in 1995 to 7% in 2005, and is expected to grow to 13% by 2025. If the Indian economy continues on its current high growth path, then the Indian pharmaceuticals market will undergo major changes in the next decade. It is expected that the market would triple to US$ 20 billion by 2020 and can easily become one of the world's top-10 pharmaceuticals markets. In terms of scale, the Indian pharmaceutical market is ranked fourteenth in the world. By 2020, it will rank among the top 10 in the world, overtaking Brazil, Mexico, South Korea and Turkey. A report by RNCOS titled "Booming Pharma Sector in India" has projected that the pharmaceutical formulations industry is expected to prosper in the same manner as the pharmaceutical industry. Indian Pharma growth has been fuelled by exports and its products are exported to a large number of countries with a sizeable share in the advance regulated markets of US and Western Europe.

Growth in the domestic pharma market would be driven by increase in the penetration of medical facilities, increase in the prevalence of chronic diseases, rising per capita income and increase in the health insurance coverage. Growth in the exports of pharmaceutical products from India would also be driven by patent expiries of the major branded drugs across the world, particularly in the US market. The growth in the US market would be led by increasing generic formulations and healthy Abbreviated New Drug Application (ANDA) stream of Indian pharma players. In the long term, growth in the exports market would be sustained by emerging markets like Russia, Brazil, South Africa etc., along with the intensified focus on the niche and complex product segments. The 'high risk high return' products offer comparatively huge entry barrier; as their clinical trials, approvals and manufacturing process are more complex and time consuming. Hence, very limited number of industries has entered these segments resulting in limited competition.

1.5 PHARMACIST

An individual who is trained and licensed to prepare, compound and dispense drugs upon written order (prescription) from a licensed veterinary, medical or dental practitioner is called Pharmacist. The scope of pharmacy practice includes compounding and dispensing of medications, and more modern services such as clinical services, reviewing medications for safety and efficacy, and providing drug information. Pharmacists work in the research and development of medicines and other health-related products and are involved in the management of pharmaceutical industries. Pharmacists, therefore, are the experts on drug therapy and are the primary health professionals who optimize use of medication for the benefit of the patients.

1.6 CAREER IN PHARMACY

Career in pharmacy is one of the best careers across the globe. Pharmacy is a part of healthcare services and today this discipline has made enormous progress in production and research. It has attained independent status as pharmaceutical sciences that include all the stages in drug product development starting from its discovery, development, formulation, quality control, packaging, storage, marketing, distribution etc. Dr. B. Suresh, the President of Pharmacy Council of India says 'Contrary to popular perception, increasing number of hospitals, nursing homes and pharmaceutical companies all over is a clear indication of the growing scope in pharmacy thus offering excellent and rewarding career opportunities both by way of jobs as well as in terms of starting own business'.

The pharmacist has various job opportunities in pharmaceutical industry, universities, teaching, hospitals, investigation and research institutes, Government departments, etc. A wide range of opportunities are available to pharmacists but if nothing, he can get going with his own business. The various positions a pharmacy professional can opt for are discussed below.

1. **As a Pharmacist**

    The Pharmacy course is considered as a paramedical programme. The pharmacy diploma/degree holders can therefore work in hospitals as hospital pharmacist, community pharmacist, consultant pharmacist or industrial pharmacist.

    (i) Hospital Pharmacy: A registered pharmacist can work in hospitals drug stores as hospital pharmacist. Pharmacist plays a key role in dispensing/compounding the prescription, maintaining patient's medical history and all patient profile. They are actively involved in counseling the patients and medical staff, maintaining patient records and history and in the usage of self-diagnostic kits by the patients.

    (ii) Community Pharmacy: Retail pharmacy in developed countries like U.S.A. and Canada as well as in developing countries is a highly demanded opportunity. In Indian healthcare services community pharmacy is also a rapidly growing concept. Registered pharmacist can start and run their own retail drug store or chemists and druggists shop to stock and sell medicines and dispense them as per physician prescriptions. Community pharmacist is a vital link between the patient and physician. In a retail pharmacy he has to perform buying and selling of related items demanded by the people. They dispense prescriptions; provide advice on drug selection and usage to doctors and other health professionals, provide primary healthcare advice, and educate customers on health promotion, disease prevention and the proper and safe use of medicines.

    (iii) Consultant pharmacist: Consultant pharmacists are either employed by hospitals, or are self-employed and contract with hospitals to provide medication reviews for residential care or ambulatory care patients and/or other medication-related cognitive services. They work as part of a healthcare team and are involved in monitoring of medicine usage, counseling patients, providing drug information and advice to health professionals and the community, conducting clinical trials and preparing products for patient use. They usually have a lot of contact with other health professionals and members of the public.

    (iv) Industrial pharmacist: Industrial pharmacists undertake research and the development, manufacture, testing, analysis and marketing activities for pharmaceutical and medical products.

2. Central and State Governments

Pharmacists are employed within the central and state government departments such as Health Protection Branch of the Department of Health and Welfare, the Pest Control Division of Agriculture, the Department of National Defense, Provincial Research Councils, and the Provincial Departments of Agriculture or the Environment and Armed forces at various positions based on educational qualifications and experience. They are employed within the food and cosmetic industries or organizations dealing with testing new products for their safe and effective use as possible. In government departments, a pharmacist maintains proper records. The Central and State Governments appoints Drugs Inspectors for controlling and regulating medicine related activities in definite areas. Drug Inspectors are public servants and are working under the control of Licensing Authority. Pharmacist as a drug inspector or government analyst has to make sure that the drugs manufactured and sold are of standard quality. He has job opportunities in government organizations such as Central Drug Research Institute (CDRI), Lucknow, National Chemical Laboratory (NCL), Pune, The Council of Scientific and Industrial Research (CSIR), Indian Institute of Chemical Technology (IICT), Hyderabad, Regional Research Laboratory (RRL), Jorhat, National Pharmacovigilance Centre. The Department of Pharmacology, AIIMS, New Delhi, Central Drug Standards Control Organization (CDSCO), New Delhi and Indian Medicines Pharmaceutical Corporation Limited (IMPCL), New Delhi. A Pharmacist has positions in the Regulatory bodies like Food and Drug Administration (FDA) at state and central level. For these government jobs the pharmacist needs to appear and pass the respective state service commission examination. Pharmacist can even find jobs in various government sectors like Railways, Hospitals, Navy and Military, and Food Inspector etc.

3. Pharmaceutical Industry

Pharmaceutical industry is another career option in pharmacy represented by production of chemicals, prescription and non-prescription drugs, and other health products. Pharmacists can do marketing, research and product development, quality control, sales, and administration. Some of the major positions in pharmaceutical industries where pharmacist is employed are discussed below.

(i) **Production and manufacturing:** India has a vast and growing pharmaceutical industry. It also has a vast market and many foreign pharmaceutical industries are opening their set-up in India. Pharma industries such as Dabur, Mylan, Microlab, Watson, Pfizer, Glenmark, Biocon, Cipla, IPCA, etc., are hiring more and more pharmacists. In these industries a pharmacist can start his career as a trainee production or chemist and grow up with becoming Production Executive, Production Officer, Production Manager, Director, Vice-President, President etc., in the production of bulk drug and intermediates or dosage forms. Pharmacists also have opportunities in production of ayurvedic preparations and veterinary products as well as in the bulk drugs. Industries manufacturing cosmetics, soaps, toiletries and dental products such as toothpaste, mouthwashes, dental cavity fillers, etc., also hire pharmacy professionals. Blood and plasma products as well as biological and biotechnological products are other areas with immense potential worldwide where pharmacists are employed on priority basis. Production of biological and biotechnological products, surgical dressings, medical devices and equipment, Ayurvedic/Homoeopathic/Unani medicines, perfumery, fragrances, nutraceuticals also involve the presence of pharmacists in its production.

(ii) Research and development: Research work is actually the most interesting aspect of pharmacy industry. Being the key to grow and sustain research or formulation and development (R&D or F&D) department is heart of any industry. The researchers in this department remain busy with synthesis of new drugs, new processes, clinical testing, etc. to justify their position and ensure the safety of medicines. They generate innovative formulas for the betterment of industry. Mainly M. Pharm. or Ph.D. degree holders are normally recruited in this department. Research scientists develop new drugs and their formulations in laboratories and scale it up to production and analyze them for purity and strength. Personnel with adequate experience in research are in great demand in the various areas of pharmacy such as novel drug delivery system (NDDS), quality control (QC), new drug discovery research (NDDR), designing of dosage form (DDF), process development (P&D), contract research (CR), formulation and development (F&D), biological products, clinical trials and bioequivalence, etc. Pharma scientists are facilitated in every way possible to carry out research work on various aspects of pharmacy.

(iii) Quality control: Pharmaceutical industry is an undisputed, ever-flourishing and biggest potential absorber of pharmacists. Excellent quality and purity of raw materials or dosage forms is requirement of pharmaceutical products for human use. Identification and characterization of these are required during production, storage and at handling of finished products. Quality control (QC) has assumed huge importance in view of current Good Manufacturing Practices (cGMP) regulations. Most people who fill this role have a B. Pharm. qualification. As Analytical Chemist or QC Manager a pharmacy graduate can play a crucial role in controlling product quality. As stated in the 'Drug and the Cosmetics Act 1940 and Rules 1945 vide No. 71(1) and 76(1), says that the manufacturing activity should be taken-up under the supervision of a technical man whose qualification should be B. Pharm., B.Sc., B.Tech. or M.B.B.S. with Biochemistry. QC chemists are responsible for the biological and chemical testing of products, raw and intermediate materials, and facilities. Their duties include performing assays and establishing and writing specifications and standard operating procedures.

(iv) Quality assurance: Quality assurance (QA) is one of the areas that get a lot of attention in pharmaceutical industries. Quality experts ensure that medicines are manufactured and tested in compliance with federal standards. QA personals ensure that in-house testing, reporting, and manufacturing are in compliance with regulatory requirements. QA personnel conduct site audits and review and analyze data and documentation. The entry-level position typically requires a B.Pharm. degree. A pharmacist can find job in big Pharma industries in the manufacturing arena. Responsibilities include designing the manufacturing process/es for drugs, ensuring the quality of finished product, creating product packaging, and planning specialized workspaces. They examine production plants, monitor investigator sites, audit study data, and validate manufacturing processes and computer systems. A person with B.Pharm. or higher education in a relevant discipline would find many opportunities in QA. Many employees in manufacturing and QA departments encounter a dual ladder in big pharmaceutical industries. QA pharmacists can get promoted doing technical work. If they have the aptitude and inclination can shift over to become a part of the management to co-ordinate the work of the technical staff.

(v) Regulatory affairs: In India Drug Control Administration is the main regulatory body governing and implementing the rules and regulations for the pharmaceutical industry. The job opportunities for pharmacy graduates in regulatory affairs (RA) are excellent but challenging. Currently pharmacy graduates and postgraduates are in high demand for patent filing and global expansion of drug manufacturing activities. A pharmacy graduate can work as Regulatory Manager (RM) in industries and contract research organizations. He can handle the job of monitoring the conduct of clinical trials that are conducted on human volunteers. He has to supervise regulatory documents such as clinical trial approval permission, marketing approval permission; etc. It is their responsibility to see that the clinical trials are carried out as per the international guidelines.

(vi) Pharmacovigilance: Pharmacovigilance is pharmacological science relating to the collection, detection, assessment, monitoring, and prevention of adverse effects with pharmaceutical products. Pharmacovigilance is more concerned with identifying the hazards associated with pharmaceutical products and with minimizing the risk of any harm that may come to patients. It is an emerging field. Drug safety and adverse effect monitoring have now been made compulsory by the Indian Government. Therefore a career into Pharmacovigilance can be fruitful on long run. Further people with experience in scientific writing can also get into Pharmacovigilance.

(vii) Business operations: Business operations include multiple standard corporate positions in finance, human resource (HR), and purchasing. If a person got an MBA in addition to B. Pharm., this is where he will find the most opportunities, in the complex industry of pharmaceuticals. Within marketing, there are abundant positions such as market research analyst, forecasting, and promotional response analyst. These are excellent entry-level positions for B. Pharm. with MBA without industry experience. One step-up with some pharma experience is assistant or associate product managers, who execute a brand's strategy under the direction of a product manager. The product manager is responsible for the overall success of a brand and works with a therapeutics-focused business director or other representatives from upper management to set performance targets and design an appropriate marketing strategy. Associate product managers primarily co-ordinate and implement campaigns for specific drugs, audiences, or both. This involves a little strategy and a lot of efforts in developing collateral pieces, working as a liaison to advertising agencies, and establishing a company presence at conventions. Product manager job requires managing a team of people and working to determine price, distribution, brand image, forecasting, and overall strategy for one or more drugs. Strategy directors develop plans for maximizing the commercial potential of a particular product or therapeutic area. They perform quantitative and qualitative analyses of disease and treatments trends, as well as assess opportunities for expanding market share and competitive positioning. These individuals typically work closely with colleagues in marketing analytics, business development, and finance. A pharmacy graduate with MBA is required but the preference is given to candidates having some industrial experience. Business development manager evaluate new business opportunities aligned with a pharma company's therapeutic product divisions and strategic goals. They examine in- and out-licensing opportunities, collaborative development deals, and joint ventures. The position requires a Pharmacy graduate with MBA, strong analytical skills, and several years of industry experience.

4. Pharmaceutical Sales

In general, the terms 'marketing' and 'selling' are synonyms but there is a substantial difference between both the concepts. Pharmaceutical selling has a product focus and mostly producer driven. It is the action part of marketing only and has short term goal of achieving market share. The emphasis is on price variation for closing the sale where the objective can be stated, as "I must somehow sell the product". Big pharmaceutical industries maintain huge staffs of pharmacists as sales representatives, who work to keep physicians, hospitals, primary health centers, and other medical institutions abreast of and partial toward their company's drugs. Registered pharmacists can sale bulk drugs as bulk drug distributor or supplier and pharmaceutical products as distributor, wholesaler and retailer.

5. Pharmaceutical Marketing

Pharmaceutical marketing is challenging job in the field of pharmacy because it is different than other businesses. The pharmaceutical marketing is a highly technical field and offers excellent opportunities for the pharmacy graduates. Ambitious people with pleasant personality and good communication skills can think of making career in pharmaceutical marketing. Pharmacy graduate with MBA degree enhances job opportunities in this field. The industries prefer pharmacy graduates for this job, as they have a good knowledge about the drug molecules, their therapeutic effects, how drug products are prepared, and stability of products as well as drug-excipient and drug-drug interactions.

Pharmaceutical marketing hierarchy defines the various levels of pharmaceutical marketing but in a pre-specified arranged manner. The pharmaceutical marketing hierarchy described below is in a descending order of pattern starting with the highest level and proceeding further describing all the lower levels. Senior level pharmaceutical marketing is the top most level which defines the entire pharmaceutical marketing and can be referred to as a strong bonding agent that ardently holds the whole pharmaceutical team well together in a well personalized manner. Middle level pharmaceutical marketing professionals have some vital experience in the field along with a degree of the same field. They work under the orders of the senior level of the pharmaceutical marketing hierarchy while taking care of the team of lower associates that is provided to them. Lower level pharmaceutical marketing is the most basic level of the pharmaceutical marketing hierarchy. These are those professionals who do not have any vital background experience of the field. They only have educational details in the wide pharmaceutical field and get appointed on their education basis. They work according to the guidelines of the middle level professionals of the pharmaceutical marketing hierarchy. Pharmaceutical marketing companies hire them and provide them with some handy training to progress in the field.

6. Academics

Academic profession is associated with job satisfaction and social status as teaching is considered to be a noble profession. Over 15,000 full-time faculty members work in the Universities and colleges of pharmacy in India. They are involved in teaching, research, public service, and patient care. Pharmacy graduate may take-up teaching as a profession as assistant professor. Becoming a member of the faculty at a college usually requires a graduate (B. Pharm.) for diploma colleges, postgraduate degree and/or Ph.D. degree (B. Pharm./M. Pharm.) for degree and post-graduate colleges. Now-a-days, most of post graduate candidates are choosing academic field as profession because of job satisfaction, facility for higher education and research, social status and comfort. Promotion scheme in academia is well defined as assistant professor, associate professor, professor and Principal/Director. Students graduate in pharmacy with first class are eligible to teaching D. Pharm. programme. Post graduate candidates with first class can work as an Assistant Professor in degree pharmacy colleges. Candidate with Ph.D. degree in any of the pharmacy specialization with 5 years of teaching experience can reach to the grade of Associate Professor. He can be Professor after 10 years of experience and 13 years to become a Principal of a college. Being in teaching profession they can do research in pharmaceutical field and can become a renowned research scientist. Besides teaching, academic related opportunities involve various positions on research posts and training programmes. After implementation of sixth/seventh pay scale and AICTE rules and regulations, most of pharmacy post graduate candidates are choosing academic field as profession.

7. Higher Education

There are many opportunities in higher education. A pharmacy student after graduation can opt for post-graduation (M.Pharm./M.S.) and Ph.D. courses. Master of Pharmacy in 10 specializations has been approved by PCI, New Delhi in 2014. Various specializations at Master in Pharmacy include Cosmeceutics, Industrial Pharmacy, Pharmaceutical Analysis, Pharmaceutical Biotechnology, Pharmaceutical Chemistry, Pharmaceutics, Pharmacognosy, Pharmacology, Pharmacy Practice, Pharmaceutical Quality Assurance and Pharmaceutical Regulatory Affairs. Today lots of Ayurvedic Pharmacies are coming up and there's an increase in craze for herbal products worldwide. In fact, it's one of the latest fields with a huge market potential and that's why Indian Government is looking forward to its growth as a breeding ground for earning foreign exchange. Recently Diploma, degree and masters and post graduate diploma courses in Ayurvedic Pharmacy are running in some of the universities in India. Biotechnology is a fast growing branch and the B. Pharm. graduates can opt for post graduate diploma programme in Bioinformatics. Various certificate courses have been offered by Government, public and private institutes and some of these courses are available on line. Theses certificate courses are P.G. Diploma in Pharmacy Management, P.G. Diploma in Pharmacy Technology, P.G. Diploma in Pharmacy Administration, Professional Diploma in Hospital Pharmacy Management, P.G. Diploma in Pharmacy Practice and Drug Store Management, MBA in Medicinal Plants, P.G. Diploma in Business Administration, Pharmacology Management, Regulatory Affairs, P.G. Diploma in Promoting Rational Drug Use, Clinical Trials and Pharmacovigilance and Bioinformatics. Students can join a foreign language course and can immigrate to other countries easily. There are three degrees courses in pharmacy education available in developed countries namely; Pharm. D., M.S. Programs and Ph.D. Program in Pharmacology, Drug Administration, Biology, Health Administration, Pharmaceutics, Pharmaceutical Engineering, Pharmaceutical Chemistry, and Pharmaceutical Administration.

8. Pharmaceutical Journalism

Pharmaceutical journalism has great potential. This requires specialist technical personnel to cover various aspects related to the field of pharmacy. Pharmaceutical journalism is for limited number of pharmacists where they can exhibit their writing and editing skills.

9. Consultancy

Pharmacists may serve as consultants for local, state, national, and international organizations. Most of experienced pharmacy professionals are providing consultancy to industry and also earning a handsome salary and popularity. Services in pharmacy are offered in various fields such as regulatory affairs, manufacturing, analytical services, documentation, approvals, research, marketing policies etc.

10. Clinical Research

In clinical research the phase of testing drug in human in product development is called the clinical trial. Pharmacy graduates have a good knowledge of therapeutic effects of drugs as well as drug-drug interaction thus can opt for career in clinical research. They are employed as clinical pharmacist or clinical research associate (CRA), clinical data manager (CDM), statistical analysis software (SAS) technician and can reach to the position of project manager in a clinical research organization. The responsibility of a clinical research associate is to help the doctors in monitoring the adverse effects of drugs under trial. The recorded data is gathered in specified formats under clinical data management and is analyzed using SAS. The CRA's works in the hospitals to assist doctors to monitor the adverse drug reactions (ADR). A CDM maintains the databases of different investigations and records them in specified formats. In the analysis of data, a person with B. Pharm. are preferred because they are familiar with terminology of ADRs. It is difficult to enter into those fields as a fresher by studying some clinical data management and SAS courses. There are huge opportunities in this field abroad. Presently salary and perks are attractive for those who know about CDM, SAS and CRA.

(i) Clinical development: The researchers in pharma companies perform the numerous investigations to take clinical compounds from the lab bench to the pharmacy shelf. Director or Vice President who are heads of company's therapeutic divisions is responsible for ensuring drug safety and to keep development programs on track. Doctorate of Medicine (MD) and sometimes Ph.D.'s or Pharm D's are responsible for product's overall clinical development plan for marketing approval. They are involved in write-up of clinical trial protocols, the instructions for an investigator that describes the objectives, design, and methods of a clinical trial. Upon approval of plans by regulatory authorities, CRAs works with investigators to conduct clinical trials. Clinical trials may be conducted in small patient group at a single site, or may involve thousands of patients at many sites worldwide. As a clinical trial proceeds, they meet with investigators and their staff to see that the study protocol is followed and they also monitor the collection of patient data. Many pharma companies outsource the conduct of clinical trials to contract research organizations (CROs). Pharma graduate with experience in clinical development within big pharma company or CROs he may find rewarding career opportunities. Clinical development offers other career opportunities like Regulatory Affairs Experts (RAE) who are the link between industry and government. Generally, pharma companies divide RA department into clinical development and formulation and quality divisions. Both these divisions communicate directly with government regulatory bodies and manage great volumes of paperwork.

(ii) **Clinical research associate**: CRA oversees clinical trials and get involved in designing protocols, enlisting physician investigators, training clinic personnel, and evaluating data. CRA has to travel a lot and manage the services of an independent CRO that runs the actual studies.

(iii) **Regulatory affairs associate:** The regulatory affairs (RA) career suits to job seekers who have a interest in documentation. A RA specialist completes and maintains documents required by regulatory agencies worldwide and communicate with these agencies to ask questions and resolve issues. Based on level of industry experience, they set regulatory strategy for a pharma company. As a Regulatory Manager (RM) he has to oversee regulatory documentation of clinical trial approval permission and marketing approval permission. A pharmacy graduate can work as RM in companies and CRO but these days M. Pharm. degree is typically the minimum qualification for entry-level positions.

(iv) **Bio-statistician:** A person with pharmacy degree and additional certificate course in statistics can work as statistician in clinical development. His duties include preparation of analysis plans for clinical studies and designing tables and figures to display information, interpretation of final data, and preparation of statistical sections of clinical study reports. A statistician titles frequently include a Class I, II, or III to indicate levels of education and experience. Entry-level positions require a M.Pharm. degree; higher levels require a Ph.D. and several years of industry experience. In most of companies' biostatisticians directly report to the head of a therapeutic division.

(v) **Clinical data manager:** Clinical data manager (CDM) supervises all aspects of clinical data. He specifies how metrics would be collected and assist to standardize data management methodology for internal operations and external reporting. CRM position requires at least a M.Pharm. degree preferably pharmacology plus several years of industry experience. A pharma graduate can seek employment as CDM to store the data in the computer and process it using software developed for the purpose.

(vi) Medical science liaison: Medical science liaison (MSL) is a field for pharmacists with Ph.D. or Pharm.D. degrees with therapeutic area specialties. They interact with physicians and researchers in the health care community, especially with those who are doing major academic research to maximize the acceptance of products.

11. Organizational Management

Organizational management offers pharmacists a national and state association and on boards of pharmacy. There is career for pharmacists in insurance sector too. They can work on managerial positions with health and welfare agencies.

12. Opportunities Abroad

In the field of pharmacy, India is one of the countries producing large number of pharmacy graduates. Pharmacy professional has golden opportunities all over globe. A registered pharmacist commands very high salary and repute in developed countries including USA and UK. There are lots of higher education and research opportunities in the developed countries. Countries like USA, Canada, UK, France, Germany, Saudi Arabia, Kuwait, Singapore, Korea, Japan and Australian continent including New Zealand have demand for pharma graduates. Pharmacists have placement opportunities in higher education, as druggist and chemist, as councilor, and manufacturing and in hospital and clinical pharmacy. The monetary job benefits to pharmacists are highly exciting and attractive.

13. Medical Transcription

Medical transcription (MT) is an allied health profession that deals in the process of transcription, or converting voice-recorded reports as dictated by practitioners or other healthcare professionals, into text format. MT is part of the healthcare industry that provides and edits doctor dictated reports and notes in an electronic form to represent the treatment history of patients. Physicians dictate what they have done after providing treatment to the patients and MT's transcribe the dictation and/or edit reports that have gone through speech recognition tools. A pharmacy graduate can work with physicians to maintain the patient treatment history, the drug to which patients are allergic etc. The approximate salary offered to a MT in India is about 2 to 5 lakh per annum. People as MT generally don't have much experience because experience strongly influences pay for this job. The highest salaries are offered if they are having experience as proofreader, in quality assurance and quality control in transcription, and editor.

1.7 PHARMACOPOEIA

The word "Pharmacopoeia" is derived from the Greek words *'pharmakon'* meaning 'drug' and *'poieo'* means 'make'. Literally it means that it is book that contains a list of medicinal substances, crude drugs and formulae for making preparations from them. These books are prepared under the authority of the Government of the respective countries. The books containing the standards for drugs and other related substances are known as the drug compendia. These books contain a list of drugs and other related substances regarding their source, descriptions, standards, tests, formulae for preparations, action and uses, doses, storage conditions etc. These books are revised from time-to-time to introduce the latest information available as early as possible. In order to keep the size of book within reasonable limit it becomes necessary to omit certain less frequently used drug information and pharmaceutical excipients from each new edition. In each new edition of these books certain new monographs are added, some are amended while the older ones are deleted. These books are prepared by the expert amongst medical practitioners, teachers and pharmaceutical manufacturers. The drug-compendia are classified as official compendia and non-official compendia. The *official compendia* are the compilations of drugs and other related substances which are recognized as legal standards of purity, quality and strength by a government agency of respective countries of their origin. Examples are British Pharmacopoeia (BP) British Pharmaceutical Codex (BPC) Indian Pharmacopoeia (IP) United States Pharmacopoeia (USP) National Formulary (NF), The State Pharmacopoeia of USSR and Pharmacopoeias of other countries. The book other than official drug compendia which are used as secondary reference sources for drugs and other related substances are known as *non-official compendia*. Examples of this type are Merck Index, The Extra Pharmacopoeia (Martindale), United States Dispensatory etc.

Pharmacopoeias are generally prepared under the authority of the government of the respective countries - these pharmacopoeias are known as national pharmacopoeias.

Example of some national pharmacopoeias are: Indian Pharmacopoeia, British Pharmacopoeia, United States Pharmacopoeia etc. The drugs used may vary from nation to nation so, the respective pharmacopoeia includes those drugs or dosage forms which are frequently used in that very country at that time. The national pharmacopoeia is recognized as the reference book by the legislative authority (by law) of the respective country, whenever a conflict arises regarding drugs these books will be referred.

Importance of pharmacopoeia

The Pharmacopoeia is very important official document for the drug industry, administration and academic people.

(i) **Pharmaceutical industry:** In the invention of a new drug molecule huge amount of money is expended for the research and development. Majority of drug industries in developing countries like India are unable to bear the expenditure. In such situations drugs or products mentioned in the pharmacopoeias can be marketed without any further research on it. This is because drugs listed in pharmacopoeia are tested, safe and efficacious. In pharmacopoeia there are various standards which should rigorously be met by the raw materials from which drugs and pharmaceuticals products prepared. Although there are other sources of information about the standard of drugs and pharmaceuticals, the pharmacopoeia is the most authentic. Assay methods and identification tests for drugs and pharmaceuticals in pharmacopoeia are approved by the authority so it becomes easy for the industry people to design the tests and use methods confidently.

(ii) Drug-administration: The major objective of every industry is 'to make profit'. So doing this some industries ignore the quality aspects of the drugs and pharmaceuticals. As drugs are related to the health of human beings and animals, this negligence is unjustifiable. Thus every nation prepared their own drug related Acts, Laws and Rules. In the conflict situations between a drug industries and the Government first reference book that is conferred, regarding the quality of the product, is the pharmacopoeia.

(iii) Academics: The pharmacopoeias are source of information regarding use of drugs and pharmaceuticals. The researchers always refer it at first hand during development of an assay methods of certain drugs and testing the quality of a dosage form. The information about microbiological and bioassays are given in details as appendices. Thus, usage of the drugs and raw materials, the adverse reaction, and many more information are provided in the pharmacopoeia. The pharmacopoeia is popular among the students, researchers and a teacher is for the reliability of the information provided in it.

1.8 HISTORY OF INDIAN PHARMACOPOEIA

Indian Pharmacopoeia Commission (IPC) is an autonomous institution of the Welfare which sets standards for all drugs that are manufactured, sold and consumed in India. A drug Enquiry Committee appointed in 1927 by the British government recommended the publication of an Indian National Pharmacopoeia. The set of standards are published under the title 'Indian Pharmacopoeia' (IP) has been modeled over the British Pharmacopoeia. The IP is an official book meant for overall quality control and assurance based on safety, efficacy and affordability of pharmaceutical products marketed in India. It contains a collection of approved methods and procedures of analysis and specifications for Drugs and products. The IP, or any part of it, has got legal status under the Second Schedule of the Drugs and Cosmetics Act, 1940 and Rules 1945 there under. The IP prescribes standards for identity, purity and strength of drugs essentially required from health care perspective of human beings and animals. The standards given in IP are authoritative in nature and are enforced by the Regulatory authorities for quality control of medicines in India.

In ancient India the sources of drugs were of vegetable, animal and mineral origin. They were prepared empirically by few experts who kept its secret within a family. There were no scientific methods of standardizing drugs. The historical developments of Pharmacopoeia in India traces back to 1563 and the credit goes to Garcia da Orta a Portuguese physician-cum-teacher. The allopathic system came into India with the British traders. Initially allopathic drugs were introduced in India by the British and were available toward the end of 19th century. The allopathic drug was not manufactured in India at that time and the requirement of the same was met from import. There was no control on manufactured or imported drugs, except London Pharmacopoeia that helped to detect and identify impurities in medicinal substances.

The history of the IP began in the year 1833 when a committee of the East Indian Company's Dispensary recommended the Publication a Pharmacopoeia. The 'Bengal Pharmacopoeia and General Conspectus of Medicinal Plants' was published in 1844. The author of this book was W. B. O'Shaughnessy and published by Calcutta, Bishop's College Press. This book listed the information about most commonly used indigenous remedies. This was followed by IP 1868, written by Edward John Waring, which covered both the drugs of British Pharmacopoeia (BP; 1867) and indigenous drugs used in India. The supplement to IP 1868 was published in 1869 incorporating the vernacular names of indigenous drugs and plants. But, from 1885 the BP was made official book of standards in India. The colonial addendum of BP 1898 was published in 1900 appeared as Government of India edition in 1901.

The Bengali and Hindi version of London Pharmacopoeia was made available in India from 1901 onwards. Drugs were mostly exported in crude form and imported in finished form. During World War-I (1914 – 1920) the imports of drugs were cut-off. Imports of drugs were resumed after the War. There was complete absence of any restrictions on the quality of drugs imported, so manufacturer abroad took advantage of the situation. The consequences led to dumping inferior quality medicines and adulterated drugs by foreign manufacturers. Markets were full of all sorts of useless and deleterious drugs and were sold by unqualified men. Some examples of maladies that happened include poisoning due to quinine, putting croton oil into eye instead of atropine solution and selling chalk powder tablets in place of quinine. Drug santonin was also badly adulterated. Some other examples were the use of potent drugs like compounds of antimony and arsenic and dispensing of digitalis without any standard. At that time few laws were there having indirect connection to drugs, but they were insufficient.

In order to take over the control of this situation a 'Drug Enquiry Committee' was appointed in 1927 by the government who recommended the publication of an Indian National Pharmacopoeia. The then Government of India on 11th August 1930, appointed an

Indian Pharmacopoeial Commission under the chairmanship of Late Col. R. N. Chopra to see into the issues of Pharmacy in India and recommend the measures to be taken. This committee report got published in 1931 with remarks that there was no recognized specialized profession of Pharmacy and a set of people so called compounders were filling the gap. Immediately after publication of the report Prof. Mahadev Lal Shroff started pharmaceutical education at the university level in the Banaras Hindu University.

In 1940 Government of India brought 'Import of Drugs Bill' which was later withdrawn. In the same year the Government brought 'Drugs Bill' to regulate the import, manufacture, sale and distribution of drugs in British India. This Bill was adopted as 'Drugs and Cosmetic Act 1940. The first Drugs Technical Advisory Board (DTAB) under this Act was constituted in 1941. In 1946 the Central Drugs Laboratory (CDL) was established at Calcutta. In 1944 Government of India asked the DTAB to prepare the list of drugs used, in India, having sufficient medicinal value to justify their inclusion in official book pharmacopoeia. The work of preparing lists of drugs in use in India at those times which were not included in British Pharmacopoeia was given to late Col. R. N. Chopra along with other nine members, by Department of Health, Govt. of India. This work was published as an 'Indian Pharmacopoeial List (IPL)'. The IPL, published in 1946 formed the foundation for the true first official Indian Pharmacopoeia.

After independence, the Indian Pharmacopoeia Committee was constituted under the chairmanship of late Dr. B. N. Ghosh in 1948 for publication of Indian Pharmacopoeia as its main function. Tenure of this committee was five years. This committee was assigned the task of preparing Indian Pharmacopoeia and to keep it up-to-date.

First Edition

For the preparation of Pharmacopoeia of India, the pharmacopoeias of other countries, like British, Europe, United States, USSR, Japan, the National Formulary (USA) and Merck Index were consulted. The persons working in pharmaceutical industry, drug control laboratories, research and teaching institutions were also actively participated. The first edition of IP was published in 1955 by The Controller of Publications, Delhi, on behalf of Govt. of India, Ministry of Health and Family Welfare. Cost was ₹ 5/- (Dollar – 8). It is written in English and official titles of monographs given in Latin. It covers 986 monographs. The IP was published in fulfilment of requirements of Drugs and Cosmetics act 1940 and rules there under. The work of revision of the Indian Pharmacopoeia as well as compilation of new edition was taken-up simultaneously under the chairmanship of Dr. B. N. Ghosh, who died in 1958. After Dr. B. N. Ghosh, Dr. B. Mukherjee, the Director of Central Drug Research Institute (CDRI) was appointed as the chairman of Indian Pharmacopoeia committee and the supplement of IP 1955 was published in 1960.

Second Edition

The second edition of IP was published in 1966 under chairmanship of Dr. Nityanand. The official titles of monographs were in English. The doses were expressed in Metric system. Usual strengths for tablets and injections were given. Formulations of the drugs were given immediately after the monograph of respective drugs. In all 274 monographs from IP 1955 and their supplement were deleted, 93 new monographs were added. The supplement to this edition was published in 1975. In this supplement 126 new monographs were included and 250 monographs were amended. Most importantly cholera vaccine was deleted.

In 1978 the Indian Pharmacopoeia Committee was reconstituted by the Govt. of India, Ministry of Health and Family Welfare, under the chairmanship of Dr. Nityanand, who was Director at Central Drug Research Institute, Lucknow.

Third Edition

The third edition of IP published in 1985 was presented in two volumes as Volume-I and Volume-II and Nine appendices, by the Controller of Publications, on behalf of Govt. of India, Ministry of Health and Family Welfare. In all total 261 new monographs were added and 450 monographs were deleted. Addendum I to IP 1985 was published in 1989 in which 46 new monographs added and 126 amended. Addendum II was published in 1991 in which 62 new monographs added and 110 amended. In the IP 1985 and its Addendums, traditional drugs were not included as publication of a pharmacopoeia. Traditional system drugs were taken-up separately and only those herbal drugs were included which had supporting definitive quality control standards.

Fourth Edition of IP

The fourth edition of IP was published in 1996 and made effective from 1st December 1996. It was presented in two volumes. The Volume-I contains Legal Notices, Preface, Acknowledgments, Introduction, General Notices, and Monographs from A to O. The Volume-II contains Monographs from P to Z, Appendices, Contents of Appendices and Index. The Appendices includes the Infra-red spectra of drugs, apparatus for tests and assays, biological tests and determinations, chemical tests and assays, chromatography and electrophoresis, spectrophotometry, clarity and color of solutions, disintegration and dissolution tests, physical tests and determinations, microbiological assays and tests, limit tests of particulate matter, other tests and determinations, general information, reagents and solutions, reference substances, tables and index. It covered 1149 monographs and 123 appendices. It includes 294 new monographs and 110 monographs have been deleted.

In view of the rapid developments is pharmaceutical sciences and technology, it became necessary to make further changes in the existing compendium. Thus, IP 1996 was updated by additions and amendments introduced through addendum. Addendum I was made effective from 31st December 2000 wherein 42 new monographs have been added.

Addendum II was made effective from 30th June 2003 with 19 new monographs have been added. Addendum 2002 amends as well as adds new drugs and preparations to the IP 1996 with a view to keeping the pharmacopoeia updated to the extent possible. Besides amending the existing monographs and appendices, it contains 19 new monographs including monographs of 12 antiretroviral drugs and 7 formulations of these substances. A new appendix on residual solvents has been incorporated. Some monographs have undergone major amendments. The appendix on high performance liquid chromatography has been replaced with a new version which also includes the ion chromatography. Following IP fourth edition and its addendums, one supplement for Veterinary Products in 2002 was also published which contains 208 monographs and four appendices. The Indian Pharmacopoeia Commission was established in year 2005, dissolving the existing I.P. Committee and started working in existing CIPL with its Director as Member Secretary. The Addendum 2005 was published by IPC which included a large number of antiretroviral drugs and raw plants commonly used in making medicinal products not covered by any other pharmacopoeias, which attracted much global attention.

Fifth Edition

The fifth edition IP was prepared in accordance with the principles and plan decided by the Scientific Body of the IPC and completed with untiring efforts made by Commission members and its Secretariat over almost two years. The fifth edition of IP was published in 2007 and presented in user friendly format in Three Volumes. Volume-I contains general notices and general chapters. Volume – II and III contains general monographs on drug substances, dosage forms and pharmaceutical aids. The General Notices, Monographs and new testing methods etc. based on the introduction of advanced technology and experimental methods widely adopted in India and abroad are being added and updated. The contents of Appendices are revised by and large in consonance with those now-a-days adopted internationally for monitoring the quality of the drugs. The monographs of special relevance to the common disease pattern of this region have been given special emphasis by incorporating such medicines. The addendum to IP-2007 was published in 2008 containing 72 new monographs.

Ministry of Health and Family Welfare, Govt. of India submerged the existing Central Indian Pharmacopoeia Laboratory along with IPC as a fully financed autonomous body from 1st January, 2009 located at NCR region in Ghaziabad. It is a 3-tier structure comprising of the General body of 25 members, Governing body of 13 members and Scientific body of 15-23 members from different related scientific fields.

Sixth Edition

The sixth edition of IP is published in 2010 by the IPC Ghaziabad in accordance with a plan and completed through the untiring efforts of its members, Secretariat and Laboratory over a period of about two years. It supersedes the 2007 edition but many monograph of the earlier edition does not figure in this edition. This edition was made effective from 1st September; 2010. This edition is presented in three volumes. The Volume-I contains the notices, preface, the structure of the IPC, acknowledgements, introduction, and the general chapters, Volume II contains the general notice, general monographs on dosage forms and monographs on drug substances, dosage forms and pharmaceutical aids (A to M), whereas, the Volume- III contains monographs on drug substances, dosage forms and pharmaceutical aids (N to Z). This is followed by monographs on vaccines and immune sera for human use, herbs and herbal products, blood and blood-related products, biotechnology products and veterinary products.

The scope of the Pharmacopoeia has been extended to include products of biotechnology, indigenous herbs and herbal products, veterinary vaccines and additional antiretroviral drugs and formulations, inclusive of commonly used fixed-dose combinations. Standards for new drugs and drugs used under National Health Programmes are added and the drugs as well as their formulations not in use these days were omitted. The number of monographs of excipients, anticancer drugs, herbal products and antiretroviral drugs were increased. Monographs of vaccines and immune sera were uP.G.raded in view of development of latest technology in the field. A new chapter on liposomal products and a monograph of liposomal amphotericin B injection was an added. A chapter on NMR is incorporated in appendices. The chapter on microbial contamination was also updated to a great extent to harmonize with prevailing international requirements. Addendum 2012 to the IP 2010 was published which had taken care of the Amendments to IP 2010 along with 52 new monographs.

Seventh Edition

The seventh edition of IP published in 2014 was presented in four volumes with DVD-ROM. IP 2014 was released by Gulam Nabi Azad, the then Health Minister at a function at the Nirman Bhawan, New Delhi. This edition was published under chairmanship of P. K. Pradhan, Secretary Health and Family Welfare, Government of India. The IP 2014 is published by the Indian Pharmacopoeia Commission (IPC) on behalf of the Government of India, Ministry of Health and Family Welfare. This edition was made effective from 1st January 2014. The scope of the Pharmacopoeia has been extended to include additional anticancer drugs and antiretroviral drugs and formulations, products of biotechnology, indigenous herbs and herbal products, veterinary vaccines. This edition incorporates 2548 monographs of drugs out of which 577 are new monographs consisting of APIs, excipients, dosage forms, antibiotic monographs, insulin products and herbal products etc. A list of 577 new monographs not included in IP 2010 and its addendum 2012 were added in this edition. In all 313 new monographs on drug substances, dosage forms and pharmaceutical aids (A to Z), 43 new drugs substances monographs, 10 antibiotic monographs, 31 herbal monographs, 5 vaccines and immune sera for human use, 6 insulin products,

7 biotechnology products etc. along with the 19 new general chapters and about 200 new IR spectrums are also added. First time 19 new radiopharmaceutical monographs and 1 general chapter are included in this edition. A separate volume of veterinary products with 143 monographs along with 16 appendices and a General chapter on veterinary products are also introduced. IP Addendum-2015 to IP-2014 has been released on 28th Nov. 2014 by Shri. Lov Verma, Secretary Health and Family Welfare and Chairman, India Pharmacopoeia Commission in the presence of senior officers of Ministry of Health & Family Welfare and Scientific Staff of IP Commission. The IP Addendum-2016 to IP-2014 has been released on 14th Nov. 2015 by Shri. J. P. Nadda, Minister of Health & Family Welfare Government of India.

Now total number of IP Standards reached almost to 3000 which are almost at par with other international Pharmacopoeias and comprises of different categories of drugs and appendices. The recent IP 2014 has 37 General Monograph on Dosage Forms and Monographs on Drug Substances, Dosage forms and Pharmaceutical Aids (A to Z) as 850 APIs, 1035 formulations and 128 excipients altogether 2013 total Standards.

Eight Edition

The preparation work for forthcoming edition of IP has already been started. The release of IP 2018 edition is scheduled on July, 2017 and it would be implemented from 1 January, 2018.

Presently the work of the IPC is performed in collaboration with members of the Scientific Body, subject experts as well as with representatives from Central Drugs Standard Control Organization (CDSCO), State Regulatory authorities, specialist from Industries, Associations, and Councils and from other Scientific and Academic Institutions.

Characteristic features of Indian Pharmacopoeia

Edition	Year	Volumes	Supp-lement	Addenda	Pages	Price (₹)	Chairman
First	1955	1	1960	--		5	Dr. B. N. Ghosh
Second	1966	1	1975	--		113.50	Dr. B. Mukherji
Third	1985	2	--	1989, 1991	858		Dr. Nityanand
Fourth	1996	2	2002 (Vet.)	2000, 2002, 2005		4000	Dr. Nityanand
Fifth	2007	3	--	2008	2328	15000	Mr. Prasanna Hota (up to 30/10/2006) Mr. Naresh Dayal (from 31/10/2006)
Sixth	2010	3	--	2012		20000	Ms. K. Sujatha Rao
Seventh	2014	4 (DVD)	--	2015, 2016	3754	25000	P. K. Pradhan

1.9 NATIONAL FORMULARY OF INDIA

The National Formulary of India (NFI) is essentially meant for the guidance to the members of the medical profession; medical students, nurses and pharmacists working in hospitals and in sales establishments. In the preparation of this Formulary, the expert opinion of medical practitioners, teachers in medicine, nurses, pharmacists and Pharmaceutical manufacturers has been obtained. The selection of drugs for inclusion in the National Formulary has been made taking into consideration the relative advantages and disadvantages of the various drugs used, the extent of their use in current medical practice and their availability in the country. Thus the NFI represents a broad consensus of medical opinion in respect of drugs and their formulations and provides the physician with carefully selected therapeutic agents of proved effectiveness which form the basis of national drug therapy.

In 1960 first edition of NFI was published by Govt. of India, Ministry of Health. In 1966 second edition was published. Third edition was published in 1979. It contains information about drug interaction, resistance, cumulative effects, drug dependence, prescription writing etc. As more than three decades have elapsed since the publication of the last edition of the National Formulary of India, it is to be expected that there would be a large number of additions and consequent deletions. The 4th edition of NFI was published in 2011. This edition has many distinct features that promoted the rational use of medicines in the country. The 5th edition of NFI is expected to be published in 2016.

The formulations included in the Formulary and the ingredients thereof should conform to the standards laid down in the current edition of the IP. If no standards are specified in the current edition but are specified in the immediately preceding edition of the IP then these standards would apply. In respect of drugs for which no standards have been laid down in the IP, these would have to conform to the standards laid down in the official pharmacopoeia of any other country wherein they are included. The provisions of the Drugs and Cosmetics Act and the Rules made there under including those relating to labelling and conditions of storage should be observed.

*Ayurvedic Pharmacopoeia of India

1.10 THE BRITISH PHARMACOPOEIA

The regulation of medicinal products by officials in the United Kingdom (UK) dates back to the reign of King Henry VIII (1491–1547). The Royal College of Physicians of London had the power to inspect 'apothecaries' products in the London area and to destroy defective stock. The first book containing list of approved drugs with their preparations was published as 'London Pharmacopoeia' in 1618. The New Latin name that had some currency at the time was Pharmacopoeia Britannica (Ph. Br.). The first edition of May 1618 was full of errors and a revised definitive edition was published on 7 December 1618. The text was in Latin because it was meant only to be used by learned physicians and apothecaries, and not for the information of the common man. The December edition described 1190 ingredients, many derived from plants, but some from animal parts and minerals such as amethyst, beryl, opal and sapphire. The preparations included waters, wines, syrups, powders, troches (lozenges), oils, ointments and plasters. Further editions were published over the years. The 1836 edition included some of the recently discovered alkaloids such as aconitine, morphine, quinine and strychnine. The 10th and final edition was published in 1851 and included chloroform and cod-liver oil. In August 1745 the College of Physicians of Ireland agreed to use the London Pharmacopoeia for their prescriptions and they continued to use it until 1806, when the first Dublin Pharmacopoeia was published. The final Dublin Pharmacopoeia came out in 1850 and was reprinted in 1856. The first edition of the Edinburgh Pharmacopoeia was published by the Royal College of Physicians of Edinburgh in 1699. This was frequently reviewed and revised. A further 11 editions were published, the last being the 1839 edition, which was published in English for the first time.

A Commission was first appointed by the General Medical Council (GMC) and the commissionerates were statutorily made responsible under the Medical Act 1858 for producing a British Pharmacopoeia (BP) on a national basis. Through an attempts to harmonize pharmaceutical standards London, Edinburgh and Dublin Pharmacopoeias were merged and the first edition of the 'British Pharmacopoeia' was published in 1864.

The BP is a collection of quality standards for UK medicinal substances and used by all those who were involved in pharmaceutical research, development, and manufacture and testing. BP is an important statutory part in the control of drugs and medicines which complements and assists the licensing and inspection processes of the Medicines and Healthcare Products Regulatory Agency (MHRA) of the UK. The BP includes general notices, general monographs, specific monographs providing mandatory standards for active pharmaceutical ingredients, excipients, formulated preparations, herbal drugs, herbal drug products and herbal medicinal products, materials for use in the manufacture of homoeopathic preparations, blood-related products, immunological products, radio-pharmaceutical preparations, infrared reference spectra, appendices, supplementary chapters and comprehensive index. The BP (veterinary) is published as a companion volume to the British Pharmacopoeia. It contains standards for substances and products used solely in the practice of veterinary medicine in the UK. The BP (vet) also incorporates monographs and texts of the European Pharmacopoeia (EuPhr).

The second edition of BP was published in 1867. The British Pharmacopoeia Commission was established in 1970 under Section 4 of the Medicines Act 1968 to carry on the work of the previous Commission appointed by the GMC. The 1874 Addendum to the BP 1867 was prepared with Attfield as the editor. The third edition was published in 1885 with Redwood, Attfield and Robert Bentley as joint editors. Another addendum was published in 1890, with

Attfield again acting as its editor. The fourth edition of BP was published in 1898. This was prepared for the GMC Pharmacopoeia Committee with Nestor Tirard as its secretary. An Indian and Colonial Addendum were published in 1900, again with Attfield as its editor. In November 1903 the Council of the Pharmaceutical Society decided to produce its own reference book. The first edition of the British Pharmaceutical Codex (BPC) was published in 1907. The BP was supplemented by BPC which gave information on drugs and other pharmaceutical substances not included in the BP, and provided standards for these. Australia and Canada are just two of the countries that have adopted the BP as their national standard alongside the UK. In November 1911 Tirard and Greenish were appointed as editors of the next fifth edition, which was published in 1914. Drugs included for the first time included aspirin, diamorphine hydrochloride and phenolphthalein. Doses were given in both the imperial and metric systems. The new sixth edition of BP became official in October 1932. There were seven Addenda to the BP 1932. A seventh edition of the BP was ready by November 1946, but it was not published until 1948 due to paper shortages. The eighth edition was published in 1953. In BP 1953 edition titles of drugs and preparations were in English instead of Latin and metric system was used to denote measures. New ninth and tenth editions of the BP were published in 1958 and 1963. The BP 1963 contained almost 1000 monographs, 200 of which appeared for the first time. In 1963 the BP Commission commented on a proposal to create a common pharmacopoeia to serve the needs of a number of European countries. This was to lead to the founding of the EuPhr in 1964. A new eleventh edition of BP was published in 1968. Another new twelfth edition was published in 1973. The 13th edition of BP was published in 1980. The 14th Edition of BP was published in 1988 which contained two volumes with 2100 monographs. In 1993, 15th edition of BP was published. In 1998 a consolidated BP NF edition was published.

In BP 2007 monographs has been introduced for material specifically used in preparation of traditional Chinese medicines. The term 'prolonged release' was replaced with the term 'slow' and the term 'gastro-resistant' was replaced with 'enteric coated' in number of monographs. The BP 2008 contains approximately 3100 monographs for substances, preparations and articles used in practice. It was made effective from 1st January 2008. The BP 2009 was published in 2009. The BP from 2007 to 2009 was given in six volumes. The Volume-I and -II contained medicinal substances while, Volume-III contained formulated preparations, blood related products, immunological products, radiopharmaceutical preparations, surgical materials and homoeopathic preparations. Volume-IV contained supplementary chapters, IR spectrums, etc. The Volume-V contains veterinary and Volume-VI contains CD ROM version.

The BP 2010 was published by The Stationery Office (TSO), on behalf of the British Pharmacopoeia Secretariat, a part of the MHRA. The standards in the BP 2010 were made legally effective in the UK from 1st January 2010. The print edition of the BP 2010 comprises four volumes of the BP 2010 and a single volume of the BP (veterinary) 2010. The BP 2012 was made legally effective from 1st January 2012. This edition of the BP comprises six volumes. The print edition of the BP 2012 comprises five volumes of the BP 2012 and a single volume of the BP (veterinary) 2012. The BP 2013 includes six volume printed edition including the BP (veterinary) 2013. This edition contained 41 new BP monographs, 40 new EuPhr monographs, 619 amended monographs and, 6 new and 1 amended infrared reference spectra. The BP 2014 edition includes about 3500 monographs which are legally enforced by the Human Medicines Regulations 2012. The BP 2014 comprises five volumes of the BP 2014 and a single volume of the BP (veterinary) 2014, along with a fully searchable CD-ROM and online access to provide flexible resources. It was legally made effective from 1stJanuary 2014. It includes 40 new BP monographs, 272 amended monographs, 3 new supplementary chapters, 4 new BP (veterinary) monographs and 1 new BP (veterinary) supplementary chapter.

The Secretariat of British Pharmacopoeia Commission published BP 2016 and the BP (Vet) 2016. All items included in the eighth edition of the EuPhr together with those from Supplements 8.1 to 8.5, were incorporated in either of the BP 2016. The BP 2016 was published in August 2015. The BP 2016 includes almost 4,000 monographs which are legally enforced by the Human Medicines Regulations 2012, and becomes legally effective on 1stJanuary 2016. This edition sees the introduction of a download format for offline use and the new integrated website pharmacopoeia.com.

Today BP is published for the Health Ministers of the United Kingdom on the recommendation of the Commission on Human Medicines in accordance with section 99(6) of the Medicines Act 1968 and notified in draft to the European Commission in accordance with Directive 98/34/EEC. It has been prepared by the British Pharmacopoeia Commission, with the collaboration and support of its expert advisory groups and panels of experts.

The BP has been providing authoritative, official standards for pharmaceutical substances and medicinal products since 1864. Today, it is used in more than 100 countries worldwide and remains an essential reference across the globe. BP, including the BP (Vet) and the Ph. Eur. are the two pharmacopoeias that have legal status within the UK. BP is published every year in August becomes effective on 1st January of the following year that incorporates all the monographs and texts of the Ph. Eur.

1.11 UNITED STATE PHARMACOPOEIA

1800-1900

The United States Pharmacopeia (USP) is a pharmacopeia for the United States published annually by the United States Pharmacopoeial Convention, a non-profit organization that owns the trademark and copyright. The USP is published in a combined volume with the National Formulary as the USP-NF. If a drug ingredient or drug product has an applicable USP quality standard, it must conform in order to use the designation "USP" or "NF". Drugs subject to USP standards include both human drugs, as well as animal drugs. A drug or drug ingredient with a name recognized in USP-NF is deemed adulterated if it does not satisfy compendial standards for strength, quality or purity. USP also sets standards for dietary supplements, and food ingredients. USP has no role in enforcing its standards; enforcement is the responsibility of FDA and other government authorities in the U.S. and elsewhere.

USP was founded in 1820 by 11 physicians in Washington DC. Dr. Spalding proposed a national pharmacopoeia in 1817. Jacob Bigelow was the primary author of the first Pharmacopoeia of the United States of America. The first Pharmacopoeia of the United States contained 217 of the most fully established and best understood medicines in the U.S. It was published by the authorities of the medical societies and colleges. In 1830 a seven member's committee for revision of USP was created. The first revision of the USP published in the same year and it was resolved to revise USP at 10-year intervals. Surgeons General of U.S. Army and Navy became first federal agencies to participate in USP revision.

In 1848 'Drug Import Act' was passed and Federal legislation recognized the USP as an official compendium. The colleges of pharmacy were invited in 1850 to participate in revision of the USP. The 1860 (USP IV) and 1870 (USP V) editions were not structurally any different from the earlier editions, but did include newer remedies and processes as well as technical methods. Charles Rice was elected as Chairman of the Committee of Revision, 1880 and soon initiated efforts to modernize USP monographs and methods. Clara Marshall appointed the first woman member of the USP Convention. The first National Formulary (NF) 1888 was published by the American Pharmacists Association. In 1880 (USP VI) and 1890 (USP VII) editions were published.

1900-2000

In 1900 USP incorporated in Washington, DC, as a not-for-profit corporation. USP Convention and Board of Trustees created. USP VIII published in 1900 became official in 1905 with significant changes. Average doses, allowable percentages of impurities, specific assays for several drugs, and nomenclature of synthetic drugs and chemicals made their way into the pharmacopoeia. Small pox vaccine was added to USP IX. The 4th edition of the NF, the first after the Act was passed, was published in 1916. The USP XV was published on 15th December 1915. In 1932 the USP Reference Standards program succeeded FDA's short-lived program with standards for Vitamin A and D content in cod liver oil. The Federal Food, Drug, and, Cosmetic Act 1938, was passed. The USPNF standards for strength, quality, purity, packaging, and labeling were recognized as official and enforced by FDA. Within this Act the "New Drug" concept was established and FDA was made approval authority for drugs safety before marketing. Revision cycle for USP was changed in 1942 and USP was published every five years. USP XII in 1942 was the first revision published under the five-year schedule and it included monographs for injections for the first time, and compressed tablets finally were included although they were in use since Charles Rice's time. USP continues international activities which began in earnest in the early 1900s. In 1949 USP Board appointed Lloyd Miller as Director of Revision. He was the USP's first salaried employee. After years of working out of the homes of its volunteers, USP purchased it first building in 1950 at Park Avenue in New York City, NY. The USP XIV and USP XV were published in 1950 and 1955, respectively. First United States Adopted Names (USAN) cumulative list was published in 1963. USAN Council was formed 1964 as joint venture of American Medical Association, USP and the American Pharmacists Association (APhA). The USP XVII was published on 1st September 1965. William M. Heller in 1970 was appointed as Executive Director. USP Convention adopts resolution calling for information to be provided to dispensers of drugs in United States. Later year USP moves to Rockville, MD, USA in 1971. In 1974 the NF was purchased by the United States Pharmacopoeial Convention. In 1977 USP and NF scope was redefined with separation as USP specified standards for drug substances and dosage forms whereas NF specified standards for excipients. USP and NF were published under same cover in 1980 as USP Dispensing Information (USP DI). Jerome A. Halperin was appointed as USP executive vice president and chief executive officer (CEO) at the 1990 USP Convention. In the convention USP Members adopted a resolution to explore establishing standards for vitamins and minerals. From 1992 USP began long-term collaboration with USADI. In 1994 USP signed an agreement with the American Medical Association (AMA) to combine the information in AMA's Drug Evaluations database with the USP DI database to develop a single product that contains drug and therapeutic information. USP members adopted a resolution in 1995 to explore establishing standards for botanical dietary supplements. The USP23NF18 has ten supplements. The first supplement was published in January 1995 and last in May 1999. USP licensed USP DI and associated products in 1998 to The Thomson Company and USP DI was published by their Micromedex subsidiary.

2000-2016

Roger L. Williams, M.D., became USP Executive Vice President and CEO at the USP Convention in April 2000. The Convention Members voted to change name of Committee of Revision to Council of Experts. The USP-USAID in collaboration made efforts that leads to evolution of DQI, a program focused on improving the quality of medicines and their appropriate uses in resource-limited countries. The USP24-NF19 appeared from 1st January 2000. In 2001 USP launched the Dietary Supplement Verification Program. From 2002 USP–NF was published annually. In 2004 USP and the Chinese Pharmacopoeia Commission collaborated for hosting first joint symposium in China to discuss key scientific and pharmacopoeial topics. The outcome of this collaboration was that USP opened its office in 2005 at Basel, Switzerland. This was followed by signing a Memorandum of Understanding

(MOU) with Chinese Pharmacopoeia Commission. In 2006 USP signed MOU with Indian Pharmacopoeia Commission to promote greater cooperation. As a result, USP opened first international laboratory facility in Hyderabad. Meanwhile USP launched the Pharmaceutical Ingredient Verification Program and acquired the Food Chemicals Codex (FCC) from the Institute of Medicine. From 2006, Spanish edition of USP is also being published. In 2007 USP opened its office and laboratory facility in Shanghai, China. In the same year USP published USP–NF as a three-volume set. The USP30-NF25 appeared from May 2007. It contains scientific standards for drugs, dietary substances, biological products and excipients used in dosage forms. It contains 4100 monographs and 200 general chapters. It has been printed in three volume set. Volume I contains general chapters and Volume II and III contains monographs. The highlights of USP30-NF25 includes complete table of contents and index in each volume, special 'Using the New USP-NF Print' tutorial CD, convenient slipcase for easy access and storage (English edition only). This edition was heavier paper stock. First supplement to USP30-NF25 appeared from August 2007 and second supplement from November 2007 which was considered official from May 2008. In 2009 USP published the USP Dietary Supplements Compendium and first Russian edition of USP–NF. The USP31-NF26 is a single-volume combination of two official compendia, the USP and the National Formulary (NF) from 1st May, 2008. Monographs for drug substances and preparations are featured in the USP, with monographs for dietary supplements and ingredients appearing in a separate section of the USP. Excipient monographs are included in the NF. The USP32-NF27 published in 2009 contained more than 4,200 monographs, over 200 general chapters, covering general tests and assays, displays helpful guides and charts that make it easy to find and focus on specific information on emerging areas of science and medicine, helps to ensure compliance with official standards, enables validation of test results against proven benchmarks, creates in-house standards for operating procedures and specifications and expedites new product development and approvals. The USP33-NF28 published on 1st October 2010 contained more than 4,400 monographs, over 200 general chapters covering general tests and assays, a new easy-to-read format, monograph layout and charts that make it easy to find focus-specific information, ensures compliance with official standards, establishes in-house standard operating procedures and specifications and facilitates new product development and approval. The USP34-NF29 published in 2011 features more than 4,500 monographs for drug substances, dosage forms, excipients, biologics, dietary supplements, and other therapeutics. USP 34-NF 29 also offers harmonized material and more than 230 General Chapters with current guidelines for the full range of laboratory tests and established processes for validating methods. The USP35-NF30 is published as a combination of two official compendia, the 'USP' and the 'NF', and was made officially applicable from 1st May, 2012 to 30 April, 2013. The USP36-NF31 is published in November 2012. The USP37-NF32 is published in November 2014. The USP38-NF33 is published in November 2015. The USP39-NF34 is published in February 2016.

Extra Pharmacopoeia

This book is a little piece of history now. Its full title was "The extra pharmacopoeia of unofficial drugs and chemical and pharmaceutical preparations" written by William Martindale. Martindale aims to cover drugs and related substances reported to be of clinical interest anywhere in the world. It provides a useful source of information for patients arriving from abroad to identify their existing medication. This may reveal that a currently taken proprietary preparation is available under another brand name. Alternatively, if the drug is not available, the class of agent can be determined allowing a pharmacist or doctor to determine which alternative equivalent drugs can be substituted. Extra Pharmacopoeia was first published in 1883 under the title 'Martindale: The Extra Pharmacopoeia'. Martindale contains information on drugs in clinical use worldwide, as well as selected investigational and veterinary drugs, herbal and complementary medicines, pharmaceutical excipients, radiopharmaceuticals, vitamins and nutritional agents, vaccines, contrast media and diagnostic agents, medicinal gases, drugs of abuse and recreational drugs, toxic substances, disinfectants, and pesticides. 'Martindale: The Complete Drug Reference' is a reference book published by Pharmaceutical Press listing some 6000 drugs and medicines used throughout the world, including details of over 180000 proprietary preparations. It also includes almost 700 disease treatment reviews.

Martindale is arranged into two main parts followed by three extensive indexes. First part is 'Monographs on drugs and ancillary substances' listing over 6,000 monographs arranged in 49 chapters based on clinical use with the corresponding disease treatment reviews. Monographs summarize the nomenclature, properties, and actions of each substance. A chapter on supplementary drugs and other substances covers some 1190 monographs on new drugs, those not easily classified, herbals, and drugs no longer clinically used but still of interest. Monographs of some toxic substances are also included. The second part is preparations that include over 180000 items from 43 countries and regions, including China. The three indexes are Directory of Manufacturers, Pharmaceutical Terms in Various Languages and General index. The directory of Manufacturers has list of some 20000 entries. Pharmaceutical terms in various languages index lists nearly 5600 pharmaceutical terms and routes of administration in 13 major European languages as an aid to the non-native speaker in interpreting packaging, product information, or prescriptions written in another language. The General index is prepared from 175000 entries which include approved names, synonyms and chemical names; a separate Cyrillic section lists nonproprietary and proprietary names in Russian and Ukrainian. The digital versions of   Extra Pharmacopoeia include an additional 1000 drug monographs, 60000 preparation names, and 5000 manufacturers. To date there have been 38 editions of 'Martindale: The Complete Drug Reference'. The 38th edition was published in June 2014 by the London Pharmaceutical Press.

MODEL QUESTIONS

1. Discuss history and development of profession of pharmacy in India.
2. Describe history of pharmaceutical education in India.
3. Explain different career options after pharmacy.
4. Write a note on Indian Pharmacopoeia/British Pharmacopoeia/United State Pharmacopoeia.
5. Write a short note on:
   (i)   National Formulary of India.
   (ii) Extra Pharmacopoeia.
   (iii) Pre and post-independence pharmacy profession.
   (iv) Indian pharmaceutical industry.

■■■

Chapter **2**...

Introduction to Dosage Forms

LEARNING OBJECTIVES

Achieving effective treatment of a disease with minimizing adverse effects of a drug requires rational selection, formulation and administration of an appropriate dosage form. This chapter is a must need for fresh pharmacy students to be explored in great enough detail to enable the student to be equipped for both literary and practical knowledge at a preliminary scale.

The objectives of this chapter include:

- Define and differentiate between the terms dose, form and delivery system.
- Enumerate and explain the properties and identify advantages and disadvantages of the major dosage forms and delivery systems for drugs.
- To understand the basics of dosage form and its types.
- To describe scientific background and technical aspects that are important in dosage form design, basic dosage forms and their therapeutic applications.
- To instruct students about in general considerations of preparation of various conventional dosage forms.
- This course will focus on the biopharmaceutical considerations and physicochemical foundation of various dosage forms.

2.1 DRUG

A 'drug' may be defined as an agent, intended for use in the diagnosis, mitigation, treatment, cure or prevention of disease in man or in animals. The "new drug" is defined as any drug the composition of which is such that it is not generally recognized, among experts qualified by scientific training and experience to evaluate the safety and effectiveness of drugs, as safe and effective for use under the conditions prescribed, recommended, or suggested in the labelling thereof.

2.2 SOURCES OF DRUGS

Records of using drug are found dating back to 2,700 BC in the Middle East and China and the most commonly used drugs were laxatives and anti-emetics. Until the last decade of 19th century, the substances used for the treatment of diseases were obtained from natural sources. Natural sources include plants, animals, and minerals. Among the natural sources, plants were mainly used. Sometimes minerals and occasionally animals were used for the same purpose. Today majority of the drugs are synthetic and are manufactured in the laboratory and large number of drugs are obtained from micro-organisms. The sources of drugs can be classified as:

I. Plants

Plants are used from a time when the leaves with shape of the liver used for the treatment of liver diseases. Various parts of the plant such as root, bark, stem, leaf, seed and flower are also used as drugs. All parts of a specific plant do not equally contain a specific drug. Today plants (with few exceptions) as such are not used as drugs for rational treatment but pharmacologically active constituents (PAC) are extracted from the plant parts and are used. The PAC of plants includes alkaloid, glycoside, oil, gum, mucilage, carbohydrate and related compounds. Some of these active constituents can be extracted by soaking the plant in suitable solvents such as ether or alcohol.

II. Animals

Chinese people used the dried skin of toad that contains adrenaline to treat toothache and bleeding in gum. The cod liver oil is obtained from cod fish contains high levels of omega 3 fatty acids, vitamin A and vitamin D. Insulin is extracted from the pancreas of bovine or porcine. Immunoglobulin G is prepared by the injecting antigen into an animal and collecting the antibody formed as a reaction to the antigen. Human immunoglobulin is prepared from pools of at least 1000 donations of human plasma containing the antibody to treat diseases such as measles, mumps, hepatitis, etc. Hepatitis B immunoglobulin, rabies immunoglobulin, tetanus immunoglobulins are prepared by pooling the plasma of selected donors with high levels of the specific antibody required. Human menopausal gonadotropin is isolated from the urine of postmenopausal women that contains a mixture of follicle stimulating hormone and luteinizing hormone. Human chorionic gonadotropin is produced by the placenta. It is isolated and purified from the urine of pregnant woman. Heparin is commonly extracted from porcine intestinal mucosa or bovine lung.

III. Minerals

The early Greek physicians used iron to treat weakness and anemia. Various clays, kaolin and activated charcoal have been used for the treatment of diarrhea. Calomel is used in the treatment of constipation and syphilis, for diuretic effect and in the treatment of congestive cardiac failure. Iodine is used for the treatment of goiter. Gold is used for the treatment for the arthritis. Sulfur is used externally in skin diseases. Aluminum hydroxide and magnesium trisilcate are widely used as antacids. Magnesium sulfide is used to relieve constipation and to control ecliptic seizure.

IV. Laboratory Sources

Today majority of the drugs are produced by chemically reacting two or more compounds or elements. Drugs produced in laboratories are safer, of high quality, less expensive, produced in large quantities within short time and more effective than drugs obtained from plants or animals. Most of the currently used analgesics, chemotherapeutic drugs, hypnotics and local anesthetics are produced in the laboratory. Some examples of these types of drugs are digoxin and salicylates, sulfonamides, apomorphine, homatropine, human insulin, etc. Antibiotics that are produced by the micro-organism actinomycetes are actinomycin, amphotericin, chloramphenicol, erythromycin, kanamycin, neomycin, gentamicin, streptomycin and tetracycline. Aspergillate group of fungi produces antibiotics such as penicillin, griseofulvin and cephalosporin. Among the bacteria, genus *Bacillus* produces antibiotic polymyxin B and bacitracin.

2.3 RATIONALE FOR DEVELOPMENT OF DOSAGE FORM

The drug also called active ingredient is the biochemically reactive component of the pharmaceutical product. An active ingredient is rarely given in pure form. Instead, one or more active ingredients are combined with one or more inactive ingredients. Most drug products contain one or more active ingredients that are dispersed to obtain solution or suspension within an inert primary base, or vehicle, that may contain other ingredients for various functions. Drugs are converted into suitable formulation called as dosage form. Pharmaceutical product is a system containing active and inactive pharmaceutical ingredients formulated into the particular dosage form, packed and labelled, appropriately. Dosage form provides unique properties, advantages, and disadvantages which may result in development of different dosage forms for one drug. For example, ibuprofen is available in tablet, capsule, suppository, syrup, suspension, oral drop, parenteral, cream, and gel formulations. Dosage forms are provided in pharmacopoeia for most of the drug substances but the processes for the preparation of many of them are beyond the scope of the Pharmacopeia.

Need of Dosage Form

1. To facilitate the administration of drug substances to have better patient compliance.
2. To enhance stability of drugs at normal storage conditions.
3. To ease transportation, distribution, production and effectiveness of therapy.
4. To protect the drug in the stomach from gastric acid upon oral administration, for example, enteric coated tablets.
5. To provide a safe and convenient delivery of accurate dosage.
6. To conceal the bitter, salty or an obnoxious taste or odor of a drug substance, for example, capsules, coated tablets and flavored syrups etc.
7. To provide for the optimum drug action through inhalation.
8. To deliver drugs into the body-cavities, for example, rectal suppositories.
9. To provide for the maximum drug action from topical administration sites, for example, creams, ointments, ophthalmic preparations etc.
10. To provide sustained release action by controlling drug release, for example, sustained release tablets.
11. To provide liquid dosage form of the drugs soluble in a suitable vehicle, for example, solutions.
12. To avoid local irritations or injury when they are present at high concentrations at the site of administration.
13. To modify pka profile of drug to enhance bioavailability.

2.4 CLASSIFICATION OF DOSAGE FORMS

Dosage forms are divided in to various types based on their states, route of administration, site of application, type of vehicle, use and sterility.

(A) Physical state

1.	Solid	Powder, tablet, capsule, caplet, cachet, pill, lozenge, cachet, capsule, insufflation, dentifrice, effervescent granule, pessary, suppository etc.
2.	Semi-solid	Gel, ointment, cream, jelly, paste etc.
3.	Liquid	Solution, emulsion, syrup, elixir, magma, suspension, lotion, application, aromatic water, collodion, draught, ear drop, eye drop, nasal drop, mixture, enema, gargle, gel, injection, irrigation, linctus, liniment, lotion mouth wash, spirit, spray, syrup, tincture, paint etc.
4.	Gaseous	Aerosol, spray, inhalation

(B) Route of administration

1.	Oral	Powder, tablet, capsule, solution, emulsion, syrup, elixir, magma, gel, cachet, pill.
2.	Parental	Solution, suspension, emulsion, tablet, implant.
3.	Rectal	Suppository, enema.
4.	Topical	Ointment, cream, powder, paste, lotion, plaster, liniment, gel, transdermal patch.
5.	Urethral	Suppository, douche, intrauterine device, pessary, vaginal ring, tablet.
6.	Sublingual	Lozenge, tablet.
7.	Intranasal	Solution, spray, inhaler.
8.	Conjunctival	Ointment.
9.	Ophthalmic	Eye drop, ophthalmic gel, ophthalmic ointment, solution.
10.	Intra-respiratory	Aerosol.
11.	Otic	Ear drop (solution or suspension).

(C) Site of application

1.	Skin	Powder, solution, emulsion, gel, ointment, cream, paste, lotion, plaster.
2.	Eye	Solution, ointment.
3.	Tooth	Powder, solution, paste, spray.
4.	Hand	Powder, solution, emulsion, gel, suspension, ointment, cream, paste, lotion, plaster.
5.	Foot	Powder, solution, emulsion, gel, ointment, cream, lotion, plaster.
6.	Hair	Solution, gel, cream.
7.	Nose	Aerosol.

(D) Based on type of vehicle

1.	Aqueous preparations	Water, diluted acid, solution, douche, enema, gargle, juice, ophthalmic, sweet viscid solution, syrup, honey, mucilage, jellies, suspension, mixture, magma, gel, lotion.
2.	Non-aqueous preparations	Solution, injection, ear drop, nasal drop, liniment, medicated body oils, medicated hair oil.

(E) Based on use

1.	Internal	Powder, tablet, capsule, solution, emulsion, syrup, elixir, magma, gel, cachet, pill, suspension, lozenge.
2.	External	Aerosol, ointment, cream, powder, paste, lotion, plaster, suppository, douche, foam, solution, spray, inhalation.

(F) Based on sterility

1. Non-Sterile Dosage Forms

I. **Solid dosage forms**				
	(A) **Powders**			
		(a) **Powders**		
			1. Internal use	Simple or compound powders, bulk powder.
			2. External use	Dusting powder, snuff, insufflation, spray, dentifrice, tooth powder.
		(b) **Compressed Dosage Forms**		
			1. Tablets	
			(i) Oral tablets	Standard compressed tablet, lozenge, buccal tablet, dental cone, sublingual tablet, dispersible tablet, multiple compressed tablet, Sustained release tablet, enteric coated tablet, sugar coated tablet, chewable tablet, film coated tablet.
			(ii) Other tablets	Vaginal tablet, soluble tablet, hypodermic tablet, effervescent tablet.
		(c) **Non-Compressed Forms**		
			1. Pills	
			2. Capsules	
			(i) Oral	Soft gelatin capsule, hard gelatin capsule.
			(ii) Topical	Ointment.
II. **Semi-solid dosage forms**				
	(A) **Ointments**			Oleaginous base, water soluble base.
	(B) **Creams**			
	(C) **Pastes**			
	(D) **Jellies**			
	(E) **Poultices**			
	(F) **Plasters**			

III.	**Liquid dosage forms**			
	(A)	**Monophasic**		
		(a)	**Internal Use**	Simple mixture, solution, draught, linctus, syrup, elixir, drop, tinctures, linctuses, mouth wash, aromatic water, gargles, injections.
		(b)	**External Use**	Liniment, lotion, collodion, application, tinctures, spirits, mouth washes.
		(c)	**Special Use**	
			1. Oral cavity	Glycerite, throat paint, gargle, mouth wash, Throat spray.
			2. Other than oral cavity	Douche, enema, ear drop, nasal drop, application, inhalation, spray, aerosol, injections, irrigations, enemas.
	(B)	**Biphasic**		
		(a)	**Emulsions**	
			1. o/w emulsions	Internal use, external use.
			2. w/o emulsions	Internal use, external use.
		(b)	**Suspensions**	Internal use, external use.
IV.	**Gaseous dosage forms**			Aerosols, inhalations.

2. Sterile Dosage Forms

I.	**Parenteral Dosage Forms**		
	(A)	**Small Volume Parenterals**	Powder to be suspended in vehicle before use, powder to be solubilized in solvent prior to use, readymade suspension, readymade solution, emulsion.
	(B)	**Large volume Parenterals**	
		(a) Large volume Parenterals	Infusions, hyperailmentation, cardioplegic solutions, peritoneal dialysis solution.
II.	**Ophthalmic Dosage Forms**		
	(A)	**Eye drops**	Ophthalmic solution, ophthalmic emulsion, ophthalmic suspension.
	(B)	**Eye lotions**	
	(C)	**Eye ointments**	
	(D)	**Controlled delivery systems**	Mucoadhesive dosage form, ocular insert, collagen shield, drug presoaked hydrogel type contact lens, ocular iontophoresis, polymeric solution.
III.	**Implants**		Tablets

(A) SOLID DOSAGE FORMS

The majority of solid dosage forms is composed of powders and is usually processed to some degree to change their form.

Advantages:

1. Solid medications are more stable than liquids and have longer shelf lives.
2. Easy to package, handle, ship and transport and requires less shelf space.
3. Generally, no need to add preservatives except containing unstable drugs.
4. Accurate single dose can be taken since the medication is already in unit measure.
5. Suitable for controlling drug release for desired delivery.
6. Patients are able to self-administer solid medications more easily.
7. Solid dosage forms have been created to release the medication over a longer period of time in the patient's body and thus allow the patient to take fewer doses.

Disadvantages:

1. The processing of solid dosage forms is complicated and requires expensive machines.
2. Children, seriously ill persons and old patients find difficulty in swallowing solid dosage form.
3. Some drugs resist flow and compression into dense compacts, owing to their amorphous nature and low density character.
4. Solid medications are not an appropriate choice for patients who are unconscious or have nasal/mouth breathing tubes for ventilation.
5. Solid medications take longer to be broken down, absorbed, and distributed in the body. The stomach has to metabolize the medication before it can take effect.
6. Solid medications are not fast enough for immediate action treatments.

POWDERS

Powders are solid dosage form of drug substances meant for internal or external use. The powder is classified as divided powder and bulk powder. A single-dose presentations of powder that are intended to be issued to the patient as such, to be taken in or with water is called as 'divided powders'. When the powders are dispensed in large quantities in a container and the patient is supposed to measure a specified quantity as a dose then these powders are known as 'bulk powders'. The powders meant for internal use are known as 'oral powders' whereas those meant for external use are known as 'dusting powders'. Dusting powders are fine medicinal (bulk) powders intended to be dusted on the skin by means of sifter-top containers. Medical dusting powders are mainly used for superficial skin conditions. Surgical dusting powders are sterilized before their use and are used in body cavities and on major wounds as a result of burns and to treat umbilical cords of infants. The mixed powders are mixtures of different drug substances stored in dry form and prepared when required for dispensing.

Examples:

(i)   Bulk powder for internal use: Compound Sodium Chloride-Dextrose Oral Powder, Compound Rhubarb Oral Powder.

(ii)   Bulk powders for external use: Talc Dusting Powders and Tooth Powder.

(iii)   Medical dusting powder: Dicophane Dusting Powder, Zinc and Salicylic Acid Dusting Powder, Zinc, Starch and Talc Dusting Powder etc.

(iv)   Mixed powders: Neosporin Powder and Canesten Powder.

Advantages:

1. Powder is most versatile and convenient form to compound and administer.

2. It provides freedom for physician to manipulate the conventional dose of drug as per requirement of the patient particularly for children and infants.

3. Powders are stable and do not enter easily into reaction in solid state.

4. Being fine in particle size powder form facilitate rapid drug absorption.

5. They are less incompatible compared to liquid dosage form.

6. Powders are rapidly dissolved in the GIT minimizing the problems of local irritation.

7. Powders can be administered by mixing with suitable liquid to make them palatable.

8. Powder manufacturing is economic and thus product cost is low.

Disadvantages:

1. Powders are time consuming to compound.

2. Inaccurate amount of drug may be delivered in powder form.

3. Individual dose wrapping for powders make them expensive.

4. Powders with volatile, hygroscopic, oxidizing and deliquescent properties are unstable.

5. Powder dosages can be inaccurate.

6. Patient may misunderstand the correct method of use if not instructed clearly. For example, correct route of administration, method of making solution of powder etc.

7. Not suitable for oral administration if drug has bitter or unpleasant taste.

GRANULES

Granules are wetted, dried, and ground coarse pieces made of powders containing drug. These are free flowing, dry conglomerates ranging from 1 to 5 mm in diameter. The drug and the excipients are mixed to form cohesive mass with a suitable moistening agent and the mass is pressed through a sieve of required granule size and dried. Granules are larger and usually more stable than the powders. Granules may be placed on the tongue and swallowed with water or are intended to be dissolved in water before administration.

Examples: Senokot® Granules used as stimulant laxative and Principen® (ampicillin) for Oral Suspension.

Advantages:

1. The segregation of the constituents of the powder mixture could be avoided by granulation.
2. Granules are more stable against humidity and atmosphere and less likely to make cake or harden upon standing.
3. They are more easily wetted by liquids than light and fluffy powders and are more preferable for dry products intended to be constituted into solution or suspension.
4. Granules are more flowable compared to powders. The easy flow characteristics are important in supplying drug materials from the hopper or feeding container into the tableting presses.
5. Granules also eliminate or control dust.
6. Granules increase compressibility.
7. Granules have smaller surface area than a comparable volume of powders. This makes granules more stable physically and chemically than the corresponding powders.
8. Granules are less likely to cake or harden upon standing than are powders.
9. Granules are more easily wetted by a solvent than certain powders thus granules are preferred in making solutions.
10. Granules produce particle-size uniformity and thus content uniformity.

Disadvantages:

1. Making granules is time consuming and its packaging is difficult.
2. They are bulky to carry about.
3. Powder particles may spill when they are being opened.
4. Sometimes granules cannot be processed to tablet or capsule and are to be formulated as suspension.
5. Drugs with an unpleasant taste cannot be formulated as granules and need to be filled in a hard capsule.
6. Volatile deliquescent, hygroscopic or oxygen-sensitive drugs are difficult formulate as granules.

EFFERVESCENT GRANULES

The effervescent granules are solid dosage form of drug substances, meant for oral administration that contain a drug mixed with citric acid, tartaric acid and sodium bicarbonate and sometimes saccharin or sucrose is added as a sweetening agent.

Examples: Andrews Liver Salts (magnesium sulphate dihydrate, sodium hydrogen carbonate and citric acid, anhydrous - laxative and antacid), Cacit D3$^{®}$ Effervescent Granules (calcium carbonate/cholecalciferol).

Advantages:

1. Attractive dosage form for the public.
2. The carbonated solution masks undesirable taste of the drug.
3. The liberated carbon dioxide is used as a therapeutic agent; it increases gastric secretions and hence facilitates digestion, and it also acts as anti-nauseant.
4. Using granules rather than powders decreases the rate of solution and prevents uncontrollable *effervescence.*

Disadvantages:

1. Requires a complex production process.
2. They are unstable in presence of moisture.
3. It has packaging problems and thus need special packaging materials and storage.

TABLETS

Tablets are defined as solid pharmaceutical dosage forms containing drug substances with or without suitable excipients prepared either by compression or moulding methods.

Examples: Crocin® Tablet (paracetamol); Analgin® Tablet (aspirin), Prozac® Tablet (fluoxetine)

Advantages:

1. Tablets are elegant in appearance and convenient to swallow.
2. They are simple and economical and provide prolonged stability to drug.
3. It is most convenient form to pack, ship, and transport.
4. The product identification mark can be printed on tablet surface.
5. A wide range of tablet types are available, offering a range of functionalities.
6. Tablets may contain more than one drug for combination effects.
7. Unpleasant taste can be masked by sugar coating enhancing patient acceptability.
8. Tablets do not require any measurement of dose and provides accurate dose.
9. They are easy to swallow and carry thus have high level of patient acceptability.
10. An accurate and small amount of drug can be incorporated.
11. Administration of minute dose of drug in accurate amount.
12. Tablets are easy to divide into halves and quarters whenever fraction dose is required.

Disadvantages:

1. Children and elders find difficulties in swallowing tablets.
2. Tablet requires many trials to find good compatibility between drug and excipients.
3. The absorption of drugs from tablets shows interpatient variation.
4. Highly amorphous and low dense substances are very difficult to compress.
5. Poor wetting and slow dissolution drugs cannot be formulated as tablets.

6. A tablet may exert irritant effects on the GI mucosa and bioavailability problems due to slow/fast disintegration and dissolution.
7. Drugs with poor wetting, slow dissolution and large dose are not suitable.
8. Many times specially designed tablets are not economical.
9. Liquid drugs are difficult to formulate in tablet.

Types of Tablets:

(i) Tablets ingested orally:

1. Compressed tablet
   For example, Crocin® Tablet (paracetamol)
2. Multiple compressed tablet
   For example, Mucinex® Tablet (guaifenesin)
3. Repeat action tablet
   For example, Trital® Tablet (phenylephrine, ascorbic acid, paracetamol)
4. Delayed release tablet
   For example, Enteric coated Bisacodyl Tablet
5. Sugar coated tablet
   For example, Becovit® Tablet (multivitamin and minerals)
6. Film coated tablet
   For example, Flagyl® Tablet (metronidazole)
7. Chewable tablet
   For example, Gelusil® Tablet (alumina, magnesium and simethicone)

(ii) Tablets used in oral cavity:

1. Buccal Tablet
   For example, Oravig® Tablet (miconazole)
2. Sublingual Tablet
   For example, Vicks® Tablet (menthol)
3. Troches or Lozenges
   For example, Difflam® plus Tablet (lignocaine)
4. Dental Cone
   For example, Parasorb® Cone (gentamicin)

(iii) Tablets administered by other route:

1. Implantation tablet
   For example, Nexplanon® Tablet (etonogestrel)
2. Vaginal tablet
   For example, Canesten® Tablet (clotrimazole)

(iv) Tablets used to prepare solution:

1. Effervescent tablet
   For example, Dispirin® Tablet (aspirin)

2. Dispensing tablet

   For example, Enzyme Tablet (digiplex)

3. Hypodermic tablet

   For example, Morphine Sulphate Tablet

4. Tablet triturates

   For example, Enzyme Tablet (digiplex)

IMPLANTS

Implants are small, sterile, cylindrical solid masses not more than 8 mm length consisting of a highly purified drug (with or without excipients) made by compression or molding and is placed under the skin by means of minor surgery. They are intended for implantation in the body (usually subcutaneously) for the purpose of providing continuous release of the drug over long periods of time. Implants are administered by means of a suitable special injector or surgical incision.

Examples: Estradiol Tablet (Hormone replacement therapy), Norplant® Tablet (levonorgestrel).

Advantages:

1. Implants have been used to administer hormones such as testosterone or estradiol.
2. They are packaged individually in sterile vials or foil strips.
3. Enhanced patient compliance and convenience.

Disadvantages:

1. Complications at the site of insertion make its limited use.
2. The insertion methods require special surgical technique for implantation and discontinuation of therapy.

PILLS

Pills are spherical dosage forms prepared by mixing drug uniformly with diluents, binders, disintegrators or other suitable excipients. Pills have now been almost completely replaced by capsules and tablets. As dosage form pills are very popular in Ayurvedic medicine and are known as 'Vati'. Today, "pills" include tablets, capsules, and variants thereof like caplets essentially any directly ingestible oral dosage forms. Some pills are designed to contain sensory and communication elements that collect and wirelessly transmit physiological information after being swallowed.

Examples: Viagra® Pill, Kamagra® Pill, Detox® Pill, Choice® Pill, Unwanted 72® Pill etc.

LOZENGES

Lozenges are solid dosage form of drugs containing a sweetening, flavouring and a strong binding agent meant for slow dissolution in the mouth prepared either by molding or by compression. They are usually intended for treatment of local irritation or infections of the mouth or throat but may contain active ingredients intended for systemic absorption after swallowing. The tablets produced by fusion or candy molding process are called lozenges.

Examples: Compound Bismuth Lozenge, Liquorice Lozenge, Nystatin Lozenge, Clotrimazole Lozenge etc.

PASTILLES

Molded lozenges are sometimes referred to as pastilles. Pastilles are softer than lozenges. The drug along with gelatin and glycerin is converted into a pastille for slow dissolution in the mouth.

Examples: Vocalzone® Throat Pastille, Rescue® Pastille.

TROCHES

Compressed lozenges are often referred to as *troches*. The compressed tablets are also called as troches. Flavors and sweeteners are added to make troches palatable.

Examples: Ketamine HCl Troche, Clotrimazole Troche

Advantages:

1. Lozenges are easy to administer to both pediatric and geriatric patients.
2. It has a pleasant taste and extends the time of contact with the oral cavity for an extended period of time.
3. It can be prepared extemporaneously by pharmacists with a minimal amount of equipment and time.
4. Formulas are easy to change and can be patient specific.
5. Lozenges have traditionally been used for local effect.
6. Recently, lozenges are being used as a way to deliver drugs systemically.
7. Useful for patients who have difficulty swallowing oral solid dosage forms.
8. To enhance patient compliance, especially in children, lozenges are formulated to taste good.
9. Reduce dose size, gastric irritation, increase bioavailability and avoid first pass metabolism.

Disadvantages:

1. Mistakenly it could be used as candy by children.
2. Preparing and forming hand-rolled lozenges requires experience and good technique.
3. Mostly hand-rolled lozenges do not have an elegant appearance.
4. Special molds are usually required to make lozenges by molding.
5. Handling of base materials requires special skill, experience, and care to obtain satisfactory preparations.

6. Caution must be used when incorporating drugs sensitive to heat.

7. Although the dosage units of molded lozenges may be determined either by weight or by volume, both methods require special equipment, calculations, or procedures.

DENTAL CONES

Dental cones are tablet dosage form intended to be placed in the empty socket following a tooth extraction. Main purpose of dental cones is to prevent the local multiplication of pathogenic bacteria associated with tooth extractions or to reduce bleeding. Main purpose behind the use of this tablet is either to prevent multiplication of bacteria in the socket by employing a slow releasing antibacterial compound or to reduce bleeding by an astringent or coagulant containing tablet. The cones may contain an antibiotic or antiseptic. It's formulated to dissolve or erode slowly in presence of a small volume of serum or fluid over 20-40 min period.

Examples: Parasorb® Dental Cone (gentamicin).

PESSARIES

Pessaries are solid unit dosage form of medicament either compressed in a suitable shape or molded with the help of a base meant for introduction into vagina. There are three types of pessaries namely molded pessaries, compressed pessaries and vaginal capsules. Molded pessaries are cone shaped and prepared in a similar way to molded suppositories. Compressed pessaries are made in a variety of shapes and are prepared by compression in a similar manner to oral tablets. Vaginal capsules are similar to soft gelatin oral capsules differing only in size and shape. The alternative term for delivery of medicine via vagina, urethra and rectum routes is pharmaceutical pessary. A therapeutic pessary is a medical device similar to the outer ring of a diaphragm. They are used to support the uterus, vagina, bladder, or rectum. A pessary is most commonly used to treat prolapse of the uterus. It is also used to treat stress urinary incontinence, a retroverted uterus, cystocele and rectocele.

Examples: Lactic Acid Pessary, Nystatin Pessary.

Advantages:

1. Some drugs can only achieve adequate concentrations in the body when administered as pessary.
2. No systemic side effects when administered as pessary.
3. Can exert local effect on rectal mucosa.
4. Used to promote evacuation of bowel.
5. Avoid any gastrointestinal irritation.
6. Can be used in unconscious patients (for example, during fitting).
7. Can be used for systemic absorption of drugs and to avoid first-pass metabolism.
8. Can be used when babies or old people cannot swallow oral medication.
9. Suitable for people suffering from severe nausea or vomiting.

Disadvantages:

1. Pessaries has problem of patient acceptability.
2. It is not suitable for patients suffering from diarrhea.
3. In some cases, the total amount of the drug given would be either too irritating or in greater amount.
4. Incomplete absorption may be obtained because suppository usually promotes evacuation of the bowel.
5. The contraindications to pessary placement include primary vaginitis, active pelvic inflammatory disease, latex sensitivity, a noncompliant patient, and lack of assured follow-up.

CAPSULES

Capsule is defined as a solid unit dosage form of medicament in which the drug or drugs are enclosed in a practically tasteless, hard or soft soluble container of shell made-up of gelatin.

(a) Hard gelatin capsules

Hard gelatin capsules are made up of two cylindrical halves, one slightly larger in diameter but shorter in length known as cap and the other slightly shorter in diameter but longer in length known as base.

Examples: Ampicillin Capsule, Multivitamin Capsule.

Advantages:

1. Easy to swallow as they are smooth and slippery.
2. Suitable for substances having bitter taste and unpleasant odor.
3. They are economic, attractive and available in wide range of colors.
4. Minimum excipients required.
5. Little pressure required to compact the material.
6. Convenient to handle as they are unit dosage forms.
7. Easy to store and transport.

Disadvantages:

1. Not suitable for highly soluble substances like potassium chloride, potassium bromide, ammonium chloride etc.
2. Not suitable for highly efflorescent or deliquescent materials.
3. Requires special storage conditions.
4. Drugs administer in capsule are exposed to first pass effects in liver.

(b) Soft gelatin capsules

Soft gelatin capsules are flexible, spherical, ovoid cylindrical or tubes. The small spherical capsules are also known as 'pearls'. Soft gelatin capsules are used to enclose solids, semisolids or liquids.

Examples: Chloramphenicol Soft Gelatin Capsule.

Advantages:

1. They are easy to swallow and release their contents very quickly.
2. They have the ability to mask odor and unpleasant taste.
3. They have an elegant appearance.
4. Readily dissolve in the gastric juices of the gastrointestinal tract (GIT).
5. They may enhance the bioavailability of the active ingredient
6. Gelatin capsules can be made into chewable, extended release, captabs etc.
7. They can be used for ophthalmic preparations, for example, Aplicaps, vaginal/rectal suppositories.
8. These capsules have dosage accuracy, uniformity and precision in dosage.
9. They are tamper-resistant and provide protection against counterfeit.
10. Provide protection from light, oxidation and degradation.

Disadvantages:

1. Water soluble materials are difficult to incorporate in capsules.
2. They are highly moisture sensitive.
3. Efflorescent material cannot be incorporated due to softening/leaching.
4. Deliquescent materials cannot be incorporated as they may cause hardening.
5. They are comparatively costlier than the soft capsules and the liquid dosage forms.
6. They have some dietary restrictions as gelatin is traditionally made out of the bones and skins of pigs and cows.

Delayed-release capsules

Delayed-release capsules may be coated, or, more commonly, encapsulated granules may be coated to resist releasing the drug in the gastric fluid of the stomach where a delay is important to alleviate potential problems of drug inactivation or gastric mucosal irritation. The term "delayed-release" is used for enteric coated capsules that are intended to delay the release of medicament until the capsule has passed through the stomach.

Examples: Omeprazole DR Capsule, Nexium® DR Capsule (esomeprazole).

Extended-release capsules

Extended-release capsules are formulated in such manner as to make the contained medicament available over an extended period of time following ingestion. Expressions such as "prolonged-action," "repeat-action," and "sustained-release" have also been used to describe such dosage forms.

Examples: Indomethacin ER Capsule, Morphine Sulphate ER Capsule.

CAPLETS

Caplet is an oblong tablet that is a hybrid of the capsule and tablet. The caplet is simply a tablet shaped like a capsule and sometimes coated to look like a capsule. The inside of the caplet is solid, whereas the inside of a capsule is often powder or granular material. The caplet offers the advantage of easier swallowing, more stability and longer shelf life than a capsule.

Examples: Relafine® Caplet (nabumetone), Ceptin® Caplet (cefuroxime), Renovit® Caplet (Multivitamin and mineral)

INSUFFLATIONS

Insufflations is a dosage form that provide a medicament intimately mixed with a dusting powder to be deeply inhaled or blown into the body cavities such as ears, nose, tooth sockets and vagina by an insufflator. The insufflations are used to produce a local effect, as in the treatment of ear, nose and throat infection with antibiotics or to produce a systemic effect from a drug that is destroyed in the GIT. Snuffs are finely divided solid dosage forms of drugs inhaled into nostrils.

Examples: Braniff® Snuff, Dentobac® Snuff etc.

Advantages:

1. Insufflator sprays the powder into stream of finely divided particles all over the site of application.
2. Produce local effect.

Disadvantages:

1. Difficulty in obtaining measured quantity of the drug as a uniform dose.
2. It gets blocked when it is slightly wet or the powder used is wet.

DENTRIFICES

Dentifrices (tooth powders) are preparations which are generally used with the help of tooth brush for cleansing the surfaces of the teeth. They are available in the form of fine powders and pastes. They contain a suitable detergent or soap, abrasive substance as fine powder, sweetening agent sodium and a suitable flavour.

Examples: Colgate® Tooth Paste and Powder, Close-up®, Miswak®.

Advantages:

1. Dentifrices help to keep teeth clean and healthy.
2. They give nice breath.
3. They provide teeth protection against plaque, cavities and gum diseases.
4. Help to keep teeth white.

Disadvantages:

1. Fluoride used in dentifrices cause health issues.
2. Flavoured dentifrices doesn't protect against plaque.
3. We find change in taste of food after brushing teeth.

CACHETS

Cachets are disc or cylinder shaped devices made from rice paper and consist of a lower and upper part, the latter having a slightly broader flange. Medication of disagreeable taste is enclosed between the two halves and sealed. There are two types of cachets.

  (i) Wet seal cachets: Lower half of the cachet is filled with powdered drug. Then the flange of the empty upper half of the cachet is moistened with water, and pressed over the lower half. The cachet is dried for 15 minutes.

  (ii) Dry seal cachets: Drug powder is filled in the lower half and the upper half is pressed over it just like a capsule.

Examples: Sodium Amino Salicylate Cachets, Sodium Amino Salicylate and Isoniazid Cachets.

Advantages

1. They are used for administering the drug with unpleasant taste
2. They are used for administering the drug in large dose.

Disadvantages:

1. Pre-use preparation is required as before administration; a cachet should be immersed in water for few seconds.
2. Tedious administration as it has to be first placed on the tongue and then swallowed with water.

BEADS

The beads are multi-particulate dosage forms that can be packaged in an outer capsule shell for oral administration. Beads can be mixed with other excipients and compressed into a tablet dosage form.

Examples: Adderall XR$^{®}$ Beads, Methylphenidate Beads.

PELLETS

These multi-particulate dosage forms can be packaged in an outer capsule shell for oral administration. Pellets can be mixed with other excipients and compressed into a tablet dosage form.

Examples: Calcium Chloride Pellets, Plantenextracten Pellets.

Advantages:

1. Round pellets have good flow behaviour and are easy to dose.
2. They have compact structure, good dispensability, high bulk density and dense surface and excellent stability.
3. They are dense and have very low hygroscopicity, uniform surface, narrow grain size distribution and low abrasion.

4. High active ingredient content possible.
5. They have optimum starting shape for subsequent coating and are suitable for controlled-release applications.
6. They can be divided into desired dosage strength without process or formulation changes.
7. When pellets containing the active ingredient are in the form of suspension, capsules, or disintegrating tablets, they offer significant therapeutic advantages over single unit dosage forms.
8. They can be blended to deliver incompatible bioactive agents.
9. They can be used to provide different release profile at the same or different sites in the GIT.
10. Pellets offer high degree of flexibility in the design and development of oral dosage form like suspension, sachet, tablet and capsule.

Disadvantages:

1. Dosing by volume rather than number and splitting into single dose units as required.
2. Involves capsule filling which can increase the costs or tableting which destroy film coatings on the pellets.
3. The size of pellets varies from formulation to formulation.
4. The risks of the local damage to the GI-tract mucosal.

PLASTERS

Plasters are solid or semisolid and medicated or non-medicated preparations that adhere to the body and contain a backing material such as paper, cotton, linen, silk, mole skin, or plastic.

Examples: Ketoclin® Plaster (ketoprofen), Hansaplast® Plaster (belladonna), Sinsin® Plaster (salicylic acid).

Advantages:

1. Bring medication in to close contact with the surface of skin.
2. Furnish on occlusive and macerating action.
3. Afford protection and mechanical support.

SUPPOSITORIES

Suppositories are special shaped semi-solid to solid molded preparations of various weights and shapes meant for insertion into the rectal, vaginal, or urethral orifice of the human body. They resemble pessaries which are meant for vagina. Drugs like hypnotics, tranquillizers, antispasmodics etc., are often given as suppositories.

Examples: Perrigo® Suppository (acetaminophen), Terconazol Vaginal Suppository.

Advantages:

1. They avoid any gastrointestinal irritation and first-pass metabolism for example, phenylbutazone and indomethacin.
2. They can have a topical effect on vaginal tissues in conditions like hemorrhoids and local infections.
3. They serve as an alternate for drug administration when oral administration of a drug is not suitable.
4. Suppositories have also been used for prolongation of drug action.
5. Absorption of drugs from rectal mucosa directly into the venous circulation may bring about a faster onset of action as compared to oral administration.
6. Can exert local effect on rectal mucosa.
7. Used to promote evacuation of bowel.
8. Can be used in unconscious patients (e.g. during fitting) and postoperative people who cannot be administered oral medication and people suffering from severe nausea or vomiting.

Disadvantages:

1. They are sometimes messy and inconvenient.
2. The problem of patient acceptability.
3. Concerns of inadvertent dosing partner when using estrogens.
4. Suppositories are not suitable for patients suffering from diarrhea.
5. In some cases, the total amount of the drug must be given will be either too irritating.
6. Greater amount cannot be given through suppository.
7. Incomplete absorption due to evacuation of the bowel.

TRANSDERMAL PATCHES

A transdermal (TD) patch or skin patch is a medicated adhesive patch that is placed on the skin to deliver a specific dose of medication through the skin and into the bloodstream. Transdermal systems include semisolid mixtures of drug substances and excipients which are used by spreading a suitable amount of the mixture on the backing layer. An advantage of a transdermal patch over other types such as oral, topical etc. is that it provides a controlled release of the medicament into the patient. The first commercially available patch was scopolamine for motion sickness.

Examples: Fentanyl TD® Patches (Analgesia), Nitroglycerine TD Patches, Nicotine TD Patch.

Advantages:

1. TD patches are elegant alternative to injectable as it is pain and stress-free.
2. No need for trained specialist for its use.

3. Long-term drug delivery with minimal fluctuations of drug concentrations.
4. These forms have good compliance.
5. Unlike other controlled drug delivery systems, drug delivery can be immediately discontinued by detaching from skin upon occurrence of adverse reactions.

Disadvantages:

1. TD patches are not feasible for all drugs.
2. A well balanced lipophilicity is required to be maintained.
3. High doses cannot be accommodated and delivered using TD patches.
4. It may exert local irritation or disrupts skin barrier function.
5. It may exhibit practical difficulties in application and cause discomfort.
6. They are not cost-effective.

VAGINAL RINGS

Vaginal rings are doughnut-shaped polymeric drug delivery devices designed to provide controlled release of drugs to the vagina over extended periods of time.

Example: Fem® Ring (estradiol-acetate) and Nuva® Ring (progesterone and estrogen).

INTRAUTERINE DEVICES

It is a birth control device placed in the uterus, also known as an IUD or a coil. The IUD is the world's most widely used method of reversible birth control. The device has to be fitted inside or removed from the uterus by a doctor. It remains in place over the entire time when pregnancy is not desired. Depending on the type, a single IUD is approved for 5 to 10 years use. There are two broad categories of IUDs namely inert and copper-based devices and hormonally-based devices that work by releasing progesterone.

Examples: Paragard® (IU copper), Mirena® (levonorgestrel).

EYE INSERTS

Eye inserts are biodegradable solid dosage forms containing soluble or insoluble drugs that are released slowly into the eye cavity.

Examples: Pilo-20® Occusert (pilocarpin), Timolol Eye Insert, Lacrisert® (hydroxypropyl cellulose).

(B) SEMISOLID DOSAGE FORMS

Semisolid dosage forms are defined as single-phase systems with the drug substance in solution in the semisolid material or drug in more complex two-phase or multiphase systems.

Advantages:

1. It is used externally.
2. Probability of side effects is low.
3. Used majority of time for local action

Disadvantages:

1. There is no dosage accuracy in this type of dosage form.
2. The base which is used in the semi-solid dosage form can be easily oxidized
3. If we go out after using semi-solid dosage form problems occur.

CREAMS

Creams are aqueous or oily viscous liquid or semisolid emulsions intended for external use.

Examples: Cetomacrogol Cream, Cetrimide Cream, Hydrocortisone Cream, Zinc Cream BPC.

Advantages:

1. Creams are more acceptable as they are less greasy and are easier to apply.
2. They interfere less with skin functions.
3. O/w type of creams (superior to w/o type) can be rubbed onto the skin more readily and are easily removed by washing.
4. W/o type of creams can be spread more evenly.
5. O/w types of cream are less likely to soil clothes.
6. Evaporation of water from o/w type of cream causes cooling sensation.
7. An o/w cream absorbs the discharges from the wound (liquid exudate) very quickly.
8. w/o creams can be used on non-weeping surfaces to prevent dehydration and to restore softness.
9. Creams release hormones into the blood exactly as formulated.
10. Can be used to avoid first pass effects of liver.

Disadvantages:

1. Creams are not used for internal use.
2. The aqueous phase is prone to the growth of molds and bacteria.
3. Preservatives are required to prevent deterioration of product.
4. Oils used in creams are susceptible to rancidification.
5. Slower onset of action.
6. Requires intermittent and daily application.
7. Extremely thin people may require more frequent dosing.

GELS

Gels are transparent or non-greasy semisolid preparations meant for external application to the skin or mucous membrane for medication or lubrication purposes.

Examples: Contraceptive jellies (spermicidal action), Ichthammol jelly, etc. The gelling agents may be gelatin, or a carbohydrate such as starch, tragacanth, sodium alginate or cellulose derivative.

Advantages:

1. Gels are used to avoid first pass effects.
2. They have less blood clotting risk than oral estrogens.
3. Gels are richer in liquid than magma.
4. Jellies are attractive as they are transparent or translucent non-greasy semisolid gels.
5. They are used for lubricating catheters, surgical gloves and rectal thermometers.

Disadvantages:

1. Gels have slower onset of action.
2. They requires daily application.
3. More frequent dosing is required.

OINTMENTS

Ointments are the soft semisolid, greasy preparations meant for external application onto the skin or mucous membrane (rectum and nasal mucosa). They usually contain a medicament dissolved, suspended or emulsified in the base.

Examples: Compound Benzoic Acid Ointment, Cetrimide Emulsifying Ointment.

Advantages:

1. Ointments are used for their emollient and protective action to the skin.
2. Handling of ointments is easier than bulky liquid dosage forms.
3. They contain very less amount of powdered solids.
4. They are soft and have smooth texture on application.
5. They are less viscous, hence spread beyond the area of application.
6. They being non-porous perspiration cannot escape through it.
7. They are chemically more stable than liquid dosage forms.
8. They are suitable for patients who find it difficult to take the drugs by other routes.
9. They prolong the contact time between the drug and effected area.
10. The bioavailability of drugs is more since it prevents passage through liver.

Disadvantages:

1. They are bulkier than solid dosage forms.
2. An application of an exact quantity of ointment to the affected area is difficult.
3. They are less stable than solid dosage forms.

Ointments are classified in to medicated ointments and unmedicated ointments.

Medicated Ointments

Medicated ointments contain drugs which show local or systemic effects. These are of several sub-types:

(i) Dermatologic ointments

These ointments are applied topically on the external skin. The ointment is applied to the affected area as a thin layer and spread evenly using gentle pressure with the fingertips. These are of three types

(a) Epidermic ointments: The drugs present in these type of ointments exert their action on the epidermis of the skin.

Example: Ketoconazole Ointment.

(b) Endodermic ointments: The drugs present in these types of ointments exert their action on the deeper layers of cutaneous tissue.

Example: Demodex® Ointment.

(c) Diadermic ointments: The drugs present in these types of ointments enter into the deeper layers of skin and finally in the systemic circulation and exert systemic effects.

Example: Nitroglycerine Ointment.

(ii) Ophthalmic ointments

Ophthalmic ointments are sterile preparations packed in sterile containers meant for application inside the lower eye lid. Only anhydrous bases are used in their preparation. The ointment is applied as a narrow band of approximately 0.25 - 0.5 inches.

Example: Sulfacetamide Sodium Ointment. Atropine Ointment, Chloromycetin Ointments.

(iii) Rectal ointments

Rectal ointments are the ointments to be applied to the perianal or within the anal canal. The bases used are combinations of PEG 300 and PEG3350, cetyl alcohol and cetyl esters, wax, liquid paraffin and white paraffin.

Example: Benzocaine Ointment.

(iv) Vaginal ointments

These ointments are applied to the vulvo vaginal area or inside the vagina. As vagina is more susceptible to infections, the ointment should be free from micro-organisms, moulds and yeasts.

Example: Candicidin Ointment.

(v) Nasal ointments

Nasal ointments are used in the topical treatment of nasal mucosa. Drugs get absorbed into the general circulation through the rich blood supply of the nasal lining.

Example: Ipratropium Bromide Ointment.

Non-medicated Ointments

Non-medicated ointments do not contain any drugs. They are useful as emollients, protectants or lubricants.

Example: Petroleum Jelly.

PASTES

Pastes are semisolid preparations meant for external application to the skin. They generally contain large amount of finely powdered solids such as starch, zinc oxide, calcium carbonate, etc.

Examples: Magnesium Sulfate Paste, Zinc and Coal Tar Paste.

Advantages:

1. They provide a protective coating over the areas to which they are applied.
2. Their stiffness makes them useful as protective coatings.
3. Pastes are less greasy, less penetrating and less macerating.
4. It forms an unbroken film on skin and the solid it contains can absorb and neutralize certain noxious chemicals before they ever reach the skin.

Disadvantages:

1. Less occlusive than ointments (can be a benefit depending on indication)
2. Due to the high solids content, pastes are often porous, allowing moisture loss from the applied site.
3. Pastes are generally applied as a thick layer at the required site and are therefore considered to be cosmetically unacceptable.
4. Staining of clothes is often associated with the use of pastes
5. The viscosity of pastes may be problematic in ensuring spreading of the dosage form over the affected site.

POULTICES

Poultice is paste-like preparations applied to skin in order to reduce inflammation and in some cases to act as a counter irritant. Poultices must retain heat for a considerable time. After heating the preparation is spread on dressing and applied to the affected area.

Example: Kaolin Poultice BPC.

(C) LIQUID DOSAGE FORMS

Liquid form of a dose of a chemical compound used as a drug or medication is intended for administration or consumption. Liquid dosage forms may be administered systematically by mouth or injected, by using different techniques, into the skin, muscles, or veins.

MIXTURES

A mixture is a dosage form made up of two or more different substances which are mixed but are not combined chemically. A mixture refers to the physical combination of two or more substances wherein the identities are retained and are mixed in the form of solutions, suspensions, and colloids.

Examples: Iromac XT$^{®}$ Mixture (ferrous ascorbate folic acid)

SOLUTIONS

Solutions are liquid dosage forms that contain one or more drug substance dissolved in one or more solvents to form a clear, homogeneous and single-phase system.

Advantages:
1. Solution are faster in action.
2. They are easier to swallow.
3. They have more flexibility in dose adjustment.

Disadvantages:
1. Drugs in solution have shorter shelf lives.
2. Most solutions are unpleasant in taste.
3. They are inconvenient to handle and may spill.
4. They require careful measuring.
5. Solutions require special storage or handling requirements.

DRAUGHTS

Draught, a liquid dosage form, is defined as the amount of liquid swallowed or inhaled of oxygen into the lungs. These are liquid oral preparations of which only one or two rather large doses of the order of 50 ml are prescribed. Each dose is issued in a separate container. The exception is Ipecacuanha Emetic Drought (pediatric) whose normal dose is 10 or 15 ml and therefore a multiple dose volume is prescribed.

Examples: Digoxin Draught Oral, Dosaflex® Draught Oral, Ex-Lax® Draught (sennosides)

FLUID EXTRACTS

A fluid extract is a liquid preparation of a vegetable drug in alcohol (solvent and preservative) that contains therapeutic constituents and a standard drug (USP). Fluid extracts are alcoholic extracts with a weight: volume ratio of 1:1, wherein, concentrated alcohol solution of a vegetable drug of such strength that each ml contains the equivalent of 1 g of the dry form of the drug.

Examples: Celery Fluid Extract, Oak Fluid Extract.

AROMATIC WATERS

Aromatic waters are clear, saturated aqueous solutions of volatile oils or other aromatic or volatile substances. They are saturated solutions of volatile oils or other aromatic or volatile substances.

Examples: Camphor Water, Rose Water and Peppermint Water, Concentrated Dill Water.

GLYCERITES

Glycerites are the viscous preparations in which the drug is dissolved in glycerin with or without heating. They are generally used as antiseptic or anti-inflammatory preparations.

Examples: Icthammol Glycerin, Tannic Acid Glycerin, Phenol Glycerin, Borax Glycerin.

LINCTUSES

Linctuses are viscous, liquid, oral preparations that are usually prescribed for the relief of cough. They contain medicaments which have demulcent, sedative or expectorant action. The viscous vehicle soothes the sore membrane of the throat. The usual dose is 5 ml.

Linctuses should be taken in small doses, sipped and swallowed slowly without diluting it with water in order to have the maximum and prolonged effect of medicaments. Simple Syrup is generally used as a vehicle. For diabetic patient's sorbitol solution is used instead of Simple Syrup.

Examples: Cocorex® Linctus (chlorpheniramine maleate), Koflet-SF® Linctus (Tulsi), Simple Linctus, Camphor Linctus, Codeine Linctus.

SYRUP

Syrups are highly concentrated, aqueous solutions of sugar or a sugar substitute that traditionally contain a flavoring agent. The syrup is actually used as a vehicle for medicine. It is usually used as a flavored vehicle for drugs.

Examples: Simple Syrup, Abpex® Sugar Free Syrup (Acebrophylline), Chericof® Cough Syrup (dextromethrophan hydrobromide), Cherry and Orange Syrups, Cocoa Syrup,

ELIXIRS

Elixirs are liquid preparations that consist of alcohol and water and are sweet in taste and have a nice flavor. There is no clear cut difference between elixirs and syrups. The amount of alcohol in elixir may vary greatly.

Examples: Compound Benzaldehyde Elixir (3 to 5%) and Aromatic Elixir USP (21 to 23%).

Dry elixirs:

These are the formulations used to enhance solubility and so the bioavailability of the non-steroidal anti-inflammatory drug (NSAID) by encapsulating in dextrin.

DROPS

Pharmaceutical drops are liquid preparations for oral use that are intended to be administered in small volumes with the aid of a suitable measuring device. They may be solutions, suspensions or emulsions.

Examples: Tempra® Drop (paracetamol), Danz® Drop (ondensetron)

GARGLES

They are aqueous solutions used in the prevention or treatment of throat infections. Usually they are prepared in a concentrated solution with directions for the patient to dilute with warm water before use. Gargling is the human act in which air from the lungs is bubbled through a liquid in the mouth. It usually requires that the head be tilted back, allowing a mouthful of liquid to sit in the upper throat.

Examples: Hexitidine Bactidol Gargles, Betadine® Gargle, Sinaseptic® Gargle (phenol, sodium borate and sodium bicarbonate).

The head can be tilted by tilting either the neck or the back, depending on what is comfortable for the gargler. Vibration caused by the muscles in the throat and back of the mouth cause the liquid to bubble and percolate through the throat and mouth cavity. A study in Japan has shown that gargling water a few times a day will lower the chance of upper respiratory infections such as colds, though some medical authorities are skeptical.

MOUTH WASHES

Mouthwashes are similar to gargles but are used for oral hygiene and to treat infections of the mouth. Mouthwash is a liquid preparation held in the mouth passively or swirled around the mouth by contraction of the perioral muscles and/or movement of the head, and may be gargled, where the head is tilted back and the liquid bubbled at the back of the mouth. Usually mouthwashes are an antiseptic solution intended to reduce the microbial load in the oral cavity. There are two main types of mouthwash: cosmetic and therapeutic. Therapeutic mouthwashes are available both over-the-counter and by prescription, depending on the formulation. There are therapeutic mouthwashes that help reduce or control plaque, gingivitis, bad breath, and tooth decay. Children younger than the age of 6 should not use mouthwash, unless directed by a dentist, because they may swallow large amounts of the liquid inadvertently. Mouthwashes might be given for analgesic, anti-inflammatory or anti-fungal action. Additionally, some rinses act as saliva substitutes to neutralize acid and keep the mouth moist in xerostomia (dry mouth).

Examples: Colgate® Mouthwash, Listerine® Mouthwash, Viodine® Mouthwash, Uniseft® Mouthwash.

GLYCERITES

Glycerites are viscous hygroscopic liquid or semisolid preparations that contain not less than 50% by weight of glycerin and dissolved medicaments. Glycerites have sweet taste and act as preservative.

Examples: Borax Glycerin (bacteriostatic), Phenol Glycerin (ulcers), Tannic acid Glycerin (ulcers)

MOUTH PAINTS

Paints are aqueous or alcoholic solutions prepared with collodion base and is applied to skin. The volatile solvent evaporates leaving behind dry or resinous film of medicament.

Examples: Candid® Mouth Paint, Dequadin® Mouth Paint, Crystal Violet Paint, Coal Tar Pain.

THROAT PAINTS

Throat paints are aqueous or alcoholic liquid preparations applied to mucous surface of throat. Throat paints are more viscous due to high content of glycerin for prolonged action of medicaments.

Examples: Mandle's Paints, Betadine® Paint, Crystal Violet paint.

THROAT SPRAY

Throat sprays are aqueous alcoholic or glycerin solutions intended to be applied in throat or nose by means of atomizer or nebulizer.

Examples: Adrenaline Spray and Atropine Spray.

DOUCHE

A douche is medicated aqueous solution for rinsing body cavity applied at low pressure. Douches have cleansing or antiseptic action, and they may promote healing or be astringent.

Examples: Feminine® Douche, Summers Eve® Douche, Messengill® Douche.

ENEMAS

An enema is a fluid injected into the lower bowel by way of the rectum for retention or evacuation. These preparations are used to deliver medication to the body bypassing the stomach while being absorbed and to evacuate the lower intestine to prepare for surgeries or for women in labor.

Examples: Sulabh Enema, Green Enema, Sodium Phosphate Enema.

EYE DROPS

Eye drops are saline-containing drops used as an ocular route to administer. Eyes drops sometimes do not have medications in them and are only lubricating and tear-replacing solutions.

Examples: Lomeflox® Eye Drops, Gentamicin Eye Drops, Sunetra® Eye Drops.

Advantages:

1. Eye drops have less of a risk of side effects than do oral medicines,
2. Eye drops are used for stopping itching and redness of the eyes.
3. Packed in smaller volumes, 10-20 ml.
4. Eye drops help to relieve dryness and irritation, promoting comfort.
5. Eye drops can be used for lubrication to minimize the chance of the eye becoming further scratched or damaged from blinking.
6. Eye drops help to heal the surface of the injured eye.

Disadvantages:

1. They are manufactured as sterile preparation.
2. Preservatives in eye drop that can trigger allergic reactions in some patients.
3. Certain medications could cause extremely dry eyes.
4. Eye drops sometimes may not work well enough to provide you long-lasting comfort.
5. Repeated application can be annoying, inconvenient and expensive.
6. Emergency cases need to be always handled immediately to preserve vision.
7. Eye drops should only be used when recommended.

EAR DROPS

Ear drops are a form of medicine used to treat or prevent ear infections, especially infections of the outer ear and ear canal (otitis externa). Bacterial infections are sometimes treated with antibiotics.

Examples: Polysporin Ear Drop, Murine Ear Drop, Ciprosine Ear Drop, Ciprodex Ear Drop.

NASAL DROPS

Nasal drops are the solutions of drugs that are instilled in to the nose with a dropper. These are usually aqueous and not oily drops since the latter inhibits the movements of cilia in the nasal mucosa and if used for the long periods may reach the lungs and cause lipoid pneumonia. They are used to treat colds and allergies and work on the specific site rather than the whole body

Examples: Otrivin® Nasal Drops (xylometazoline HCl), Nozolin® Nasal Drops (sodium chloride), Xylomet® Nasal Drops (xylometazoline HCl).

NASAL SPRAYS

Nasal sprays are liquid preparations used in local treatments for conditions such as nasal congestion and allergic rhinitis. Other applications include hormone replacement therapy, treatment of Alzheimer's disease and Parkinson's disease.

Examples: Otosan® Spray (hypertonic solution), Azelastine Hydrochloride Spray.

Advantages:

1. Nasal sprays provide an agreeable alternative to injection or pills.
2. Nasal sprays deliver drug to the systemic administration.
3. They help the drug substances to be assimilated extremely quickly and directly.
4. Nasal sprays more efficient way of transporting drugs with potential use in crossing the blood–brain barrier.
5. They help combat irritation caused by dust and pollen.
6. Some reduce congestion, swelling and inflammation in the sinuses.
7. Help treat an itchy and runny nose.
8. Helps to relieve stuffiness and congestion.
9. Some are effective in loosening mucus in nasal passages and moisten the nose.

Disadvantages:

1. Most nasal sprays need to be used with caution if you have heart problems.
2. The majority of them have not been proven safe to use during pregnancy.
3. Some cause swelling of the nasal membranes, stinging, sneezing, dry mouths and headaches.
4. They have a bitter and unpleasant taste and are not liked by children.
5. Most can lead to increased irritation, nasal burning and nose bleeds.
6. They can lead to addiction and chronic swelling of the nasal passages.
7. Most give temporary relief or relief that last a few hours.
8. Most are not effective in relieving rhino-sinusitis or some common colds.

INJECTABLES

Injectables are liquid formulation for administration using a hypodermic (hollow pointed) needle and are formulated as liquids or powders/lyophilisate for preparation of the solution.

Examples: Laennec[®] Injection (human placental extarct), Orfenac[®] Injection (diclofenac)

(a) Irrigations: Wound irrigation solutions are used to hydrate the wound, to remove debris and bacteria, to assist in visual inspection, to prevent infection, and to improve healing and cosmesis. Wound irritation solutions includes normal saline, sterile water, diluted 1% povidone-iodine.

Examples: 0.25% Acetic acid Irrigation, 5% Mannitol Irrigation

(b) Injections: Pharmaceutical injections are sterile, pyrogen-free liquids (solutions, emulsions, or suspensions) or solid dosage forms containing one or more active ingredients, packaged in either single-dose or multidose containers. An injection is an infusion method of putting fluid into the body, usually with a syringe and a hollow needle which is pierced through the skin to a sufficient depth for the material to be administered into the body.

Examples: Calcium Gluconate Injection, Carboplatin Injection, Midoryx[®] (Midazolam) Injection BP.

Advantages:

1. Injections can be used for drugs that are poorly absorbed, inactive or ineffective if given orally.

2. Injections by i.v. route provides immediate onset of action as there is absence of absorption.

3. The i.m. and s.c. routes can be used to achieve slow or delayed onset of action.

4. Patient concordance problems can be avoided.

Disadvantages

1. Healthcare staffs need additional training and assessment.

2. Injections can be costly.

3. They can be painful.

4. Aseptic technique is required for preparing injections.

5. They may require additional equipment, for example programmable infusion devices.

(c) Infusions

Infusions (plasma-substituting preparations) are sterile, aqueous solutions or emulsions with water as the continuous phase. They are free from pyrogens and are usually made isotonic with respect to blood. They are delivered by infusion therapy that involves the administration of medication through a needle or catheter. Typically, "infusion therapy" means that a drug is administered intravenously or subcutaneously.

Examples: Cloxatine® Infusion (benzathine and cloxacillin), Amphotercin B Infusion.

Advantages:

1. Today infusions are available as pre-filled ready to use, dose-specific products.
2. They are available in hermetically sealed containers that allows predictable sterility, ease of use, improved control and lower total costs.
3. They deliver drug directly in to systemic circulation.

LINIMENTS

Liniments are liquid, semi-liquid or occasionally semi-solid preparations intended for application on the skin. They may be alcoholic or oily solutions or emulsions. Counter-irritant liniments are massaged onto the skin whereas analgesic and soothing liniments are applied on warm dressing or with a brush. Liniments must not be applied to broken skin because they would be very irritating. Alcohol is used as main vehicle as it increases the penetration of counter-irritant molecules through skin.

Examples: Soap Liniment, Camphor Liniment, Methyl Salicylate Liniment.

LOTIONS

Lotions are liquid preparations for external application without friction. They are either dabbed on the skin or applied on a suitable dressing and covered with water proof material to reduce evaporation.

Examples: Copper and Zinc Sulfate Lotion (impetigo), Zinc Sulfate and Salicylic Acid (ulcer), Salicylic Acid Lotion (dandruff), Salicylic Acid and Mercuric Chloride Lotion (follicular infection).

APPLICATIONS

Applications are liquid or viscous preparations intended for application to the skin. Usually, they are suspensions or emulsions. Most of the official preparations contain paraciticides and are intended for only a limited number of applications. They are dispensed in coloured fluted bottles in order to distinguish them from preparations meant for internal use. The container is with instruction "For External Use Only".

Examples: Lactocalamine Application (calamine), Dicophane Application BPC.

COLLODIONS

Collodions are liquid preparations meant for external application to the skin. They are convenient for application on small cuts and abrasions and are used when a prolonged contact between the skin and the medicament is required. The vehicle is volatile and evaporates on application to the skin, leaving a flexible, protective film covering the site.

Examples: Kryolam® Collodion, Collodium® Collodion, Mehron® Collodion.

TINCTURES

These are alcoholic preparations containing the active principles of vegetable drugs. They are weaker than extracts. They are usually prepared by maceration and percolation, or may be prepared by dissolving the corresponding liquid extract of chemical substances (e.g. iodine) in alcohol or hydroalcohol solvent.

Examples: Belladonna Tincture, Aromatic Cardamom tincture, Iodine tincture.

SPIRITS

Spirits are alcoholic or hydroalcoholic solutions of volatile substances. Most spirits are used as flavouring agents but a few have medicinal value.

Examples: Chloroform Spirit, Lemon Spirit, Compound Orange Spirit.

EMULSIONS

An emulsion is essentially a liquid preparation containing a mixture of oil and water that is rendered homogeneous by the addition of an emulsifying agent. The pharmaceutical emulsion is solely used to describe preparations intended for internal use. Emulsion for external use is always given a different title that reflects their use such as application, lotion and cream. Emulsions are of three types namely; o/w, w/o and w/o/w or o/w/o.

Examples: Frelax® Oral Emulsion (magnesium hydroxide and liquid paraffin), Flatameal® DS (aluminium hydroxide, magnesium hydroxide and simethicone), Liquid Paraffin Emulsion, Castor Oil Emulsion.

Advantages:

1. Emulsions are used to administered unpalatable oils and unpalatable oil-soluble drugs in palatable form.

2. The aqueous phase of emulsion is easily flavored.

3. The oily sensation is easily removed.

4. The rate of drug absorption is increased.

5. It is possible to include two incompatible ingredients, one in each phase of the emulsion.

Disadvantages:

1. Emulsion preparation needs to be shaken well before use.
2. A measuring device is needed for administration of emulsion.
3. A degree of technical accuracy is needed to measure a dose.
4. Storage conditions may affect stability of emulsion.
5. They are bulky, difficult to transport and prone to container breakages.
6. They are susceptible to microbial contamination which can lead to emulsion cracking.

SUSPENSIONS

A pharmaceutical suspension is a coarse dispersion in which internal phase consisting of insoluble solid particles having a specific range of size is dispersed uniformly throughout the external aqueous or organic or oily liquid phase with aid of single or combination of suspending agent.

Examples: Brufen® Oral Suspension (ibuprofen), Ceftef® Oral Suspension (cefixime)

Advantages:

1. Suspension can improve chemical stability of certain drug.
2. Drug in suspension exhibits higher rate of bioavailability than other dosage forms.
3. Duration and onset of action can be controlled.
4. Suspension can mask the unpleasant/ bitter taste of drug.

Disadvantages:

1. Physical stability, sedimentation and compaction can cause problems.
2. Susceptible to degradation and the possibility of chemical reaction between the ingredients in the solution where there is water as a catalyst.
3. It is bulky sufficient care must be taken during handling and transport.
4. It is difficult to formulate.
5. Uniform and accurate dose cannot be achieved unless suspension are packed in unit dosage form

LEMONADES

Lemonades are sweet, sour, and usually clear liquid preparations intended for oral use. Lemonades are usually prepared by dissolving hydrochloric acid, citric acid, tartaric acid, or lactic acid, in simple syrup and purified water, and filtering, if necessary. These are prepared before use and stored in tight containers for preservation.

Examples: Somatomax® Ultra Concentrate Lemonade, Creatine HCl Raspberry Lemonade.

FOAMS

An emulsion packaged in a pressurized aerosol container that has a fluffy, semisolid consistency when dispensed is called as foam. Foams can also be classified as two-phase liquid dispersion as they consist of a gas phase dispersed with in a liquid. Pharmaceutical foams are useful for the topical, rectal and vaginal delivery of drug substances.

Example: Vaginal Foam (antibacterial, antimycotic, antiprotozoal), Vaginal Contraceptive Foam.

(D) GASEOUS DOSAGE FORMS

MEDICAL GASES

Compressed medical gases include gaseous and liquid (cryogenic) forms stored in high-pressure cylinders that are administered as a gas. Pharmaceutical and medical gases are fluids manufactured specifically for the medical, pharmaceutical manufacturing, and biotechnology industries. They are frequently used to synthesize, sterilize, or insulate processes or products which contribute to human health. Pharmaceutical gases are also inhaled by patients in a technique known as gas therapy. Within medical facilities, gases are introduced to a patient's airway most often by the use of a medical ventilator and/or continuous-flow anaesthesia machine. Other means of introducing the gas to the patient's lungs include tracheostomy tubes, laryngeal masks, and endotracheal tubes.

Examples: Oxygen, Carbon Dioxide, Helium, Nitrogen, Nitrous Oxide, Medical Air, and combinations of these gases.

AEROSOLS

An aerosol is defined as a disperse phase system, in which very fine solid drug particles or liquid droplets get dispersed in the propellants (gas), which acts as continuous phase.

Examples: Oral B Foam (fluoride), Solarcaine Spray (lidocaine)

Advantages:

1. Dose from aerosol can be easily withdrawn from the package without contamination.
2. Aerosols are easy and convenient and can be administered without the help of others.
3. The onset of action is faster compared to other dosage forms.
4. The dispersion of medicament is very good.
5. Aerosol form can avoid decomposition of drug by the pH or enzymatic action of the stomach or intestine.
6. Stability of drugs affected by atmospheric oxygen or moisture can be enhanced.
7. Products sterility is maintained.
8. Controlled and uniform use of dose is possible using metered valve.

9. The aerosol containers protect the photosensitive medicaments.

10. The rapid volatilization of the propellant provides a cooling, refreshing effect.

11. Aerosols are rapid in action and provide best drug efficacy.

12. They form uniform thin layer to the skin without touching the affected area.

Disadvantages:

1. Aerosols are costly.

2. Disposal of empty aerosol containers are difficult.

3. Due to volatility of the propellant/s can irritate the injured skin.

4. Patients sensitive to the propellant/s it may show carcinotoxic effects on repeated use.

5. Aerosol packs must be stored away from temperature and fire to avoid its explosion.

6. Formulation as aerosol is difficult for the drugs insoluble in the propellant.

7. If therapy is continued for a long period of time propellants may cause toxic reactions.

METERED DOSE

A metered-dose inhaler (MDI) is a device that delivers a specific amount of medication to the lungs, in the form of a short burst of aerosolized medicine that is usually self-administered by the patient via inhalation. It is the most commonly used delivery system for treating asthma, chronic obstructive pulmonary disease (COPD) and other respiratory diseases. The medication in a metered dose inhaler is most commonly a bronchodilator, corticosteroid or a combination of both for the treatment of asthma and COPD.

Examples: Ashtalin® Inhalation (salbutamol sulphate BP), QVAR® (beclomethasone dipropionate)

DRY POWDER INHALERS

A dry powder inhaler is a handheld device used to administer medications in the form of a dry powder to deliver it to the lungs as you inhale through it. It doesn't contain propellants or other ingredients but just the medication.

Examples: Ventolin® (salbutamol), Xopenex HFA® (levalbuterol), Atrovent HFA® (ipratropium), Pulmicort® (budesonide) Dry Powder Inhalers.

MODEL QUESTIONS

1. Define drug. Give different sources of drug.
2. What is rationale for development of dosage form?
3. Define dosage forms and give its classification with examples.
4. Discuss advantages and disadvantages of different dosage forms.

■■■

Chapter 3...

Prescription

LEARNING OBJECTIVES

Prescription order being an important therapeutic transaction between physician and patient, it brings into focus the diagnostic acumen and therapeutic proficiency of the physician with instructions for palliation or restoration of the patient's health. The most carefully conceived prescription order may become therapeutically useless, however, unless it communicates clearly with the pharmacist and adequately instructs the patient on how to take the prescribed medication. Thus,

The objectives of this chapter include:

- To understand the professional way of handling the prescription.
- Learning about writing, reading and understanding prescription and improve upon the prescription filling and refilling skills.
- To emphasize on the importance of error free prescription writing.
- To increase awareness about the problems caused by errors in prescription writing and ways to minimize the same.
- To know the pattern or rate of prescription errors and assess the causes and devise novel interventions for the practicing to prevent prescription errors.

3.1 INTRODUCTION

A patient treatment by doctor assumes his physical evaluation and diagnosis of any ailments. The doctor can select a method to treat patient from variety of therapeutic approaches. Treatment using drug is most commonly chosen approach. This, in most cases requires the writing of a prescription.

3.2 PRESCRIPTION

The prescription order is the most important therapeutic transaction observed between a doctor and a patient. A prescription order may be written and issued by a physician, dentist, veterinarian, or other properly licensed medical practitioner.

A medical prescription is a written order from a doctor to a chemist/pharmacist that includes instruction for preparing and dispensing medicines to a certain patient. The prescription represents a mechanism in the form of written information through which a treatment modality is provided to the patient. The prescription for each patient is a unique entity that designates a specific medication or medications for a specific patient at a specific time.

The prescription is generally written on paper but these days it can be usually written on specific printed form. The form possesses blank spaces for the necessary information. Such blanks are often supplied to the doctors in the form of a pad containing 100 blank forms.

This is a typical printed form for outpatients. In hospitals, drugs are prescribed on a particular page in the patient's hospital chart. A prescription order follows a definite pattern that facilitates its interpretation. The definite functions of the prescription are given below.

Functions of the prescription:

1. Prescription can be used as legal document.
2. It can be a record source.
3. It acts as means of communication.
4. It is needed in case of therapy modality.
5. It is means of medical control of therapy.
6. It is means of clinical trial.

All prescription orders should be correct, unambiguous, without cross-outs and signed clearly for optimal communication between prescriber, pharmacist, and nurse. It is required that a medical prescription in India be written in English or Latin.

3.3 PARTS OF PRESCRIPTION

A complete prescription should have the following parts:

1. Prescribers details

Prescriber's details include the name and the surname of the doctor, the hospital, clinic or polyclinic medical center, their address, doctor's name, designation, registration number, phone number, e-mail and the date. Information about physician is essential so that the doctor could be contacted in emergency to seek clarification and necessary instruction, missing words, confirmation, etc. Prescription number is required for a refill or for insurance purposes. The date is important from the standpoint of ascertaining for determining the life of the prescription. Date must be written on the prescription by the prescriber at the same time when it is written. The date on the prescription helps a pharmacist to find out the cases where prescription is brought for dispensing long time after its issue. The prescription of narcotics and controlled substances are governed by special laws and regulations and thus it cannot be filled after more than 10 days from the date of issuance; but an order for children can be reissued 7 days after the date on which such prescription was issued. Thus, prescriptions containing narcotic or other habit-forming drugs must bear the date.

2. Details of Patient

This part of prescription includes the name, address, age and sex of the patient. Patient's full name must be written instead of only surname or the family name. This information helps in identifying the prescription and thus must be written on the prescription. If it is not written then, the pharmacist himself should ask the patient about these particulars and put down at the top of the prescription. The prescribed medication is only for the patient whose name is on the prescription. Medications should not be given to another patient even if the other patient has similar symptoms. This avoids the possibility of giving the finished product to a person other than the one it is meant for. Age and sex of the patient especially in the case of children helps the pharmacist in checking the medication and the dose. Therefore, there will be less danger of its being administered to the wrong member of the family or the hospital ward having similar names. Age and weight is important for calculation of dose, dose frequency and route of administration. The address of the patient is recorded to help for any reference at a later stage, to contact the patient or to deliver the medication personally.

3. Superscription

Superscription consists of the specific direction to the chemist on how to compound the medication. The superscription is represented by a symbol, Rx, which is always written at the beginning of the prescription. In the days of mythology and superstition the symbol was considered as a prayer to Jupiter, the God of healing, for quick recovery of the patient but now this symbol is understood as an abbreviation of the Latin word recipe, meaning "take thou" or "you take". Most of direction is usually expressed in contracted Latin or in the form of abbreviation. Instructions for preparation are also given such as: 'make a mixture', 'mix and make 10 tablets', or 'dispense 10 capsules'.

4. Inscription

Inscription is the main part of the prescription, because this is the doctor's order. It contains the names, the medicinal forms and quantities of the prescribed drugs. The names of the drugs are written each on a separate line, followed by the quantity ordered and the last item written is generally the vehicle or diluent.

In complex prescriptions containing several drugs and additives the inscription is divided into three parts:

1. The base or the active medicament which is intended to produce the therapeutic effect.
2. The additive which is included either to enhance the action of the medicament or to make the product more palatable, and
3. The vehicle which is either used to dissolve the solid substances and/or to increase the volume of the preparation for ease of administration.

In addition, for following three parts enough care is taken by the prescriber.

1. Use of brand name (proprietary name) or generic name (INN – international nonproprietary name). The medicinal substances are required to begin with a capital letter and to be in the Genitive case.
2. The dosage form is placed at the beginning or after the drug/s name/s.
3. The dose is noted after the medicinal product name. The strength of the medication is written in metric units.

Example: Tab. Paracetamol .... 500 mg.

5. Subscription

This part of the prescription contains prescriber's instructions to the pharmacist regarding the dosage form to be prepared and number of doses to be dispensed or medicinal forms to be supplied to the patient. Since, now a day only a few prescriptions are compounded therefore such directions are less frequent.

6. Transcription/Signatura/Signa

The transcription gives instructions to the patient on how, how much, when, and how long the drug is to be taken. It is usually abbreviated as "Sig" from the Latin, meaning 'mark' on the prescriptions. It provides instructions as to how the medicine should be taken by the patient. It usually indicates the quantity of medicament or number or dosage units to be taken, how many times in a day or at what time it should be taken; if the drug has to be used externally only, or to be shaken well before use, or whether it is a poison, and other such facts are included. The Signatura should always be written in English; however, physicians continue to insert Latin abbreviations. For example,

(i) '1 Cap t.i.d. pc' which the pharmacist translates into English as 'take one capsule three times daily after meals'.

(ii) 1 Tab. t.i.d.' for 'one tablet three times a day'.

7. Renewal

The number of times a prescription is to be repeated is written by the doctor under renewal instructions. It may also contain special instructions, warnings, followed by the signature of the prescriber who in most cases a doctor.

8. Signature

Finally, the prescription must bear the signature of the prescriber to justify its legal validity.

9. Other important instructions

(a) Refills: the prescription must include the number of refills permitted /no refills.

(b) Qty: "quantity" or how much is in the package.

(c) Mfg.: "manufacturer" or who makes the medication.

(d) Expiry date: do not use the medication past this date. Do not save unused medications. If same patient gets sick again, prescriber should be consulted.

(e) Take complete /full course: patient should finish taking the entire contents of the prescription even if feeling better especially patient taking antibiotics. This is to avoid recurrence of infection and development of resistance.

(f) Take with / without food: means medication is to be taken after a meal or empty stomach. Some medications work better when the stomach is full while some medications work better when the stomach is empty.

(g) Take four times a day: means to take the medication four times in 24 h with equal time interval. It is different than 'Take every four hours'. If any confusion occurs about when to give the medications, one should consult doctor or pharmacist. Most medications do not have to be precisely timed to be effective, but some do.

(h) Take as needed as symptoms persist: means the medication can be taken when symptoms are present, without consulting the prescriber.

(i) The package may also have bright colored warning labels with additional information. The following are examples:

1. Safe storage instructions, such as 'keep refrigerated'.

2. Instructions for use, such as 'shake well before use'.

3. Possible side effects, such as 'may cause drowsiness'.

Prescriptions are difficult to interpret and understood by a layman. Even a pharmacist at beginning requires some effort and training. It is only after considerable experience he can read the prescription. The reason is that, the busy doctor always writes very swiftly and uses too many abbreviations, which a pharmacist alone has to interpret. In many cases the doctors are known for their bad and illegible handwriting. The process of swiftness at times crosses all limits and doctors writing a letter or two only for the name of a drug are common and the use of Latin in prescription writing is traditional. These days teaching of Latin has slowly gone out of the curricula of medicine and pharmacy. Some of the Latin words and abbreviations have very deep roots and thus doctors still use them frequently. Infact, at old times prescription was a secret between the doctor and the pharmacist and was mystery for the patient. The increasing awareness about drugs and ready access to drug related information no secrecy is now warranted. As such the patient has a right to know what medication has been prescribed and his interest is protected under the Consumer Protection Act.

All other parts of the prescription may be printed or type-written but the prescriber's name must be hand-written and should be signed with ink. This eliminates the danger of dispensing medicament on a spurious order and it authenticates the prescription. The prescriptions containing narcotic or other habit-forming drugs must bear the address and registration number of the prescriber. This identifies the special license which a prescriber must have to prescribe the narcotic and other habit-forming drugs.

Prescription Types

Prescriptions can be classified as compounded and non-compounded.

(i) Compounded prescription

Compounded prescriptions are also called as extemporaneous prescription. It is an order that requires mixing of one or more drugs with one or more pharmaceutical excipients. The doctor selects the drugs, doses, and dosage form that he/she desires and the pharmacist prepares the medication accordingly. The name of each drug is placed on a separate line right under the preceding one.

Model Prescription

NAME OF HOSPITAL Doctor's Name: ________________________ Qualification (MBBS, MD etc.)   Registration No. _________ (Allopathy/Ayurvedic/Homeopathy) Full address: _______________________________ Contact No. _________(Tel), _______(Mobile), E-mail id: _____________
Date: / / Name of patient: ____ Postal address: ____ Contact No. __________________ E-mail id: ___________________ Age: _____ Years.   Sex: _______.   Height: ______.   Weight: ___Kg. **℞** 1.   Name of medicine 1   Strength, dosage instructions, duration and total quantity

> 2.   Name of medicine 2
>   Strength, dosage instructions, duration and total quantity
> 3.   Name of medicine 3
>   Strength, dosage instructions, duration and total quantity
>
>   Doctor's signature
>   Stamp
>
> Dispensed by:
> Date: /   /   Name of Pharmacist: _____________________
> Name of Pharmacy: _____________________ City: _______

(ii) Non-compounded prescription

Non-compounded prescription does not require mixing of two or more ingredients to obtain a finished product. A pre-compounded order consists of a drug or a mixture of drugs supplied by a pharmaceutical company by its official or proprietary name and, if it contains more than one substance, the specific ingredients do not have to be listed.

Units of measurement used in the prescription

The strength of the drugs should be written in metric units. The quantities of drugs are measured in grams, milligrams, and micrograms. The gram (g) is the basic unit of weight in the metric system. One one-thousandth of a gram is 1 milligram (mg). One one-thousandth of a milligram is 1 microgram (µg) or 1 mcg. One thousand grams is one kilogram. The liter is the basic unit of volume in the metric system. We commonly use the milliliter (ml), which is one one-thousandth of a liter. The unit cubic centimeter, or cc, is used as an equal to ml. The strength of a solution is usually expressed as the quantity of a solute in a sufficient solvent to make 100 ml; for example, Potassium Chloride Solution 20% is 20 grams of KCl per 100 ml (g/100 ml). The gram is equal to the weight of 1 ml distilled water at $4°C$ in vacuum.

3.4 HANDLING OF PRESCRIPTION

Patient must be made to feel attended and comfortable by friendly gesture and ambience as soon as they come into the pharmacy. Communication should be opened in such a way that it encourages the patient to convey his/her needs by producing a prescription or by asking for other products or advice.

1. Upon receiving the prescription, the pharmacist should confirm identity of the patient and whether the prescription is presented by the patient himself or by someone on the patient's behalf.
2. The patient may be politely requested to wait while the pharmacist review the prescription for therapeutic aspects (Pharmaceutical and pharmacological), appropriate for an individual, social, legal and economic aspects and legality and completeness of prescription.
3. Prescription should be complete with regard to name of the doctor, his /her address and registration number, name, address, age, sex, height and weight of the patient,

name(s) of the medicine(s), potency, dosage, total amount of the medicines to be supplied, instruction to the patient, refill information if any and prescribed doctors' usual signature.

Any ambient, confusion, shortcoming or anomalies should be brought to notice of the prescribing doctors.

The prescription should be checked for:

(i)   **Dosage**: Whether the dosage prescribed is within the standard minimum and maximum dose range.

(ii)   **Double medication:** Double medication (same drug or different drug with same pharmaco-therapeutic effect) concurrently prescribed by the same Doctor or by two or more doctors to the same patients undergoing concurrent treatment by more than one doctor.

(iii) **Interaction:** Interaction between the currently prescribed medicines, Over The Counter (OTC) medicines being taken by the patient and the medicines being taken from any past prescription (records of which may be available in the Patient's Medication Records) should be checked. Any drug interaction that likely to render the therapy ineffective or cause undesirable effects to the patients should be brought to the notice of the prescribing doctor.

(iv)   **Contraindication**: Age, sex, disease(s), conditions or other characteristics of a patient that may cause certain prescribed medicines to be contraindicated.

(v)   **History:** History of overuse, under use, or misuse of medicines by the patient.

Any of the above as well as handwriting legibility problem should be brought to the notice of the prescribing Doctors. Any necessary change made by the doctor should be recorded on the prescription, with the words "Changes made over the telephone in consultation with the Dr. (name) at (time) on (date)" and should be signed and stamped by the pharmacist. This exercise necessitates a trust based professional relationship with the prescribing doctor incise of any doubt the prescription should be got suitably amended from the doctor.

3.5 ERRORS IN PRESCRIPTION

A medication (a medicinal product) is 'a product that contains a active pharmaceutical ingredient with proven biological effects and excipients or excipients only. The active compound is usually a drug or prodrug. Medication may also contain contaminants. Medicinal product is one that is intended to be taken by or administered to a person or animal for one or more of the following reasons:

1. As a placebo;
2. Prevent a disease;
3. Make a diagnosis;
4. Test for the possibility of an adverse effect;
5. Modify a physiological, biochemical or anatomical function or abnormality;
6. Replace a missing factor;

7. Ameliorate a symptom;

8. Treat a disease;

9. Induce anesthesia.

Medication (the process) is the act of giving a medication (the object) to a patient for any of these purposes.

An error

An error is 'something incorrectly done through ignorance or inadvertence; a mistake, For example, in calculation, judgment, speech, writing, action, etc. or 'a failure to complete a planned action as intended, or the use of an incorrect plan of action to achieve a given aim'.

A medication error

A medication error can be defined as 'a failure in the treatment process that leads to, or has the potential to lead to, harm to the patient'. Medication errors include prescribing errors, dispensing errors, medication administration errors, and patient compliance errors. Specific types of medication errors are categorized in Table 3.1.

Table 3.1: Types of medication errors

Type	Definition
Prescribing error	Incorrect drug selection (based on indications, contraindications, known allergies, existing drug therapy, and other factors), dose, dosage form, quantity, route, concentration, rate of administration, or instructions for use of a drug product ordered or authorized by physician (or other legitimate prescriber); illegible prescriptions or medication orders that lead to errors that reach the patient
Omission error	The failure to administer an ordered dose to a patient before the next scheduled dose, if any
Wrong time error	Administration of medication outside a predefined time interval from its scheduled administration time (this interval should be established by each individual health care facility)
Unauthorized drug error	Administration to the patient of medication not authorized by a legitimate prescriber for the patient
Improper dose error	Administration to the patient of a dose that is greater than or less than the amount ordered by the prescriber or administration of duplicate doses to the patient, i.e., one or more dosage units in addition to those that were ordered

contd. ...

Wrong dosage-form error	Administration to the patient of a drug product in a different dosage form than ordered by the prescriber
Wrong drug-preparation error	Drug product incorrectly formulated or manipulated before administration
Wrong administration-technique error	Inappropriate procedure or improper technique in the administration of a drug
Deteriorated drug error	Administration of a drug that has expired or for which the physical or chemical dosage-form integrity has been compromised
Monitoring error	Failure to review a prescribed regimen for appropriateness and detection of problems, or failure to use appropriate clinical or laboratory data for adequate assessment of patient response to prescribed therapy
Compliance error	Inappropriate patient behaviour regarding adherence to a prescribed medication regimen
Other medication error	Any medication error that does not fall into one of above predefined categories

A potential error is a mistake in prescribing, dispensing, or planned medication administration that is detected and corrected through intervention before actual medication administration. Potential errors are reviewed and tabulated as separate events from errors of occurrence (errors that actually reach patients) to identify opportunities to correct problems in the medication use system even before they occur. Detection of potential errors is a component of the hospital's routine quality improvement process. Documentation of instances in which an individual has prevented the occurrence of a medication error help to identify system weaknesses and to reinforce the importance of multiple checks in the medication use system.

Medication Error - Prevention

The best way to understand how medication errors happen and how to avoid them is to consider their classification, which can be contextual, modal, or psychological. Contextual classification deals with the specific time, place, medicines and people involved. Modal classification examines the ways in which errors occur (for example, by omission, repetition or substitution). Psychological classification is to be preferred, as it explains events rather than merely describing them. Its disadvantage is that it concentrates on human rather than systems sources of errors. The following psychological classification is based on the work of reason on errors in general. There are four broad types of medication errors.

1. Knowledge-based errors (through lack of knowledge)

Communication problems with senior staff and difficulty in accessing appropriate drug-dosing information contributed to knowledge based prescription errors. Example - giving penicillin without having established knowledge for whether the patient is allergic. These types of errors should be avoidable by being well informed about the drug being prescribed and the patient to whom it is being given. Computerized prescribing systems, bar-coded medication systems, and cross-checking by others (for example, pharmacists and nurses) can help to intercept such errors. Education is important.

2. Rule-based errors (using a bad rule or misapplying a good rule)

Example - injecting diclofenac into the lateral thigh rather than to the buttock. Proper rules and education help to avoid these types of error, as do computerized prescribing systems.

3. Action-based errors (called slips)

Example - picking up a bottle containing diazepam from the pharmacy shelf when intending to take one containing diltiazem. It has been observed that most errors are due to slips in attention that occurred during routine prescribing, dispensing or drug administration. These can be minimized by creating conditions in which they are unlikely (e.g. by avoiding distractions, by cross-checking, by labeling medicines clearly and by using identifiers, such as bar-codes has been proposed as a way to avoid misreading of labels. A subset of action-based errors is the technical error e.g. putting the wrong amount of potassium chloride into an infusion bottle. This type of error can be prevented by the use of checklists, fail-safe systems and computerized reminders.

4. Memory-based errors (called lapses)

Memory-based errors are hard to avoid; they can be intercepted by computerized prescribing systems and by cross-checking. For example, giving penicillin, knowing the patient to be allergic, but forgetting.

Latent factors

Mistakes (knowledge- and rule-based errors), slips (action-based errors) and lapses (memory-based errors) are called 'active failures'. There are several 'latent factors' that make prescribers susceptible to error. For example, working overtime with inadequate resources, poor support, and low job security all contributed to an increased risk of medication errors by nurses. Among doctor's depression and exhaustion are important. Errors are more likely to occur when tasks are carried out after hours by busy, distracted staff, often in relation to unfamiliar patients. There is a particular risk of errors when doctors first arrive in hospital, because of shortcomings in their knowledge, and presumably also because they are unfamiliar with local prescription charts and other systems. Improved education and improved working conditions, including better induction processes, should reduce the risk of errors that are due to these factors; a national prescription form would help.

Detecting and reporting errors

There is pharmacist who make them fear of disciplinary procedures and do not want to report them is one of the major difficulty in detecting errors. The establishment of a blame-free, non-punitive environment can obviate this. The reporting of errors, including close-misses, should be encouraged, using error reports to identify areas of likeliest occurrence and simplifying and standardizing the steps in the treatment process. However, some systems for voluntarily reporting medical errors are of limited usefulness, because reports often lack details and there is incomplete reporting and underreporting. A medication error reporting system should be readily accessible, with clear information on how to report a medication error, and reporting should be followed by feedback; detection may be improved by using a combination of methods.

Prescribing faults and prescription errors

Errors in prescribing can be divided into irrational prescribing, inappropriate prescribing, ineffective prescribing, under prescribing and overprescribing, and errors in writing the prescription. The inadequacy of the term 'error' to describe all of these is obvious. Failing to prescribe an anticoagulant for a patient in whom it is indicated (under prescribing) or prescribing one when it is not indicated (overprescribing) are different types of error from errors that are made when writing a prescription. Therefore, it is preferred to use the terms 'prescribing faults' and 'prescription errors'. The term 'prescribing errors' is ambiguously encompassing both the types.

(i) Prescribing faults

Irrational and inappropriate prescribing 'Rational' is defined in the Oxford English Dictionary as 'based on, derived from, reason or reasoning' and 'appropriate' as 'specially fitted or suitable, proper'. One would expect rational prescribing to be appropriate, but that is not always true. A rational approach can result in inappropriate prescribing, if it is based on missing or incorrect information. If, for example, one does not know that another prescriber has already prescribed paracetamol unsuccessfully for a headache, a prescription for paracetamol might be rational but inappropriate. Consider an example of a woman with Liddle's syndrome presented with severe symptomatic hypokalemia. Her doctor reasoned as: she has potassium depletion. The spironolactone is a potassium-sparing drug and thus if prescribed it will help her to retain potassium and thus her serum potassium concentration will normalize. She took a full dose of spironolactone for several days, based on this logical reasoning, but still had severe hypokalemia. Her doctor should have reasoned that she has potassium depletion due to Liddle's syndrome, a channelopathy that affects epithelial sodium channels. There is a choice of potassium-sparing drugs such as spironolactone acts via aldosterone receptors where as amiloride and triamterene via sodium channels. Unfortunately, for Liddle's syndrome an action via sodium channels is required. When she was given amiloride instead of spironolactone her serum potassium concentration rapidly rose to within the reference range. This signifies the importance of understanding the relation between the pathophysiology of the problem and the mechanism of action of the drug.

(ii) Ineffective prescribing

Ineffective prescribing is prescribing a drug that is not effective for the indication in general or for the specific patient; it is distinct from under prescribing. In a study of 212 patients, 6% of 1621 medications were rated as ineffective. Of 196 US out-patients aged 65 and older who were taking five or more medications, 112 (57%) were taking a medication that was ineffective, not indicated, or duplicative. And in a Scottish study, 49% of general practices prescribed homoeopathic remedies, 5% of practices accounting for 50% of the remedies prescribed. One would expect ineffective prescribing to be minimized by the use of guidelines, but there is conflicting evidence; prescribing guidelines may be ineffective unless accompanied by education or financial incentives.

(iii) Under prescribing

Under prescribing is failure to prescribe a drug that is indicated and appropriate, or the use of too low a dose of an appropriate drug. The true extent of under prescribing is not known, but there is evidence of significant under prescribing of some effective treatments, such as angiotensin converting-enzyme inhibitors for patients with heart failure and statins for hyperlipidemia. The sources of under prescribing include fear of adverse effects or interactions, failure to recognize the appropriateness of therapy, and doubts or ignorance about likely efficacy. Cost may play a part. There is a tendency to avoid treatment in older people, and this can lead to unwanted effects, including the so-called risk-treatment mismatch, in which those who are at greatest risk are less aggressively treated, an effect that may be partly associated with age. However, other factors may contribute to this type of mismatch, such as distraction by co-morbidities, miscalculation of the true benefit to harm balance and a reluctance to undertake or exacerbate multiple drug therapy. In a study of the relation of under prescribing to polypharmacy in 150 elderly patients, the probability of under prescribing increased significantly with the prescribed number of drugs. This resulted in failure to use β-adrenoceptor antagonists after myocardial infarction, ACE inhibitors for heart failure, anticoagulants in atrial fibrillation and bisphosphonates in osteoporosis.

(iv) Overprescribing

Overprescribing is prescribing a drug in too high a dosage (too much, too often or for too long). In some cases, treatment is not necessary at all. For example, among hospital patients who were given a proton pump inhibitor treatment was indicated in only half. Poly pharmacy is defined as the use of five or more drugs, occurs in >10% of people aged over 65 years. Although not all poly pharmacy is inappropriate, some undoubtedly leads to ADRs and drug-drug interactions. Overuse of antibiotics is well known and much discussed. A systematic review of 55 trials showed that no single strategy or combination of strategies was better than any other and none was highly effective. It is suggested to undertake active education of clinicians as a strategy to pursue. In a Spanish study, those who overprescribed were more likely to be in rural practices, further from specialist centers, caring for children, lacking postgraduate education and in part-time or short-term work. Doctors' income may have an effect on prescribing medications.

(v) Prescription errors

In general, all the factors that lead to medication errors contribute towards prescription errors. They include lack of knowledge, using the wrong drug name, dosage form, or abbreviation, and incorrect dosage calculations. In a one of the studies of about 900 medication errors in children, 30% were prescription errors, 25% were dispensing errors and 40% were administration errors. In one study the most common form of prescription error was writing the wrong dose. In hospitals the most common errors on prescription charts were writing the patient's name incorrectly and writing the wrong dose, which together accounted for 50% of all errors. In a hospital study of 192 prescription charts, only 7% were correctly filled; 79% had errors that posed minor potential health risks and 14% had errors that could have led to serious harm.

Achieving balanced prescribing:

Each item given below relates to an important process in prescribing, and in the absence of evidence that following this schedule improves prescribing; it makes sense to use it. Nine questions should be asked before writing a prescription:

1. Indication: is there an indication for the drug?
2. Effectiveness: is the medication effective for the condition?
3. Diseases: are there important co-morbidities that could affect the response to the drug?
4. Other similar drugs: is the patient already taking another drug with the same action?
5. Interactions are there clinically important drug–drug interactions with other drugs that the patient is taking?
6. Dosage: what is the correct dosage regimen (dose, frequency, route, formulation)?
7. Orders: what are the correct directions for giving the drug and are they practical?
8. Period: what is the appropriate duration of therapy?
9. Economics: is the drug cost-effective?

The mnemonic for this list is 'i.e. do I dope?'.

Improvement in prescribing would help reducing medication errors. Following five prescription rules help to improve prescription writing.

1. Education, to be taken as often as possible (a repeat prescription—learning should be lifelong).

2. Special study modules for graduates and undergraduates, to be taken as required.

3. Proper assessment: in the final undergraduate examination, to be taken once or twice; in postgraduate appraisal, to be taken occasionally; this could be linked to a license to prescribe.

4. A national prescription form for hospitals: to be applied uniformly and used as a training tool.

5. Guidelines and computerized prescribing systems: to be taken if indicated (their roles and proper implementation).

MODEL QUESTIONS

1. Define prescription. Explain different parts of prescription.
2. Explain handling of prescription.
3. Discuss different errors in prescription.
4. Write a note on:
   (i) Compounded and non-compounded prescriptions
   (ii) Medication errors

Chapter 4...

Posology

LEARNING OBJECTIVES

Posology is a branch of medical science which deals with dose quantity of drug which can be administered to a patient to get the desirable pharmacological action. The objective of drug therapy is to bring drug plasma concentration within the therapeutic window.

The objectives of this chapter include:

- To study of the dosages of drugs, especially the determination of appropriate dosages.
- To obtain relevant information to guide the posology recommendation taking into account patient and product specificities.
- To identify and understand the factors affecting drug dosages.
- To know various methods of dose calculation for pediatric patients.

4.1 INTRODUCTION

Posology term is derived from the Greek word *'posos'* meaning 'how much' and *'logos'* meaning 'science'. Posology is the branch of medicine/pharmacy which deals with dose quantity of drug which can be administered to a patient to get the desirable pharmacological action. In simple terms the term posology is the science of doses. All Pharmacopoeias prescribe the doses of drugs for internal use. These days the term posology is not commonly used in medical practice. This term is existing only in books. Directly the professionals use the term DOSE and DOSAGE which are directly self-explanatory. Posology is study of dose and dosage. Dose is the quantitative amount of drug administered or taken by a patient for the intended medicinal effect. It is a mere table of standardized minimum and maximum dose like a directory. The dependent factors are age, sex, body weight, constitution, life style, pregnancy, lactation, old age, children, infants, drugs already taken, being taken, occupation and the type of formulation.

The dose is usually expressed as a range. The minimum dose or the lower limit of the dose is essential for eliciting an intended therapeutic response whereas the maximum dose or the higher limit of the dose is the amount of the drug substance that can be tolerated by an average individual. These doses are prescribed for the guidance of the prescriber. The pharmacist is much concerned with the maximum limit of the doses which, if exceeded, may cause untoward effects in the patient. The actual dose of a drug is to be decided by the prescriber depending on patient's age, sex, symptoms, his medication history and the factors like tolerance, idiosyncrasy, route of administration, etc.

4.2 FACTORS AFFECTING POSOLOGY

1. Age

Age is the most common factor that influences the amount of drug to be given. An infant would require much less dose than an adult. Children under 12 years require fraction of adult dose. The adult dose is for people between 18 and 60 years of age. Elderly patients may require more or less than the average dose, depending upon the action of the drug and the condition of the patient.

(i) **Newborns:** A newborn infant has high total body water, low fat, immature renal and hepatic function and different protein binding. The drug dosage of newborn is low because gastric acid secretion are not adequate (GIT absorption of ampicillin and amoxicillin is greater in neonates due to decreased gastric acidity), liver microsomal enzymes (glucuronyl transferase) are deficient (administration of chloramphenicol may lead to Grey baby syndrome because of inadequate glucouronidation of chloramphenicol resulting in drug accumulation), plasma protein binding is less, glomerular filtration rate and tubular secretions are not adequate. In addition, there is immaturity of blood brain barriers in neonates (sulfonamides may lead to hyper bilirubinemia and kernicterus). Infants have an immature renal tubular transport system. Penicillin, streptomycin and amino glycosides are not administered. After one year of age, elimination by kidneys is increased. Hepatic metabolizing capacity is also underdeveloped.

(ii) **Children:** The tissues of an infant and child are highly sensitive to large number of drugs. Thus they require fewer doses. Children under 12 years require fraction of adult dose because drug metabolizing enzyme system is inefficient in them (Glucuronidation takes 3 months to develop). Their blood brain barriers (BBB) are not fully developed, thus are more sensitive to CNS stimulants. All parts of the body are affected by the drug. In children tetracyclines may cause permanent teeth staining, corticosteroids may lead to growth and development retardation and antihistaminics may cause hyperactivity. The dose for a child is calculated from the adult dose up to 8 years of age.

(iii) **Adult:** The average adult dose is for an individual of medium built with age 18 to 16 years and weight 70 kg. For very thin or obese individual the dose may be modified using either the body surface area or body weight. Surface area is found from height and weight, and is around $1.7\text{-}1.8/m^2$.

(iv) **Geriatric:** The geriatric age group is age more than 60 years. These patients require special consideration because physiological changes occur with age are to be kept in consideration such as reduced body weight, reduced body fat, reduced intestinal motility and mesenteric blood flow, reduced renal and hepatic functions and altered mental functions. In elderly patients, aging and renal and hepatic dysfunction issues results into requirement of fewer doses. Elderly often require lesser doses than adults because they are prone to suffer from adverse drug reactions. If liquid preparations are available, they should be preferred as are convenient for absorption. Liver functions are impaired. Drugs like diazepam, theophylline having lower therapeutic index, may have much larger half-lives (2 h in normal 90 h in old). Kidney functions are also impaired. Drugs like digoxin, lithium and amino glycosides have decreased excretion. Plasma protein binding is decreased leading to greater amounts of active drugs. Increased sensitivity to CNS depressants like diazepam, morphine also occurs.

2. Sex

Patient sex is particularly important in the case of treatment with sex hormones. Female adults generally require smaller doses than males due to the presence of more body fat. Testosterone increases the rate of biotransformation of drugs. Decreased metabolism of some drugs in female (Diazepam) occurs. Females are more susceptible to autonomic drugs (estrogen inhibits choline esterase). Drugs used for ulcer may cause increased prolactin. During menstruation, salicylates and strong purgatives should be avoided as they may increase bleeding. During lactation, drugs may be excreted through milk and may affect the infant, e.g. some purgatives, penicillin, chloramphenicol and oral anticoagulants. Morphine normally depresses CNS but may produce excitation in some individuals, especially women.

3. Pregnancy

In pregnancy cardiac output, Glomerular Filtration Rate (GFR) and renal elimination of drugs, volume of distribution and metabolic rate of some drugs are taken in to consideration. Lipophilic drugs cross placental barrier and are slowly excreted. During pregnancy, uterine stimulants, strong purgatives and drugs likely to have teratogenic effects and thus should be avoided, especially during first trimester no drug should be given unless absolutely necessary. During labour, morphine should be avoided as it crosses placental barrier and depresses respiration in newborn.

4. Weight

Weight of patient has a more direct bearing on the dose than any other factor. The dose is given per kg body weight. Average muscular weight is between 50 and 100 kg. Being the average, the usual doses for drugs are mentioned generally for 70 kg adult. The drug concentration at site of action is based on the ratio between the amount of drug administered and size of the body. The dose calculations for abnormally thin or obese patients are required to calculate on the basis of body weight.

5. Severity of disease

It is a common experience that dull headache may be relieved by a single tablet of aspirin whereas severe headache may necessitate administration of 2-3 tablets of the same drug. But this is no true in all cases. For example, in case of iron deficiency anemia, the dose of iron salt administered orally remains the same irrespective of severity because there is a limit to which iron can be absorbed from the intestine daily and incorporated in hemoglobin.

6. Health and nutrition

Debilitated and anemic patients are more sensitive to the toxic effects of drugs and hence are given in smaller doses. Persons with severe anemia associated with hookworm infestation are more susceptible to the toxic effects of tetrachloroethylene. Myxoedematous patients are known to show less response to drugs like amphetamine because of low cellular metabolism.

7. Pathological state

Smaller dose is indicated if the organs, through which biotransformation or excretion takes place, are diseased. For example, in case of renal insufficiency, phenobarbitone (mainly excreted by the kidneys) is given in smaller dose and in case of patients suffering from liver diseases, morphine is given in smaller dose (morphine is mainly inactivated in liver). Aspirin has no effect on normal body temperature but lowers the body temperature in fevered patients. Quinine precipitates black water fever more often with falciparum malaria than otherwise.

8. Tolerance

Some children can tolerate relatively large doses of arsenic, belladonna and calomel. Tolerance can be acquired as a result of repeated administration of some drugs e.g., morphine, heroin and cocaine.

9. Simultaneous administration drugs

(a) **Synergism:** Synergism is the facilitation/potentiation of pharmacological response by simultaneous use of two drugs. In synergism, the effect produced is greater than the algebraic sum of the effects of individual drugs e.g., adrenaline and cocaine.

   (i) **Addition:** When two or more drugs given together produce the same resulting effect is the algebraic sum of their individual effects. The response is not more than their total algebraic sum. For example,

   1. Aspirin and paracetamol as analgesic/ antipyretic

   2. Ephedrine and theophylline as bronchodilator

   3. Nitrous oxide and ether as general anesthetic

   (ii) **Potentiation:** The total effect is more than the sum of their individual effects.

   1. Acetylcholine and physostigmine: Physostigmine inhibits the action of esterase prolonging the effect of acetylcholine.

   2. Levodopa (Parkinsonism) and carbidopa/Benserazide: Levodopa is decarboxylated peripherally, carbidopa inhibits the decarboxylase.

   3. Sulfonamide (effective against some microorganisms) when combined with trimethoprim is effective against a wider range of microorganisms.

(b) Antagonism: When two drugs having opposite effect e.g. the use of amphetamine to correct partially the sedation caused by anticonvulsant doses of phenobarbital and the administration of ephedrine to correct hypotension resulting from spinal anesthesia.

(i) Chemical antagonism: It involves reduction of the biological activity of a drug by a chemical reaction with another agent.

Example: Acids and alkalies: British anti-Lewisite (dimercaprol; BAL) and arsenic.

Antacids, used for dyspepsia involve administration of sodium bicarbonate to react with hydrochloric acid. In cases of heavy metal poisoning chelating agents like dimerzapam are used. In iron poisoning deproxamine is given which binds sulphydral groups forming insoluble complexes which can be easily detoxified.

(ii) Pharmacological antagonism: Pharmacological antagonism is of two types:

(a) Competitive or reversible antagonism: In this type of antagonism the agonist and antagonist compete with each other for the same receptors. The extent of antagonism depends on the relative number of receptors occupied by the two compounds. Other features of competitive antagonism are:

1. Antagonist has chemical resemblance with agonist.

2. Antagonism can be overcome by increasing the concentration of the agonist at receptor site. It means the maximal response to agonist is not impaired.

3. Antagonist shifts the dose response curve to right

4. E_{max} of agonist is obtained with high concentration of agonist

5. Duration of action is short and is depends on drug clearance

Example: Acetyl choline and atropine antagonism on muscarinic receptors.

In presence of antagonist, log dose response curve of agonist shifts to right, indicating a higher concentration of agonist is required for same response. Maximum height of the curve can be attained by overcoming the action of antagonist. This leads to a parallel shift of log dose response curve towards right.

(b) Non-competitive antagonism: Here an antagonist inactivates the receptor in such a way so that the effective complex with agonist cannot be formed irrespective of the concentration of the agonist. This can happen by various ways:

1. The antagonist might combine at the same site in such a way that even higher concentration of the agonist cannot displace it.

2. The antagonist might combine at a different site of receptor in such a way that agonist is unable to initiate characteristic biological response

3. The antagonist might itself induce a certain change in receptor so that the reactivity of the receptor site where agonist should interact is abolished.

Other features of this antagonism are:

1. Antagonist has no chemical resemblance with agonist.

2. Maximum response is suppressed

3. Although antagonist shifts the dose response curve to right, the slope of the curve is reduced.

4. The extent of antagonism depends on the characteristics of antagonist itself and agonist has no influence upon the degree of antagonism or its reversibility

5. E_{max} of agonist is decreased even with high concentration of agonist

6. Duration of action is long which depends upon new receptor synthesis.

Example: Phenoxybenzamine and adrenaline at alpha adrenergic receptors.

(c) Physiological antagonism: In this type of interaction of two drugs, both are agonists, so they act at different receptor sites. They antagonize the action of each other because they produce opposite actions.

Example: Adrenalin and histamine. The former cause bronchodilatation while later bronchoconstriction. So adrenalin is a lifesaving drug in anaphylaxis.

10. Route of administration

In general, the rate of absorption of a drug decreases with route of administration in the order of i.v. > i.m. > s.c. > oral. Thus, in general, i.v. dose of a drug is smaller than its i.m. or s.c. or oral dose.

Example: Ergotamine dose for oral route is 2 to 5 mg, i.m. route is 1 mg (about to 1/2 of oral dose) and for i.v. route is 0.25 mg (about to 1/8 of oral dose and % of i.m. dose).

11. Time and frequency of drug administration

Biological half-life of a drug (the time required for the blood level to drop down to 50 % of the initial peak level), is the main factor that governs frequency of drug administration.

Example: The biological half-life of sulphadiazine is 4 hours, thus 1 g of the drug has to be given every 4 hours after initial dose of 2 g. On the contrary, reserpine a tranquilizer, biological half-life of a drug has no relation to frequency of administration.

12. Allergy

Allergy is the abnormal response of drug resulting from antigen-antibody reaction, leading to liberation of histamine and histamine-like substances. Therefore, there may be skin rashes, urticaria, bronchoconstriction and fall of blood pressure. Allergic reactions may occur immediately or may be delayed for many days. Immediate and acute allergic reactions lead to acute anaphylactic shock which is dangerous for patient and may even be fatal e.g. penicillin, sera, vaccines. Penicillin may produce anaphylactic shock (sudden fall of blood pressure) in allergic patient, but not in normal patients. Sometimes skin rashes or urticaria along with fever and pain in joints and swelling of lymph nodes may occur after a few days. This is delayed type of allergy called serum sickness type reaction. Thus, prior to dose calculation patient history of previous allergic reactions, preliminary test dose and drugs to deal with emergency should be kept ready.

13. Plasma Protein Binding

Malnutrition causes decreased amino acids, decreased proteins leading to decreased binding sites for drugs.

14. Food

Drugs are better absorbed in empty stomach. To prevent gastric irritation most drugs are taken after or between foods, which affects the outcomes.

Example: Anti-motion drugs are taken on empty stomach. Helminthes (for evacuation of worms) are also taken on empty stomach.

15. Drug Dependence (Drug addiction)

Drug dependence is a state of periodic or chronic intoxication which is detrimental to person and society. It becomes almost impossible to carry out normal physical functions without the drug. The components of phenomenon of addiction include euphoria (sense of happiness and forgetfulness), tolerance (due to increased production of enzymes), psychic dependence/habituation (person desires but in absence of drug no harm occurs), physical dependence and withdrawal symptoms/abstinence syndrome (symptoms opposite pharmacological actions of drug develop in absence of drug).

4.3 PEDIATRIC DOSE CALCULATIONS

Children are more sensitive than adults to medications because of their weight, height, physical condition, immature physiological systems, and metabolism. Nurses who administer medications to infants and children must be vigilant in determining whether the patient is receiving the correct medication. The correct dose is one of the six rights of drug administration: right patient, medication, route, time, dose, and documentation. The physician or provider will prescribe the medication to be delivered. However, the nurse is responsible for detecting any errors in calculation of dosage, as well as for preparing the medication and administering the drug. The nurse needs to be aware that pediatric dosages are often less than 1 mL; therefore, a tuberculin syringe is used for accurate dosing. Pediatric medications are calculated using the infant or child's kilogram weight. The dosages have been established by the drug companies. Safe and therapeutic dosages are readily available from a reliable source such as 'The Harriet Lane Handbook'. In general, pediatric dosages are rounded to the nearest tenth. For infants and young children, doses may be rounded to the nearest hundredth. The child who weighs more than 50 kg may receive adult dosages. If the calculated dose is greater than the recommended adult dose, DO NOT administer the medication. A child should not receive higher doses than those recommended for the adult, ever. Many drugs have a "do not exceed" or "max. dose" in 24 hours listed; this must always be considered. Additionally, the physician or pharmacist may use the child's body surface area (BSA) to calculate a dosage of medication to administer. The BSA calculation may be used when an established dosage has not been determined by the drug company, as with some anticancer or specialized drugs.

In pharmacy accurate dosage calculations are very important. Pharmacists has to calculate standard and non-standard dosages every day. However, a pharmacist is ultimately responsible for all medications and takes the final decision on which methods, formulas and calculations are to be used. Patient always needs to consult a licensed medical doctor or pharmacist before determining any dosage calculation.

Most drugs in children are dosed according to body weight (mg/kg) or body surface area (BSA) (mg/m^2). Care is taken to properly convert body weight from pounds to kilograms (1 kg = 2.2 lb) before calculating doses based on body weight. Doses are often expressed as mg/kg/day or mg/kg/dose, therefore orders written "mg/kg/d" is confusing and requires further clarification from the prescriber. Chemotherapeutic drugs are commonly dosed according to body surface area which requires an extra verification step (BSA calculation) prior to dosing. Medications are available in multiple concentrations; therefore, orders written in "mL" rather than "mg" are not acceptable and require further clarification. Dosing also varies by indication; therefore, diagnostic information is helpful when calculating doses. The following examples are typically encountered when dosing medication in children.

Most reference manuals for medications focus primarily on the adult dosages. But children can require very different medication doses compared to adults. In order to calculate pediatric dose, several different rules such as Nomogram method, Fried's rule, Young's rule and Clark's rule may be used to determine the correct dosage of medication for a pediatric patient.

(a) Age

Clark's rule and Young's rule are used when either the manufacturer has not recommended dosages for children or the prescriber has requested them to be used. The best explanation for these is simply that children vary so much in weight, size, tolerances, etc. Clark's rule uses weight in pounds (lbs) and never in kg.

1. **Young's rule:** Young's rule is a rule for evaluating the dosage of medicine for a child by adding 12 to the child's age, and dividing the sum by the age of the child, then dividing the adult dose by the result obtained. Thus;

$$\text{Dose for Child} = \text{Adult dose} \times \frac{\text{Child Age}}{\text{Child Age} + 12} \qquad \dots (4.1)$$

    Example: A 10 year old girl weighing 60 lbs. Average adult dose given for the girl is 300 mg. Calculate the child's pediatric dose.

    Solution: Given, age of child = 10 year, average adult dose = 300 mg.

$$\text{Child's pediatric dose} = \left[\frac{\text{Age of child}}{\text{Age of child} + 12}\right] \times \text{Average adult dose}$$

$$= [10 / (10 + 12)] \times 300 \text{ mg}$$

$$= (10 / 22) \times 300 \text{ mg}$$

$$= 0.4545 \times 300 \text{ mg}$$

$$= 136.36 \text{ mg}$$

2. **Cowling's Rule:** Cowling's Rule is used to calculate doses for children two years of age or older.

$$\text{Dose of child} = \text{Adult dose} \times \frac{\text{Age at next birthday (in years)}}{\text{Age} + 12} \qquad \dots (4.2)$$

3. **Fried's Rule (for infants):** Fried's Rule is for calculating doses for infants younger than one year of age. This rule is a method, to estimate the medicine dosage for a child, by dividing the age of the child (in months) by 150 lbs. The result is multiplied by the adult's dosage.

$$\text{Dose for infant} = \text{Adult dose} \times \frac{\text{Age (in months)}}{150} \qquad \dots (4.3)$$

Example: Calculate the child dose for 1-year-old baby, if the adult dose of the medicine is 400 mg.

Solution: Given, age of child in month = 12 months and average adult dose = 400 mg.

$$\text{Child dose} = (\text{Age of child in month} / 150 \text{ lbs}) \times \text{Average adult dose}$$
$$= (12 / 150 \text{ lbs}) \times 400 \text{ mg}$$
$$= 32 \text{mg}$$

(b) Body Weight

Drugs are often prescribed based on an adult or child body weight in order to more accurately dose. The calculation is very simple and easy to perform. However, you must pay close attention to whether the dosage has been prescribed per kg or lbs. The official usual doses for drugs are considered suitable for 70 kg (150 pounds) individuals. The ratio between the amount of drug administered and the size of the body influences the drug concentration at the site of action. Thus, drug dosage may require adjustment from the usual adult dose for abnormally lean or obese patients. The determination of drug dosage for children on the basis of body weight is more accurate than that based on age.

4. **Clarks rule:** Clark's Rule is an obsolete rule for an approximate child's dose, Clark's Rule is not used clinically but it is a favorite dosage calculation formula for pediatric nursing instructors. It determines the approximate dose of medicine appropriate for a child two years of age or older by dividing the child's weight in pounds by 150 and multiplying the result by the adult dose.

$$\text{Dose for child} = \text{Adult dose} \times \frac{\text{Weight in pounds}}{150 \text{ (averge weight of adult in lbs)}} \qquad \dots (4.4)$$

(c) Body Surface Area

Many physicians believe that doses for children should be based upon body surface area (BSA), since the correct dosage of drugs seems more proportional to the surface area. But there exist a close relationship between a large number of physiological processes and BSA. Many physiological factors such as plasma volume, oxygen consumption, and body electrolyte are proportional to the BSA. The BSA used to calculate dose, e.g., anticancer drug methotrexate is administered on mg/mm^2 of body surface. The average BSA of a 70kg adult is 1.7 to 1.8 m^2. The dose for child based on BSA is calculated using formula:

$$\text{Approximate dose for child} = \text{Adult dose} \times \frac{\text{BSA of child (in m}^2\text{)}}{1.8 \text{ m}^2 \text{ (average adult BASA)}} \qquad \dots (4.5)$$

1. **Nomogram Method:** The Nomogram method is used to determine the correct pediatric medication dosage based on BSA. It takes into consideration the person's body surface area in square meters with 1.73 m^2 being the surface area of the average adult (weighing 150-154 lbs). Since, it is based on the patient's height and weight, the Nomogram method is the best method.

$$\text{Child's dose} = \text{Child's BSA} \times \left(\frac{\text{Adult dose}}{1.73}\right) \qquad \ldots (4.6)$$

Example 4.1: Calculate the dose of amoxicillin suspension in mL for otitis media for a 1-year-old child weighing 22 lbs. The dose required is 40 mg/kg/day divided as b.i.d. The suspension has concentration of 400 mg/5 mL.

Solution:

1. Convert pounds to kg: 22 lb × 1 kg/2.2 lb = 10 kg

2. Calculate the dose in mg: 10 kg × 40 mg/kg/day = 400 mg/day

3. Divide the dose by the frequency: 400 mg/day ÷ 2 (b.i.d.) = 200 mg/dose b.i.d.

4. Convert the mg dose to mL: 200 mg/dose ÷ 400 mg/5 mL = 2.5 mL b.i.d.

Example 4.2: Calculate the dose of ceftriaxone in mL for meningitis for a 5-year-old weighing 18 kg. The dose required is 100 mg/kg/day given i.v. once daily. The drug has concentration of 40 mg/mL.

Solution:

1: Calculate the dose in mg: 18 kg × 100 mg/kg/day = 1800 mg/day

2: Divide the dose by the frequency: 1800 mg/day ÷ 1 (daily) = 1800 mg/dose

3: Convert the mg dose to mL: 1800 mg/dose ÷ 40 mg/mL = 45 mL once daily

Example 4.3: Calculate the dose of vincristine in mL for a 4-year-old with leukemia weighing 37 lb and is 97 cm tall. The dose required in 2 mg/m^2. The drug has 1 mg/mL concentration.

Solution:

1: Convert pounds to kg: 37 lb × 1 kg/2.2 lb = 16.8 kg

2: Calculate BSA (see BSA Nomograms): 16.8 kg × 97 cm/3600 = 0.67 m^2

3: Calculate the dose in mg: 2 mg/m^2 × 0.67 m^2 = 1.34 mg

4: Calculate the dose in mL: 1.34 mg ÷ 1 mg/mL = 1.34 mg

Converting Pounds to Kilograms

The formula: 2.2 lbs = 1 kg

Infants and young children's weight in pounds must be converted to kilograms to accurately calculate medication doses and daily fluid requirements. Safe and Therapeutic (S&T) drug dosages have been established using kilogram weights. Always round the kilogram weight to the nearest tenth, NOT a whole number.

MODEL QUESTIONS

1. Define Posology. Explain different factors affecting posology.
2. How pediatric dose is calculated on the basis of age, body weight and body surface area?
3. Write a note on:
   (i)   Young's rule
   (ii) Fried's rule

   (iii) Clarks rule

UNIT II

Chapter 5...

Pharmaceutical Calculations

LEARNING OBJECTIVES

The dosage regimen is the modality of drug administration that is chosen to reach the therapeutic objective. This depends on the drug used, the condition to be treated, and the patient's characteristics. For most drugs, a usual dosage regimen is proposed by the manufacturer and approved by registration authorities. This regimen should suit the average patient's needs. As a principle, individualization of the dosing regimen should be considered systematically, leading in selected cases to apply unusual dosing decisions in order to tailor the treatment to a patient condition.

The objectives of this chapter include:

- To review various systems and methods of dose measurement and expressing doses and dosage regimens.
- Learn to calculate the amount of drug product to prescribe or dispense or supply.
- Learn methods to calculate doses with suitable examples
- To discuss various ways to express solution strengths.
- To know proper methods of calculating proof spirit and its strength.

5.1 MEASUREMENT SYSTEMS

The most crucial steps in compounding any pharmaceutical product are the accurate calculation and measurement of the component ingredients of the formulation. In order to carry out these critical functions, the pharmacist must have a working knowledge of three systems of measurement namely; the metric system, the apothecary system, and the avoirdupois system. There are two main systems for measurement of distance and weight, the Imperial System of Measurement and the Metric System of Measurement. Most countries use the Metric System, which uses the measuring units such as metres and grams and adds prefixes like kilo, milli and centi to count orders of magnitude. In some of the countries like United States, they use the older Imperial system, where things are measured in feet, inches and pounds.

5.2 THE IMPERIAL SYSTEM

The Imperial System is also called The British Imperial because it came from the British Empire that ruled many parts of the world from the 16th to the 19th century. After the U.S gained independence from Britain, the new American government decided to keep this type of measurement, even though the metric system was gaining in popularity at the time. The Imperial system is more complicated than the metric system, as it does not work in multiples of 10 as the metric system does. Imperial system has two other systems of measurements.

(5.1)

(i) The Apothecary System

The Apothecary system was commonly used in the past by pharmacists and physicians as the system of weights and measures for prescribing and dispensing medications. Although it has largely been replaced by the less complex metric system, the pharmacist still encounters these symbols in his/her routine practice. Indeed, the apothecary system of fluid measure is still commonly used in a variety of products, both pharmaceutical and non-pharmaceutical. Everyone should be familiar with the fluid ounce, pint, quart, and gallon.

(ii) The Avoirdupois System

The Avoirdupois system is a system of weight measurement only. Its basic unit, 'grain', is the same as in the Apothecary system. The Avoirdupois ounce and pound differ in weight and symbols from those in the Apothecary system. The Avoirdupois pound is the pound to which we are all accustomed in our daily lives. It is also the weight measure in which bulk chemicals and over the counter pharmaceuticals are bought and sold. It is important to make this distinction from weights in the Apothecary systems, which are used only in the prescription or medication order.

In the Imperial system the base units are:

(i)   Length, commonly measured in inches (in), feet (ft), yards and miles;

(ii) Time, commonly measured in seconds (s), hours (hr), days (d), weeks and years (yr);

(iii) Weight, commonly measured in pounds (lb); and

(iv) Temperature, measured in Fahrenheit (°F).

The Imperial system commonly uses weight, rather than mass. Weight refers to the gravitational pull on an object, whereas mass refers to the amount of matter in the object. An object would have the same mass on the moon as it does on the earth, but it would weigh less on the moon as the gravitational pull of the moon is less than the gravitational pull of the earth. Conversions between the common units of length used in the Imperial system are listed below

12 in = 1 ft

3 ft = 1 yard

1760 yards = 1 mile

The units of time are generally accepted for use with the metric system, as well as the Imperial system. Conversions between the common units of time are listed below:

60 s = 1 min

24 hrs = 1 day

7 days = 1 week

52 weeks = 1 yr

The most common imperial units of measurement are:

Quantity	Unit	Symbol
Length	foot	ft
Weight	pound	lb
Volume	gallon	gal

Here are the most common conversions of imperial units of measurement:

Length	**Weight**	**Volume**
1 foot (ft) = 12 inches (in.)	1 pound (lb.) = 16 ounces (oz)	1 pint (pt) = 2 cups
1 yard (yd) = 3 feet	1 ton = 2000 pounds (lbs)	1 quart (qt) = 2 pints
5280 feet (1760 yards)		1 gallon (gal) = 4 quarts

The standard unit for capacity is gallon and is same for both the Avoirdupois and the Apothecary systems.

1 gallon (c)	=	160 fluid ounces
$1/4^{th}$ of gallon	=	1 quart
$1/8^{th}$ of gallon	=	1 pint(O)
$1/160^{th}$ of gallon	=	1 fl. ounce
1 quart	=	40 fl. ounces
1 pint	=	20 flounces 1 fl. ounce = 480 minims
1 fl drachm	=	60 minims

5.3 THE METRIC SYSTEM

The metric system is the preferred and most frequently used system of measurement in pharmacy. Since it is a decimal system, other denominations of measure in the system are easily and quickly generated as a 10th multiple of the basic unit. To convert from larger to smaller units one only needs to move the decimal, the appropriate number of places to the right. The decimal is moved to the left to convert from smaller to larger units.

The metric system or SI (International System) is easiest system to use in practice. The base units for the metric system are the units of:

(i)   Length, measured in metres (m);
(ii) Time, measured in seconds (s);
(iii) Mass, measured in grams (g); and
(iv) Temperature, measured in Celsius (°C).

Various units in the metric system are related to one another through the use of prefixes, each of which has a specific numerical value. Some of the more commonly used prefixes and their numerical values (written in a variety of forms) are listed below.

Prefix	**Conventional**	**Decimal**	**Exponential**
kilo– (k)	1,000	–	10^3
hecto– (h)	100	–	10^2
deka– (da)	10	–	10^1
deci– (d)	1/10	0.1	10^{-1}
centi– (c)	1/100	0.01	10^{-2}
milli– (m)	1/1000	0.001	10^{-3}
micro– (μ)	1/1,000,000	0.000001	10^{-6}
nano– (n)	1/1,000,000,000	0.000000001	10^{-9}
pico– (p)	1/1,000,000,000,000	0.000000000001	10^{-12}

LENGTH

In pharmaceutical practice, metre, centimetre, millimetre, and smaller are commonly used metric units for length. However, the decimetre is rarely used. The micrometre is often referred by the non-SI term micron. In some fields of chemistry, the angstrom, which is equal to 0.1 nm, historically competed with the nanometer is used.

Using the base unit for length:

1 nanometre (nm)   = 1 m / 100,000,000 = 0.000 000 001 m

1 micrometre (μm) = 1 m / 1,000,000 = 0.000 001 m

1 millimetre (mm) = 1 m / 1,000 = 0.001 m

1 centimetre (cm) = 1 m / 100 = 0.01 m

1 decimetre (dm)   = 1 m / 10 = 0.1 m

1 decametre (dam) = 1 m × 10 = 10 m

1 hectometre (hm) = 1 m × 100 = 100 m

1 kilometer (km)   = 1 m × 1,000 = 1,000 m

1 megametre (Mm) = 1 m × 1,000,000 = 1,000,000 m

1 gigametre (Gm)   = 1 m × 1,000,000,000 = 1,000,000,000 m

VOLUME

The litre, millilitre, microlitre, and smaller are commonly used metric units for volume. In Europe, the centilitre is often used for packaged products and the decilitres less frequently. Larger volumes are usually denoted in kilolitres, megalitres or gigalitres, or else in cubic meters. For scientific purposes the cubic meter is usually used. Litre is the volume of the cube of 1/10th of a meter (1 dm^3). The units for volume in metric system are as follows:

Prefix	Conventional
1 Kilolitre (kl)	1,000 Litres
1 Hectolitres (hl)	100 Litres
1 Dekalitres (dal)	10 Litres
1 Litre (l)	1 Litre
1 Decilitre (dl)	0.10 Litre
1 Centilitre (cl)	0.01 Litre
1 Millilitre (ml)	0.001 Litre
1 Microlitre (μl)	0.0000001 Litre

WEIGHT

The unit of weight in metric system is gram. It is weight of 1 cm^3 of water at 4°C.

1 kilogram (kg)	=	1000 grams
1 hectagram (hg)	=	100 grams
1 dekkagram (dg)	=	10 grams
1 gram (g)	=	1 gram
1 decigram (dg)	=	0.1 gram
1 centigram (cg)	=	0.01 gram
1 milligram (cg)	=	0.001 gram
1 microgram (mcg)	=	0.000001 gram
1 nanogram (ng)	=	0.000000001 gram
1 picogram (mcg)	=	0.000000000001 gram

The kilogram, gram, milligram, microgram and smaller ones are fairly common in pharmacy practice.

1 milligram	=	1000 micrograms
1 gram	=	1000 milligrams
1 kg	=	1000 grams

5.4 PERCENTAGE SOLUTIONS

The concentration of a solution is a macroscopic property which represents the amount of solute dissolved in a unit amount of solvent or of solution. It can be expressed in a different way. The percentage concentration in solution is commonly expressed as weight/volume per cent or mass/volume percent. This variation measures the amount of solute in grams but measures the amount of solution in millilitres. For example, 5%w/v NaCl solution contains 5 grams of NaCl in 100 mL of solution.

$$\text{Volume per cent} = \frac{\text{Weight of solute (in grams)}}{\text{Volume of solution (in mL)}} \times 100 \qquad \qquad \text{... (5.1)}$$

Since; different units are used in the numerator and denominator, this type of concentration is not a true percentage. It is used as a quick and easy concentration unit because volumes are easier to measure than weights and because the density of dilute solutions is generally close to 1 g/mL. Thus, the volume of a solution in mL is very nearly numerically equal to the mass of the solution in grams.

In pharmacy practice, generally two types of per cent solution concentrations are used namely; per cent by weight and per cent by volume. Whenever we say weight or volume of the solution, we need to add the respective weights and volumes of all the components of the solution. Do not commit the error of taking the weight or volume of only the solute or solvent in the denominators of the above expressions.

Per cent by Weight

Per cent by mass (w/w) is the weight of solute divided by the total weight of the solution, multiplied by 100 %.

$$\% \ w/w \ = \ \frac{\text{Weight of solute}}{\text{Total weight of solution}} \times 100\% \qquad \ldots (5.2)$$

Example 5.1: What is the per cent by mass of a solution that contains 20 g of glucose in 200 g of solution?

Solution: Per cent by mass $= \dfrac{\text{Mass of glucose}}{\text{Total mass of solution}} \times 100\%$

$$= \frac{20 \ g}{200 \ g} \times 100\%$$

$$= 10\% \ w/w \qquad \ldots (5.3)$$

Per cent by Volume

Per cent by volume (v/v) is the volume of solute divided by the total volume of the solution, multiplied by 100%.

$$\text{Per cent by volume} \ = \ \frac{\text{Volume of solute}}{\text{Total volume of solution}} \times 100\% \qquad \ldots (5.4)$$

Example 5.2: How would you prepare 200 ml of 60 % (v/v) of rubbing alcohol ?

Solution: $60\% = \dfrac{\text{Volume of rubbing alcohol}}{\text{Total volume of solution}} \times 100\%$

$$\text{Volume of rubbing alcohol} \ = \ \frac{60\%}{100\%} \times \text{Volume of solution}$$

$$= \frac{60\%}{100\%} \times 200 \ mL$$

$$= 120 \ mL$$

You would add enough water to 120 mL of rubbing alcohol to make a total of 200 mL of solution.

In addition to w/v and v/v, other ways to express solution percentages include v/w and w/w. There are other ways to express concentration. The concentration of a solution is most of the time expressed as molarity. Some expressions for concentration are temperature dependent. The concentration of the solution changes as the temperature changes.

Molarity

Molarity is the number of moles of solute in exactly one litre of a solution. It is spelled with an "r" and is represented by a capital letter M. To calculate the molarity of a solute in a solution we need to know the moles of solute present in the solution and the volume of solution (in litres) containing the solute. Molarity is calculated using equation:

$$\text{Molarity (M)} = \frac{\text{Moles of solute}}{\text{Volume of solution in litres}} \qquad \ldots (5.5)$$

Molality

Molality (m), is the number of moles of solute dissolved in exactly one kilogram (1000 grams) of solvent. Note that molality is spelled with two letters 'l' and represented by a lower case 'm'. To calculate the molality of a solute in a solution we need to know the moles of solute present in the solution and the mass of solvent (in kilograms) in the solution. To calculate molality, we use the equation:

$$\text{Molality (m)} = \frac{\text{Moles of solute}}{\text{Volume of solvent in kilograms}} \qquad \ldots (5.6)$$

Mole Fraction

The mole fraction (X), of a component in a solution is the ratio of the number of moles of that component to the total number of moles of all components in the solution. To calculate mole fraction, we need to know the number of moles of each component present in the solution. The mole fraction of component A, X_A, in a solution consisting of components A, B and C is calculated using the equation:

$$X_A = \frac{\text{Moles of A}}{\text{Moles of A + Moles of B + Moles of C + }\ldots} \qquad \ldots (5.7)$$

To calculate the mole fraction of B, X_B, use:

$$X_B = \frac{\text{Moles of B}}{\text{Moles of A + Moles of B + Moles of C + }\ldots} \qquad \ldots (5.8)$$

5.5 ALLIGATION METHOD

Alligation is an old and practical method of solving arithmetic problems related to mixtures of ingredients. A method by which we may calculate the number of parts of two or more components of a given strength when they are mixed to prepare a mixture of desired strength is called alligation method. Allegations are used when mixing two products with different per cent strengths of the same active ingredient. The strength of the final product will fall between the strengths of each original product. A final proportion permits us to translate relative parts to any specific denomination. There are two types of alligation methods.

(i) Alligation medial

Alligation medial is used to find the quantity of a mixture given the quantities of its ingredients. In other words, this method is used to calculate the amount of active ingredient in each substance in the compound and to calculate what per cent of active ingredient is present in whole compound. The quantities are expressed in a common denomination, whether of weight or volume.

Example 5.3: What is the percentage strength v/v of alcohol in a mixture of 3000 mL of 40% v/v alcohol, 1000 mL of 60% v/v alcohol, and 1000 mL of 70% v/v alcohol? Assume no contraction of volume after mixing. (What per cent of 5000 is 2500 ?)

Solution: 0.4×3000 mL = 1200, or 40% alcohol in 3000 mL

                 0.6×1000 mL = 600, or 60% alcohol in 1000 mL

                 0.7×1000 mL = 700, or 70% alcohol in 1000 mL

Totals: 3000 + 1000 + 1000 = 5000 mL (total amount of alcoholic solution)

             1200 + 600 + 700 = 2500 mL (total amount of alcohol in solution)

Therefore, 2500 mL/5000 mL = 0.5×100 = 50%

Thus, 50% is the strength (v/v) of alcohol present in a mixture of 5000 mL.

Example 5.4: What is the percentage of zinc oxide in an ointment prepared by mixing 250 g of 10% ointment, 100 g of 20% ointment, and 150 g of 5% ointment?

Solution: 0.10×250 = 25 g

                       0.20×100 = 20 g

                       0.05×150 = 5 g

Totals: 500 g = 50 g

Therefore,   50 g/500 g = 0.1×100 = 10%,

Example 5.5: What is the percentage v/v of alcohol in a mixture containing 400 mL of terpene hydrate elixir (40% v/v alcohol), 300 mL of theophylline sodium glycinate elixir (21% v/v alcohol), and sufficient simple syrup to make 1000 mL?

Solution: 0.40×400 mL = 160 mL

                0.21×300 mL = 63 mL

                   0×300 mL = 0 mL

Totals: 1000 mL = 223 mL

Therefore,   223 mL/1000 mL = 0.223×100 = 22.3%

(ii) Alligation Alternate

Alligation alternate is a method used to find the amount of each ingredient needed to make a mixture of a given quantity. A final proportion permits the technician to translate relative parts to any specific denomination. The strength of a mixture must lie somewhere between the strengths of its components; that is, the mixture must be somewhat stronger than its weakest component and somewhat weaker than its strongest. As indicated previously, the strength of the mixture is always a weighted average; that is; it lies nearer to that of its weaker or stronger components, depending on the relative amounts involved. Alligation alternate is more complicated and involves organizing the ingredients into high and low pairs which are then traded-off.

Example 5.6: In what proportion should alcohol 95% and 65% strengths be mixed to make 80% alcohol?

Solution:

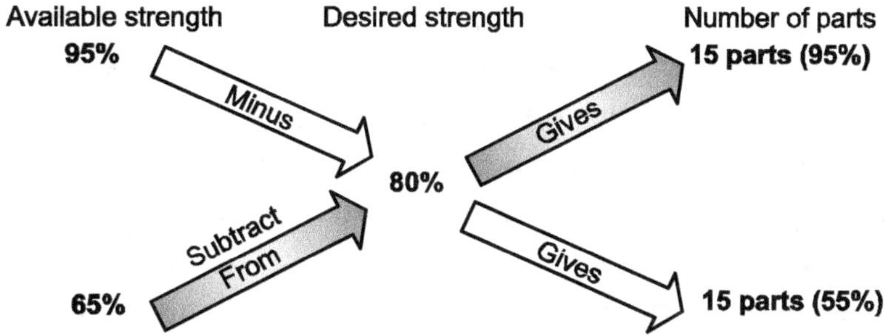

Thus, 15 parts of 65% alcohol and 15 parts of 95% alcohol is to be mixed to obtain 80% alcohol.

Example 5.7: In what proportion should 30% benzocaine ointment be mixed with an ointment base to produce a 5% benzocaine ointment?

Solution:

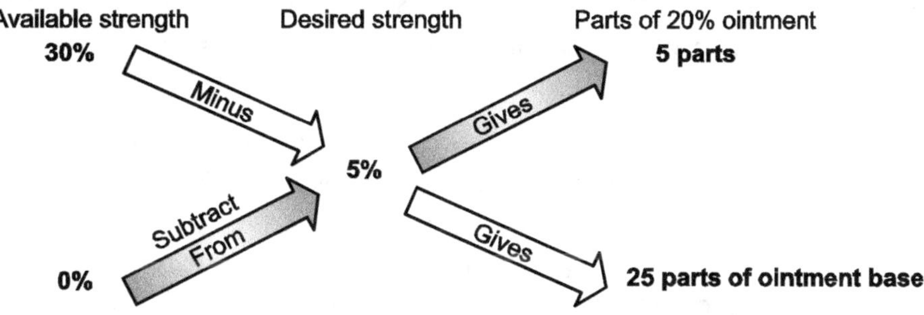

The 30% benzocaine ointment and an ointment base should be mixed at 5:25 ratio or 1:5.

Example 5.8: How much 3.5% hydrocortisone cream (in grams) should be mixed with 360 g of 0.2% cream to make a 2% hydrocortisone cream?

Solution:

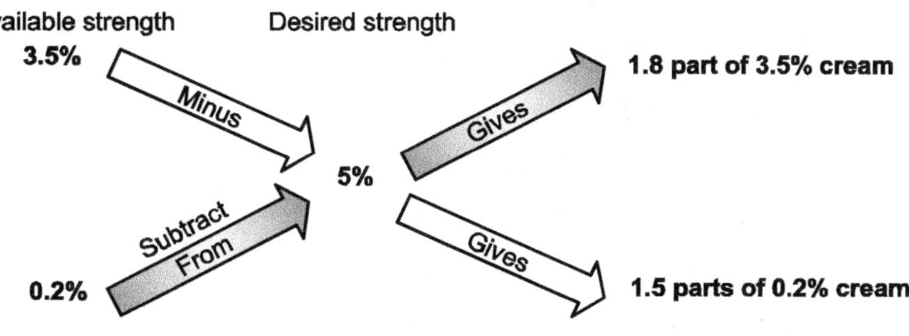

5.6 PROOF SPIRIT

Spirit is the alcohol beverage which is produced by the distillation of alcohol. The difference between alcohol and spirit is that the strength of the spirit is measured by the amount of alcohol they contain. Spirit mainly contains ethanol (alcohol). Commonly beverages are known as alcohols, all the alcohols are not consumable. Spirits are the group of consumable beverages. Alcohol can be made from fermentation, but the spirit is made from distillation. Spirit mainly consists of ethanol and is a very strong beverage.

Alcohol proof is a measure of the content of ethanol (alcohol) in an alcoholic beverage. The term was originally used in the United Kingdom and was equal to about 1.75 times the alcohol by volume (ABV). The UK now uses the ABV standard instead of alcohol proof. In India and UK 57.1% v/v or 49.28 w/w ethanol is taken as proof strength (100 proof spirit). In USA system proof spirit is 50% alcohol by volume (or 42.49% by weight). In British/Indian system proof spirit is 57.1% alcohol by volume (or 48.24% by weight).

Proof spirit is that mixture of alcohol and water, which at 510F weighs 12/13th of an equal volume of water. The density of proof spirit = 12/13 of density of water at 51°F = 0.923 g/mL. This means that any alcoholic solution that contains 57.1% v/v alcohol is a proof spirit and is said to be 100 proof. Therefore, 100-degree proof alcohol is equal to 57.1% v/v alcohol.

Proof spirit is an aqueous solution containing 50% v/v of absolute alcohol (100% v/v ethanol). Alcohols of other % strengths are said to be over proof (o/p) and below or under proof (b/p; u/p), depending on whether they contain more or less than 50% v/v of absolute alcohol. Proof strength is twice the percentage strength of alcohol and thus 50% v/v alcohol is 100 proofs. In reverse, 90 proofs alcohol is equivalent to 45% v/v ethanol. Alcohol for manufacturing purpose may be purchased by the proof gallon. A proof gallon is a gallon by measure of proof spirit; that is, a gallon of 100 proof or 50% v/v absolute alcohol.

Example 5.9: Calculate proof strength of 65%v/v and 35% v/v alcohol.

Solution: 1% alcohol = 1.75 proof spirit

65%v/v alcohol = ? Proof spirit

65 × 1.75 = 113.75 proof

Therefore, proof strength = 113.75 – 100 = 13.75° u/p.

1% alcohol = 1.75 proof spirit

35% v/v alcohol = ? Proof spirit

35 × 1.75 = 61.25 proof

Therefore, proof strength = 61.25 – 100 = – 38.75° u/p.

Example 5.10: Calculate proportion of 65%v/v alcohol and 35%v/v alcohol needed to prepare 5 litres of 25° u/p alcohol.

Solution: The 25° u/p proof strength = 65 proof spirit

1% v/v alcohol = 1.75 proof spirit

? % v/v alcohol = 65 proof spirit

= 65/1.75

= 37.14% v/v

Example 5.11: Calculate % strength of 55° o/p and 45° u/p.

Solution: (a) 55° o/p is 155 proof spirit.

Since,   1% v/v alcohol = 1.75 proof spirit

? % v/v alcohol = 155 proof spirit

= 155/1.75

= 88.57% v/v

(b) 45° u/p is 55 proof spirit

1% v/v alcohol = 1.75 proof spirit

? % v/v alcohol = 55 proof spirit

= 55/1.75

= 31.42% v/v

5.7 ISOTONIC SOLUTIONS

An isotonic solution refers to two solutions having the same osmotic pressure across a semipermeable membrane. This state allows for the free movement of water across the membrane without changing the concentration of solutes on either side. In the context of pharmaceutical dosage form, isotonic means dosage forms isotonic with body fluids. For example, saline solutions are isotonic with blood and lachrymal fluid. When the formulation is isotonic with body fluids, it causes no discomfort and irritation upon administration. But if the formulations are not isotonic, it causes either swelling or shrinkage of cells.

The solutions with low osmotic pressure than body fluids are called as *hypotonic solution*. When such solution is administered it causes swelling and burst of cells called haemolysis. Haemolysis is result of high osmotic pressure on the cells that pushes solvent inside them to achieve equilibrium, which leads to swelling and finally its rapture. This effect cannot be reversed and is permanent damage to the cells. The solutions with high osmotic pressure than body fluids are called as *hypertonic solution*. In this case, solution being highly osmotic takes away water from cells causing them to shrink. This effect is reversible as there is no bursting of cells. When the osmotic pressures of administered solution and body fluids are same, the shrunk cell regains an original shape. Thus, parenteral formulations, viz. all injectables and fluids for eye and nasal administration, need to be made isotonic.

Calculation of Isotonicity

Freezing point (FP), osmotic pressure, boiling point and vapor pressure are colligative properties of non-electrolytic solution. These properties are depending on number of particles present in solution.

1. Freezing point method

The lachrymal fluid contains solutes in it and has a FP of − 0.52°C. Thus, all solutions, which freeze at − 0.52°C, will be isotonic with the lachrymal fluid. Similarly, human blood plasma also freezes at this temperature and hence all solutions having FP at − 0.52°C will be isotonic with blood plasma. Solutions can be made isotonic if the freezing points of the drug and the inert salt (adjusting substance) present in solution are known. FP is usually expressed in terms of 1% solutions and the quantity of solute needed to be calculated by multiplying the FP with the factor.

The following equation is useful in calculating amount of solute needed to make solution isotonic. The amount of adjusting substance required may be calculated from the equation:

$$w = \frac{(0.52 - a)}{b} \qquad \qquad \dots (5.9)$$

Where,   w = weight, in g, of the added substance in 100 mL of the final solution;

a = depression of the freezing point produced by the medicament already present in solution, calculated by multiplying the value for the medicament by the strength of the solution expressed as a percentage w/v; and

b = depression of the freezing point of water produced by 1% of the adjusting substance.

Example 5.12: Calculate the amount of sodium chloride that should be added to 100 mL ephedrine hydrochloride 0.5 g nasal drop in order to make the final solution isotonic. The freezing point depression of 1% ephedrine hydrochloride and 1% sodium chloride solutions are 0.169°C and 0.576°C, respectively.

Solution: We know, 1% w/v = 1g/100 mL. We need 0.5 g, so the freezing point depression will decrease by half of 0.169°C to 0.0845°C. This means that ephedrine hydrochloride will depress the freezing point to 0.0845 below 0°C (i.e. − 0.0845°C).

Freezing point of an isotonic solution (0.9% saline) = − 0.52 °C.

Hence, the added NaCl will need to depress the freezing point of the ephedrine solution by a further 0.4355°C.

Since,

Sodium chloride (%w/v)	1	x (to be calculated)
Freezing point depression	0.576	0.4355

Therefore, $x = \dfrac{0.4355}{0.576} = 0.756$

This means that 0.756% w/v of NaCl should be added to make sure the final solution is isotonic.

Example 5.13: Calculate amount of NaCl required to prepare 200 mL of eyewash containing 1% boric acid. (Given: FP of 1% boric acid = − 0.29°C and FP of 1% solution of NaCl = 0.576°C).

Solution: The working formula for 200 mL of the eyewash will be:

$$\text{FP of solution} = 1 \times (-0.29) = -0.29°C$$

Thus,   amount of NaCl (w) required $= \dfrac{(0.52 - a)}{b}$

$$= \dfrac{(0.52 - 0.29)}{0.576} = 0.39\%.$$

For 200 mL, Boric acid (1%, for 200 mL) $= 1\,g \times 2 = 2\,g$

NaCl (0.39%, for 200 mL) $= 0.39 \times 2 = 0.78\,g$

Purified water q.s. 200 mL

2. Molecular Weight Method

Freezing point of a solute depends on the concentration of the solute dissolved therein. Greater the concentration of the solute, lower is the freezing point. In other words, it depends on the number of ions (more correctly, the number of effective ions), the weight of the substance and its molecular weight. The concentration for 0.9% NaCl solution can be expressed in the following manner:

% w/v of adjusted substance needed (w) = (0.03 × M) / n   ... (5.10)

Where, w = Concentration (g/L) of solution

n = No. of effective ions (n)

M = Molecular weight of NaCl (isotonicity factor for NaCl = 0.03)

Since 0.9% solution of NaCl (normal saline) is isotonic with body fluids, 0.03 will be the isotonicity or tonicity factor for tear secretion and blood plasma as well. Thus quantities for making eye solutions can be calculated by equating the value of 0.03 with the tonicity contributed by the drug and the additive(s).

The osmotic pressure is proportional to molar concentration which is expressed as g/L.

Gram moles = (Weight in g/L/Molecular weight)

This equation is applicable to all un-ionisable substances.

Gram moles = (Weight in g/L)/Molecular weight × n

The following equation is employed for calculating the quantity of the additive(s):

Quantity of the additive = (G/M) × n ... (5.11)

Where, G = weight in gram,

n = effective ion concentration and,

M = molecular weight of the medicament respectively.

The 'n' in equation (5.10) is number of ions formed by dissociation of substance. Only ionic species effective can be ascertained from the following generalizations;

n = 1 for non-ionisable substances, e.g. dextrose

n = 1.5 for partially ionisable solutes in two ions, e.g. silver nitrate

n = 2 for highly ionisable solutes in two ions e.g. sodium chloride

n = 2 for partially ionisable solutes in three ions, e.g. sodium sulfate

On the basis of above discussion, 0.9% NaCl is required to make solution isotonic. It can be described as:

0.9% NaCl = 9 grams/1000 mL of solution

Gram moles of NaCl required to make it isotonic = (9/58.5) × 2 = 0.31

Example 5.14: Calculate amount of NaCl required to produce 5% dextrose injection isotonic. (Given molecular weight of dextrose = 180 g/mol)

Solution: We know dextrose being non-electrolyte, is un-ionisable.

5% dextrose = 50 g/1000 mL

Therefore,

$$\text{Gram moles of dextrose} = \frac{50}{180} = 0.277$$

Required gram moles of NaCl = Gram moles of NaCl – Gram moles of drug

$$= 0.31 - 0.277$$

$$= 0.033$$

Thus,

$$\text{Gram moles} = \frac{x \text{ gram/L}}{58.5} \times 2$$

$$x \text{ gram/L} = \frac{0.277}{2} \times 58.5$$

$$= 8.10 \text{ g/L}$$

Thus, quantity of NaCl required = 0.81%.

The following equation is employed for easy calculating the quantity of the additive(s):

$$\begin{array}{l}\text{% of isotonicity} \\ \text{adjusting substance}\end{array} = \left[0.31 - \left(\frac{x \text{ gram/L}}{\text{Molecular weight}} \times n\right) \text{ of drug}\right] \times \qquad \ldots (5.12)$$

$$\left[\left(\frac{\text{Molecular Weight}}{n}\right) \begin{array}{l}\text{of a isotonicity} \\ \text{adjusting substance}\end{array}\right]$$

Example 5.15: Calculate amount of NaCl required to produce 200 mL, 0.5% procaine hydrochloride solution isotonic. (Given: molecular weight of procaine hydrochloride = 272.77 g/mol)

Solution: We know dextrose being non-electrolyte, is un-ionisable.

$$\text{% NaCL} = \left[0.31 - \left(\frac{5}{277.77} \times 2\right)\right] \times \left[\frac{58.5}{2}\right]$$

$$= \left[(0.31 - 0.0360) \times 29.25\right]$$

$$= 8.0145 \text{ g/L} = 0.801\%$$

Therefore, 200 mL, 0.5% procaine hydrochloride solution can be isotonic by adding 0.799% NaCl.

MODEL QUESTIONS

1. Classify systems of measurements.
2. Discuss various ways to express solution strengths.
3. Discuss alligation method with suitable example.
4. What is proof spirit?
5. Calculate proof strength of 75 % v/v and 25 % v/v alcohol.

6. What are isotonic solutions? Differentiate between hypotonic and hypertonic solutions.
7. Enlist methods of isotonicity adjustments.
8. Discuss freezing point method to calculate amount of isotonicity adjusting substance.
9. Discuss molecular weight method to calculate amount of isotonicity adjusting substance.
10. Write a note on:
    (i) Alligation method.
    (ii) Proof spirit.
    (iii) Isotonic solutions.

■■■

Chapter 6...

Powders

LEARNING OBJECTIVES

Powders are intimate mixtures of dry, finely divided drugs and/or chemicals that may be intended for internal or external use. Because of their greater specific surface area, powders disperse and dissolve more readily than compacted dosage forms. Children and those adults who experience difficulty in swallowing tablets or capsules may find powders more acceptable. Drugs that are too bulky to be formed into tablets or capsules of convenient size may be administered as powders. Thus,

The objectives of this chapter include:

- To understand the concept of powder and know about its classification, advantages and disadvantages.

- To know about variety of types of powders and granules.

- To know appropriate uses of pharmaceutical powders and granules.

- To understand manufacturing of divided and bulk powders and granule preparations.

- To get acquainted with principle and procedures of general formulations.

- To understand physical properties of powders and granules in formulation research and development.

6.1 INTRODUCTION

Historically, powders represent one of the oldest dosage forms. A pharmaceutical powder is solid dosage form which contains mixture of finely divided drugs or chemicals in a dry form meant for internal or external use. It is a preparation in which drug is blended with other powdered substances and used for internal or external purpose. Powder as a dosage form permits drugs to be reduced to a very fine state of division, which often enhances their therapeutic activity or efficacy by an increase of dissolution rate and/or absorption. Divided powders are also found to be convenient for administering drugs that are excessively bitter, nauseous, or otherwise offensive to the taste.

Although powders are not used now-a-day's extensively as a dosage form, they are widely used in preparation of various dosage forms. Powdered drugs can be blended with other powdered materials (additives) prior to fabrication into other solid dosage forms such as tablet and capsule. Powdered drugs are frequently added to other ingredient to make ointments, pastes, suppositories, and others.

Powder properties relevant to pharmaceutical formulations are single particle (fundamental) properties and bulk (derived) properties. Collectively these includes particle–particle interactions, powder morphology (particle size, specific surface area, porosity, and particle shape), and mixing and blending properties (types of mechanism of mixing, types of mixing equipment, and minimizing segregation tendencies). It is also important for preparing powder formulation to understand hoppers and powder transfer methods, mechanisms of particle size reduction, and various types of mills used. Powders are subdivided solids which are classified in the BP according to the size of their constituent particles ranged from 1.25 mm to 1.7 mm in diameter.

A good powder formulation has a uniform particle size distribution. If the particle size distribution is not uniform, the powder can segregate as per to particle size which may result in inaccurate dosing or inconsistent performance. A uniform particle size distribution ensures a uniform dissolution rate if the powder is to dissolve, a uniform sedimentation rate if the powder is used to remain in a suspension, and minimizes stratification when powders are stored or transported.

Reduction in particle size of a powder results in a uniform distribution of particle size. The process of reducing the particle size is called comminution. In extemporaneous compounding, there are three methods of comminution:

(i) **Trituration:** Trituration is the continuous rubbing or grinding of the powder in a mortar with a pestle. This method is used when working with hard, fracturable powders.

(ii) **Pulverization by intervention:** Pulverization by intervention method is used with hard crystalline powders that do not crush or triturate easily, or gummy-type substances. The first step is to use an "intervening" solvent (such as alcohol or acetone) that will dissolve the compound. The dissolved powder is then mixed in a mortar or spread on an ointment slab to enhance the evaporation of the solvent. As the solvent evaporates, the powder will recrystallize out of solution as fine particles.

(iii) **Levigation:** Levigation reduces the particle size by triturating it in a mortar or spatulating it on an ointment slab or pad with a small amount of a liquid in which the solid is not soluble. The solvent should be somewhat viscous such as mineral oil or glycerin. This method is also used to reduce the particle size of insoluble materials when compounding ointments and suspensions.

6.2 ADVANTAGES AND DISADVANTAGES

(a) Advantages:

(i) Drugs that have to be given in bulk can be best administered in powder form by mixing them with food or drinks.

(ii) Useful for bulky drugs with large dose.

(iii) Powders are more stable than liquid dosage form; hence many antibiotics and injections are manufactured as powder for reconstitution in respective vehicle.

(iv) More convenient to swallow than tablet or capsules.

(v) Powder possesses good chemical stability.

(vi) Since powders are in the form of small particles; they offer a large surface area and are rapidly dissolved in the gastrointestinal tract minimizing the problems of local irritation.

(vii) Rapid dissolution of powder facilitates rapid absorption.

(viii) Highly compatible compared to liquid dosage forms.

(ix) Manufacturing of powder is economic hence product cost is quite low as compared to other dosage forms.

(b) Disadvantages:

(i)   Bulk powders are not suitable for administering potent drugs with a low dose.

(ii) Not suitable for drugs which are unstable in normal atmospheric conditions.

(iii) Powder form is not suitable for drugs that are inactivated in, or cause damage to stomach; these should be presented as enteric-coated tablets.

(iv) Not suitable for bitter, nauseating and corrosive drugs, if are meant for oral administration.

(v)   The masking of unpleasant tastes may be a problem with this type of preparation. A method of attempting this is by formulating the powder into a pleasantly tasting or taste-masked effervescent product, whereas tablets and capsules are a more common alternative for low-dose products.

(vi) Inaccuracy of dose in case of bulk powder.

(vii) Inconvenient to carry.

(viii) They are susceptible to physical instability.

6.3 CLASSIFICATION OF POWDERS

1. **Powders for Internal use**

    (a) Divided powders

        (i)   Simple powders

        (ii) Compound powders

        (iii) Powders enclosed in cachet

        (iv) Tablet triturates

    (b) Bulk powders

        (i)   Antacid

        (ii) Laxative

2. **Powders for external use**

    (a) Dusting powders

        (i)   Medicated dusting powders

        (ii) Surgical dusting powders

    (b) Insufflations

    (c) Douche powder

    (d) Dentifrices

3. **Special powders**

    (a) Eutectic mixtures

    (b) Effervescent powders

1. Powders for Internal use/Oral powders

According to Indian Pharmacopoeia 2007, oral powders are finely divided powders that contain one or more medicaments with or without auxiliary substances including, where specified, flavouring and coloring agents. However, addition of saccharin or its salts is not permitted in the preparations meant for pediatric use. They are intended to be taken internally with or without the aid of water or any other suitable liquid.

(a) Divided powders: Divided powders (or charta) are single doses of powdered drugs individually wrapped in cellophane, metallic foil, or paper. The divided powder is a more accurate dosage form than bulk powder because the patient is not involved in measurement of the dose. Cellophane and foil-enclosed powders are better protected from the external environment until the time of administration than paper-enclosed powders. Divided powders are commercially available in foil, cellophane or paper packs.

(i) Simple powder: It consists of only one active ingredient and suitable inert substances. If powder is in crystalline form, then it is reduced to fine. Example: Aspirin Powder, Calcium Gluconate Powder etc.

Aspirin powder   300 mg

Procedure: Triturate aspirin so as to get fine powder. Weigh the calculated amount of aspirin powder. Wrap each dose in individual powder paper and pack it.

(ii) Compound powder: It consists of mixture of more than one active ingredient and other constituents.

Example:

1. Aspirin, Paracetamol and Caffeine Powder

Aspirin	300 mg
Paracetamol	150 mg
Caffeine	50 mg

Procedure: Triturate all the ingredients separately so as to get fine powder. Weigh the calculated amount of aspirin powder; paracetamol powder and caffeine powder and mix them in ascending order of their weight. Wrap each dose in individual powder paper.

2. Macrogol Compound Oral Powder

Each sachet contains the following quantitative composition of active ingredients:

Sodium chloride	0.3507 g
Sodium hydrogen carbonate	0.1785 g
Potassium chloride	0.0466 g
Macrogol 3350	13.125 g

Use: Macrogol Compound Oral Powder is a laxative prescribed for the treatment of long-term constipation.

(iii) Powders enclosed in cachet: Cachets consist of a dry powder enclosed in a shell, usually prepared from a mixture of rice flour and water by molding into a suitable shape and drying. They are quite useful for administering the drugs with nauseating and unpleasant taste and a large dose can be enclosed in a cachet than in a tablet or capsule. A cachet offers little protection against light and moisture. Now-a-days cachets are replaced by capsule. There are two types of catches:

- **Wet cachets**: Lower half of the cachet is filled with powdered drug. Then the flange of the empty upper half of the cachet is moistened with water, and pressed over the lower half. The cachet is dried for 15 minutes.
- **Dry cachets**: Drug powder is filled in the lower half and the upper half is pressed over it just like a capsule. They are used for administering the drug with unpleasant taste and a large dose.

Before administration, a cachet should be immersed in water for few seconds and then placed on the tongue and swallowed with water.

Example: Sodium Amino salicylate Cachets, Sodium Amino salicylate with Isoniazid Cachets.

(iv) Tablet triturates: Tablet triturates are powders molded into tablets. Tablet triturates are generally prepared by mixing the active drug with lactose, dextrose, sucrose, mannitol, or some other appropriate diluent that can serve as the base. This base must be readily water soluble and should not degrade during the tablet's preparation. Lactose is the preferred base but mannitol adds a pleasant, cooling sensation and additional sweetness in the mouth.

The base ordinarily used for molded tablet triturates is lactose containing 10% - 20% sucrose, the latter being added to make a firmer tablet. Drugs that react chemically with sugars require special bases such as precipitated calcium carbonate, precipitated calcium phosphate, kaolin, or bentonite. A liquid is added to moisten the powder mixture so it will adhere while being pressed into the mold cavities. Mixtures of alcohol and water in varying proportions (typically about 50 - 80% alcohol) are employed; the alcohol will speed-up the drying of the liquid and the water will cause the sugars to dissolve and bind the tablet. If the tablet contains ingredients that are very soluble in water, water can be omitted altogether and alcohol alone can be used.

Tablet triturates are used for oral administration or sublingual use (For example., nitroglycerin tablets). They may also be used in compounding procedures by pharmacists in the preparation of other solid or liquid dosage forms. They can be inserted into capsules, and this eliminates the problems of measuring the accurate amount of potent drugs in the powder form.

Example: Propranolol Scopolamine Tablet Triturate

Propranolol hydrochloride   40 mg

Scopolamine hydrobromide   0.5 mg

(b) Bulk powders: Bulk powders are non-potent and can be dosed with acceptable accuracy and safety using measuring devices such as the teaspoon, cup, or insufflators. The mixed ingredients are packed into a suitable bulk container, such as a wide-mouthed glass jar. Because of the disadvantages of this type of preparation the constituents are usually relatively non-toxic medicaments with a large dose. This practically limits the use of orally administered bulk powders to antacids, dietary supplements, laxatives, and a few analgesics.

(i) Antacid

Example: Magnesium Trisilicate Compound Oral Powder BP

Magnesium trisilicate	250 mg
Chalk	250 mg
Heavy magnesium carbonate	250 mg
Sodium bicarbonate	250 mg

All powders are sieved using 250 µm sieve and mixed well by triturating them in mortar. The final product is packed in amber colored glass jar or plastic container with screw cap.

Use: For relief of the symptoms of indigestion, heartburn and dyspepsia.

(ii) Laxative

Example: Polyethylene Glycol 3350 NF Powder for Oral Solution

Polyethylene glycol 3350	13.125 g
Sodium chloride	350.7 mg
Sodium hydrogen carbonate	178.5 mg
Potassium chloride	46.6 mg

Polyethylene glycol 3350 NF powder for oral solution is an osmotic agent which causes water to be retained with the stool and used for the treatment of constipation. It is supplied in powdered form, for oral administration after dissolution in water, juice, soda, coffee, or tea.

2. Powders for external use

(a) Dusting powders

Dusting Powders are externally used bulk powders. They are free flowing very fine powders containing antiseptics, antipruritics, astringents, antiperspirants, absorbents, lubricants etc.

(i) Medicated dusting powders: Medicated dusting powders are sterile ones and meant for application on superficial skin. Body dusting powders have a wide appeal because of smooth feel and cooling effect, which they impart while they temporarily absorb moisture. The cooling effect is due to extra heat loss due to large surface area of talc particles.

Talc	51 g
Kaolin	15 g
Precipitated chalk	21 g
Zinc stearate	3 g
Boric acid	5 g
Salicylic acid	5 g
Perfume	Quantity sufficient

Talc in a major ingredient in medicated dusting powder formulation, which should have good slip characteristics, covering power and body adhesion. The slip and adhesion properties of medicated dusting powder essentially depend on talc. It is essential to use grid and alkali free high quality cosmetic talc in preparation of medicated dusting powder. Talc should be free from bacteria and therefore sterilized grades should only be used.

In order to improve adhesion properties, metallic stearates such as zinc stearate or magnesium stearate and kaolin are incorporated. To improve absorbency, magnesium carbonate, starch, kaolin and precipitated chalk are used in combination. Zinc oxide and titanium dioxide, at low levels along with earth colors can be incorporated and should be sufficiently powerful to cover the base odour. Other ingredients sometimes included are boric acid to act as skin buffering agent and fused silica to give powder a lower density; salicylic acid for antibacterial action. Aluminum chloride is also incorporated as an antiperspirant.

(ii) **Surgical dusting powders:** Surgical dusting powders are intended to be used into deep layer of skin and also on major wounds as a result on burns and umbilical cords of infants. Surgical dusting powders must be free from pathogenic micro-organism and hence it must be sterilized before their use.

The dusting powders are mainly used for their antiseptic, astringent, absorbent, antiperspirant, and antipruritic action. It mainly contains antimicrobial agents like chlorhexidine and hexachlorophene. They are generally prepared by mixing two or more ingredients one of which must be starch, talc or kaolin as one of the ingredients of the formulation. Talc is more commonly used because of its chemical inertness. However, since such ingredients are readily contaminated with pathogenic bacteria, these must be sterilized by dry heat method before use. Dusting powders are dispensed in sifter-top container or aerosol containers. It may also be applied with powder puff or sterilized gauze pad.

Example: Neosporin Dusting Powder

Neosporin dusting powder is composed of the following active ingredients (salts)

Bacitracin (5000 IU)

Neomycin (3400 IU)

Polymyxin B (400 IU)

Bacitracin topical is used alone or in combination with neomycin and polymyxin to treat and prevent superficial and minor skin infections due to wounds, cuts or burns. Bacitracin belongs to the class of medications called polypeptide antibiotics. It acts by inhibiting the growth of bacteria in the wounds thereby relieving associated symptoms. Neomycin belongs to the class of medications called as antibiotics. It prevents the bacterial growth by stopping the production of essential protein in the bacterial cells, thereby relieving the associated symptoms. Polymyxin B belongs to a group of medications called as polypeptide antibiotic. It works by killing the bacteria that causes the infection.

(b) Insufflations

Insufflations are medicated dusting powders meant for introduction into the body cavities such as nose, throat, ears, etc. with the help of an apparatus known as insufflators (powder blower). It sprays the powder into a stream of finely divided particles all over the site of application. The insufflations are used to produce a local effect, as in the treatment of ear, nose and throat infection with antibiotics or to produce a systemic effect from a drug that is destroyed in the gastrointestinal tract. As like aerosols, uniform dose may not be obtained by insufflations.

Examples: Cromolyn Sodium Powder, Compound Clioquin Powder USP

(c) Douche Powder

Douche powders are intended to be used as antiseptics or cleansing agents for a body cavity; most commonly for vaginal use, although they may be formulated for nasal, otic or ophthalmic use also. As douche powder formulation often include aromatic oils, it becomes necessary to pass them through a sieve 40 or 60 to eliminate agglomeration and to ensure complete mixing. They can be dispensed either in wide mouth glass bottles or in powder boxes but the former are preferred because of protection afforded against air and moisture.

Example: Douche powder

    Zinc sulphate

    Magnesium sulphate

    Boric acid

    Lemon oil

    Purified water

(d) Dentifrices

Dentifrices are preparations meant to clean the teeth and other parts of oral cavity (gums) using a finger or a toothbrush. They are available as tooth powder, toothpastes, gels, dental creams and even as dental foams. They are meant to enhance the personal appearance of the teeth (daily removal of pellicles) by maintaining cleaner teeth, reduction of bad odour (removal of putrifying food particles from spaces between teeth) and also make the gum healthy. They contain a suitable detergent or soap, some abrasive substance and a suitable flavour. The abrasive agents such as calcium sulphate, magnesium carbonate, sodium carbonate and sodium chloride are used in fine powder form. A strong abrasive substance should not be used as it may damage the tooth structure.

The main components of toothpowders are solid particles of very fine size and the end product is also a very dry powder. Since the main components like abrasives, surface active agent are solid powders, it is required that they all are in very fine particle size, comminuted, if desired, passed through a sieve and mixed in a mortar in the lab scale and in blenders on an industrial scale. The flavoring oils are added at the end either by spraying on the powder mixture or first blending with one of the components and then mixing this blend to the rest of the mixture by the method of dilution or geometric proportion.

Hard soap (in fine powder)	50 g
Precipitated calcium carbonate	935 g
Saccharine sodium	2 g
Peppermint oil	4 ml
Cinnamon oil	2 ml
Methyl salicylate	8 ml
To make about	1000 g

3. **Special powders**

    (a) **Eutectic mixtures:** Eutectic mixtures are defined as mixtures of low melting point ingredients which on mixing together turn to liquid form due to depression in melting point of the mixture below room temperature. They are mixtures of substances, that liquefy when mixed, rubbed or triturated together. The melting points of many eutectic mixtures are below room temperature. Examples of the substances which tend to liquefy on mixing are camphor, thymol, menthol, salol. Any two of these drugs turn to liquid when mixed. This problem during formulation of powders of such material can be solved by using inert adsorbent such as starch, talc, lactose to prevent dampness of the powder and dispensing the components of the eutectic mixture separately.

    (b) **Effervescent powders:** Effervescent powders contain materials which react in presence of water evolving carbon dioxide. This class of preparations can be supplied either by compounding the ingredients as granules or dispensed in the form of salts. For evolution of the gas two constituents are essential, a soluble carbonate such as sodium bicarbonate and an organic acid such as citric or tartaric acid. The preparation can be supplied either as a bulk powder or distributed in individual powders.

There are three alternative methods of dispensing effervescent powders based upon the nature of prescription.

(i) If the effervescent salts are prescribed to be dispensed in bulk form, no granulation is necessary. The ingredients are mixed uniformly and directions stated on the label to add the prescribed quantity to water, before use.

(ii) If the effervescent salt is prescribed in divided doses, the ingredients which cause effervescence on mixing with water are enclosed separately in papers of different color. The patient is advised to take one powder of each color and add to water, before use. Quantities of the sodium bicarbonate and the organic acid, citric or tartaric, are equimolecular in proportion.

(iii) In the third case, the product contains all the ingredients mixed together in a granular form. Preparation of granular products requires pharmaceutical technique. If sodium bicarbonate and citric acid are taken in equimolecular proportion and mixed to make granules, the quantity of water of crystallization liberated from the citric acid is large enough to make the mass wet and carbon dioxide may be liberated during the preparation itself. If one tries to substitute citric acid by tartaric acid, which contains no water of crystallization; it may not be possible to form a mass necessary for granulation.

Therefore, both citric and tartaric acids are taken in suitable proportions leaving a little acid in surplus than the quantity required to neutralize sodium bicarbonate. This surplus is necessary to give the final preparation an acidic taste that is more palatable. There is a certain loss in weight of such a preparation due to the loss of water in drying the granules and partial loss of carbon dioxide due to its release during preparation.

Chemical reaction:

$$3NaHCO_3 \; + \; C_6H_8O_7.H_2O \; \rightarrow \; C_6H_5Na_3O_7 + 3CO_2 + 3H_2O$$

Sodium bicarbonate   Citric acid

$$2NaHCO_3 \; + \; C_4H_6O_6 \; \rightarrow \; C_4H_4Na_2O_6 + 2CO_2 + 2H_2O$$

Sodium bicarbonate Tartaric acid

Example: Paramax[®] Effervescent Powder

Paracetamol	500 mg
Metoclopramide hydrochloride	5 mg
Sodium carbonate	
Saccharin sodium	
Lemon flavour	
Sodium dihydrogen citrate, anhydrous	
Sodium bicarbonate	
Gelatin	

Metoclopramide hydrochloride belongs to a group of medicines called anti-emetics. It works on muscles in the upper part of the digestive system causing stomach to empty. It also works on a part of brain that prevents from feeling sick (nausea) or being sick (vomiting). Paracetamol belongs to a group of medicines called painkillers (analgesics). It works by stopping substances that naturally occur in body called prostaglandins from being made. Prostaglandins cause pain. If they are blocked, pain is relieved. Paramax is used to treat the signs of migraine, such as headache, feeling sick (nausea) or being sick (vomiting) in adults 18 years and over. Paramax must not be given to patients under 18 years of age.

6.4 PREPARATION OF POWDER

(i) **Particle size reduction:** For preparation of powder, each ingredient should be needed in finely ground form; hence manufacturer must use a number of procedures and equipment to reduce the particle size of powder ingredients, this process is called as comminution. The most common method used for particle size reduction in powder formulation is trituration, which involves placing the solid in a mortar and continually grinding the chemical between the mortar and the pestle using a firm, downward pressure. The powder must be frequently scraped from the sides of the mortar to ensure that all particles are evenly reduced and mixed. A levigating agent, such as glycerin, may be added to the solid and processed by either continued trituration or by placing the mixture on an ointment slab and using spatulation to wet the solid and further reduce the particle size. A small mesh sieve can be used to determine the prevalent particle size of a powder after it has been triturated.

(ii) **Preparing a homogenous mixture:** Particle size reduction is followed by homogeneous mixing of all powder ingredients. Many times processes similar to those used for particle size reduction are used for obtaining homogenous mixture. Powders that have been blended with a protectant to prevent the formation of a eutectic mixture must be mixed carefully with little or no pressure. Spatulation, or the mixing of particles with a spatula on an ointment slab, results in a light, well-mixed powder without interfering with the protectant. Trituration serves the dual purpose of reducing particle size and mixing powders. It is especially effective for mixing small quantities of potent drugs with larger amounts of diluents. Hazardous substances can be effectively mixed by a process called tumbling. The powders are sealed in zipper-sealed bags or clear bottles with a lid and tumbled until they are well mixed. The addition of a coloring agent can assist in determining homogeneity in the mixture. If powders being combined are unequal in quantity, then geometric dilution method is used.

(iii) Geometric dilution: Geometric dilution is the process by which a homogenous mixture or even distribution of two or more substances is achieved. This method is used when potent substances must be mixed with a large amount of diluent. The potent drug and an approximately equal volume of diluent are placed in a mortar and thoroughly mixed by trituration. A second portion of diluent, equal in volume to the powder mixture in the mortar is added, and trituration is repeated. The process is continued; equal volumes of diluent are added to the powder mixture in the mortar until all of the diluent is incorporated. For example, if dose of potent drug is 120 mg, while mixing entire quantity (120 mg) of potent drug is taken and to it 120 mg of the diluents are added and mix thoroughly. The resulting 240 mg mixture of potent drug and diluents is again mixed with further 240 mg of diluents and the process is repeated until all the diluents are incorporated.

(iv) Packaging of powders: Bulk powders for external use (sometimes called dusting powders) are often dispensed in a shaker-top container to facilitate topical application. They may also be dispensed in a wide-mouth jar or a plastic container with a flip-top lid. The jar or plastic container can be closed tightly to provide increased stability and protection from light and moisture, especially for compounds that contain volatile ingredients. Package should contain label as "For external use only".

Bulk powders intended for internal use should be dispensed in an amber colored, wide-mouth powder jar with a tight-fitting lid. They should be accompanied by an appropriately sized dosing spoon or cup and adequate directions for removing and administering a correct dose. Bulk powders for internal use should be labelled with the strength of the active ingredient per dose (e.g., Potassium chloride 600 mg per tablespoonful).

6.5 PROBLEMS ENCOUNTERED IN POWDER FORMULATION

1. Efflorescent powders:

Efflorescent powders contain drugs or chemicals that contain water of hydration, which may be released when the powders are manipulated, or when they are stored under conditions of relatively low humidity. The liberated water converts the powder to a paste or to a liquid. Examples of efflorescent powders are caffeine, citric acid, cocaine, codeine and codeine phosphate.

Problems pertaining to efflorescent powder include: water liberated when the drug or chemical is triturated may cause the powders to become damp or pasty. If water is released to the atmosphere because of low relative humidity, the drug loses its crystallinity and becomes powdery. Water of hydration is given off; a given weight of the resulting powder no longer contains the same amount of the drug. Hence strategies for handling efflorescent powders includes: storage and dispense of these powders in airtight containers. The anhydrous form of the drug may be substituted for the hydrate, but be sure to make appropriate dose corrections.

2. Hygroscopic powders and deliquescent powder

Some ingredients in powder form having the property of absorbing moisture from surrounding are called as hygroscopic materials. Absorption of moisture from air leads to partial or complete liquefaction of material. To avoid this problem while preparing powder, following precautions are taken:

(i)   Powders are applied in a granular form to decrease the exposed surface to air.

(ii) They are packed in aluminium foil or in plastic film packets.

(iii) Light magnesium oxide is added to reduce the tendency to damp.

(iv) Adsorbent materials such as starch are incorporated.

Examples of such materials are halide salts (e.g. sodium iodide) and certain alkaloids (physostigmine hydrochloride).

3. Incorporation of liquids

In some powders along with solids; liquid ingredients are necessary to add. Proper distribution of liquid in entire powder is necessary. In this case liquid is triturated with an equal weight of the powder and then remaining powder is added in several portions with trituration. Adsorbent such as light kaolin is incorporated to avoid this problem.

4. Incorporation of extracts

Some plant extracts are available as powders or as semisolid (for example, liquid extract of liquorice). In this case, powdered extracts have no problems and treated generally as powders. Semisolid extract should be mixed with an equal quantity of lactose and reduced to a dry powder by evaporation before incorporation with other ingredients. Careful heating, if present, to save potency of the extract is required.

5. Incompatible salts

Chemically incompatible salts when triturated together produce discoloration, chemical deterioration or loss of potency. To avoid this problem; minimum pressure is used while compounding such materials. Use a convenient method for mixing the powder like tumbling in a jar or spatulation on a sheet of paper. Each substance should be powdered separately in a clean mortar and then combined with other ingredients gently. Otherwise such materials are powdered and dispensed separately.

6. Explosive mixtures

Oxidizing agents such as potassium salts of chlorate, dichromate, permanganate and nitrate- sodium peroxide- silver nitrate and silver oxide explore violently when triturated in a mortar with a reducing agent such as sulfides- sulfur- tannic acid- charcoal. To avoid this problem, each salt is triturated separately or minimum pressure is used during trituration.

6.6 EVALUATION OF POWDER

Pharmaceutical powders are evaluated for following quality control parameters:

(i)   Content uniformity
(ii) Particle size and size distribution
(iii) Flow property:
    (a) Angle of repose
    (b) Flow rate
(iv) Density
    (a) Bulk density
    (b) Tapped density
    (c) True density
(v)   Hausner's ratio
(vi) Moisture content
(vii) Tensile and cohesive strength measurements
(viii) Safety and efficacy
(ix) Stability

MODEL QUESTIONS

1. Define and classify powders. Give advantages and disadvantages of powder dosage form.
2. Define and give example of simple and compound powder.
3. Give preparation of dusting powders and effervescent powder.
4. Explain methods of preparation of powder.
5. Explain problems encountered in powder formulation.
6. Write a note on
    (i)   Hygroscopic powders
    (ii) Eutectic mixtures
    (iii) Geometric dilutions

■■■

Chapter 7 ...

Liquid Dosage Forms

LEARNING OBJECTIVES

There is several liquid dosage forms used in pharmacy. The most common are syrups, suspensions and elixirs. These solutions are sometimes referred to as a "vehicle" which delivers the active drug dose.

The objectives of this chapter include:

- To understand the basic concept, principle and procedure of manufacturing liquid formulations.
- To formulate and describe various physical properties of liquid dosage forms.
- To understand the excipients and their applications in manufacturing of liquid dosage forms.

7.1 MEANING

The pharmaceutical dosage forms are means to deliver drug to the patient in the needed amount, at the required rate, consistently within a batch, from batch-to-batch, and over the product's shelf life. Liquid dosage forms provide better patient compliance for those with swallowing difficulties and offer unique advantages to many patients to better dosage control compared to solid and semisolids. There are several liquid dosage forms used in pharmacy. Liquids dosage forms are formulated as either, solutions, suspensions and emulsions depending on the nature of the drug, its solubility and stability. They are also formulated as ready to use liquids and powders for reconstitution into liquids. Liquid dosage forms are generally formulated for use in geriatric and paediatric patients. Liquid dosage forms needs various excipients including vehicle, stabilizer, and viscosity builder, preservatives, sweeteners, colour and flavour. In addition, solubilizers are required in case of clear liquids; suspending agents are needed for suspensions and emulsifying agents for emulsions. The most common are syrups, suspensions and elixirs. These solutions are sometimes referred to as a "vehicle" which delivers the active drug dose. Although they are used for multiple reasons, liquid dosage forms are especially desirable for the elderly as well as young children who have difficulty swallowing tablets or capsules. Other benefits of these liquid forms is that they may contain flavors that make them palatable and help to disguise the awful taste of the actual medicine, and can have more of a soothing feel on the way down.

7.2 ADVANTAGES AND DISADVANTAGES

Advantages:

1. Liquids dosage forms are pourable and are better for patients who have trouble in swallowing.

2. Faster absorption and rapid action than solids as they require no dissolution time.
3. More flexibility in achieving the proper dosage of the medication.
4. Liquid dosage forms are used fairly commonly by young children or the elders who have trouble swallowing the solid oral dosage forms.
5. The products like adsorbents and antacids are more effective in liquid dosage form.
6. The liquid dosage form is expected for certain types of products like cough medicines.

Disadvantages:

1. Shorter life before expiration than other dosage forms.
2. More difficult to administer and may have special storage requirements
3. Less dosage accuracy.
4. Problem occurs in preservation.
5. Transport is very much difficult.
6. No recovery is possible if it is lost one time.

7.3 EXCIPIENTS : SELECTION, PROPERTIES AND FUNCTIONS

An excipient is a natural or synthetic substance combined with the drug (active ingredient), for the purpose of long-term stability, making-up formulation that contain drug, or to confer a therapeutic enhancement on the drug in the final dosage form. In brief it can be defined as **"The components of a formulation other than the active ingredient"**. Excipients are non-active agents or inactive ingredients added into the pharmaceutical compositions during the development of the dosage forms and don't have any therapeutic value but are needed to affect the functioning of the drug and the dosage form. Being inert they generally have no pharmacological effect. Excipients are useful in the manufacturing process, to aid in the handling of the drugs concerned such as by facilitating flowability or non-stick properties and to maintain *in vitro* stability such as prevention of denaturation or aggregation over the shelf life. Therefore, excipient is indispensable component of pharmaceutical dosage forms and in most of the formulations, they are present in greater proportion in comparison to the drug.

(a) Selection of Excipient

The proper choice of excipients depends upon its physico-chemical properties and characteristics of active drug and route of drug administration. The selection of proper excipients depends upon regulatory acceptance, consistency of the material, sources, cost and availability, stability and compatibility issues, pharmacokinetic parameters, permeation characteristics, segmental absorption behaviour, drug delivery platform, intellectual property issues etc. The key to a successful pharmaceutical formulation is to have knowledge of API, excipients, their interaction and process parameters. The selection of excipients is of major concern to design stable, effective and palatable oral liquid formulation. The final selection of excipient for particular application is based upon compliance of compatibility tests that gives the manufacturer an idea to avoid any interaction.

The major challenges in design and developing liquid dosage forms are drug stability in solution, required level of solubility and an acceptable taste. These challenges can be overcome by effective selection and use of excipients.

(b) Ideal Properties of Excipients

1. Excipients have efficient functionality for intended use.
2. They must be physiologically inert.
3. They must have good physical and chemical stability.
4. They should be less sensitive to equipment and process.
5. They must be non-toxic.
6. They must be acceptable with regards to organoleptic characteristics.
7. No influence on drug bioavailability.
8. Excipients needs to be free from pathogenic microorganisms.
9. They must be in conformance with the regulatory agency requirements.
10. They must be economical.

(c) Functions of Excipients

Excipients used in the liquid dosage forms may have a variety of function to perform.

1. They may be added to maintain the integrity of the dosage form.
2. They provide protection, support or stability to the formulation.
3. They help to make-up enough formulation size in case of potent drug for assisting in accurate dose and handling.
4. They help to improve patient acceptance.
5. They contribute for improving bioavailability of drug.
6. They work to enhance and maintain overall safety and effectiveness of the formulation during its storage and use.

Although excipients are inert substances but this has been found wrong as some of the excipients have shown direct influence in dissolution rate and drug absorption. Furthermore, some excipients had been found to encounter some activity regarding the facilitation of penetration inside the tumor cell. On the other hand, some studies confirmed the doubts on presence of some side effects associated with presence of certain types of excipients, for example, the presence of sucrose, lactose, parabens, and menthol are associated with diabetes mellitus, stomach cramps, hypersensitivity reaction, spasms of the larynx in infants, respectively.

7.4 EXCIPIENTS USED IN FORMULATION OF LIQUID DOSAGE FORMS

Excipients are classified based upon the function they perform; however, several excipients behave differently at different concentrations and one excipient can be used for multiple purposes depending upon the need of the dosage form.

Oral liquid formulations are prepared by combining different ingredients to perform functions like wetting and solubilisation, stabilization and to impart suitable colour, taste and viscosity. The formulation should be compatible, non-reactive and stable. The common excipients generally required for any liquid formulation are:

(a) Vehicles (solvents/co-solvents), for example, Aqueous vehicle, propylene glycol, glycerol.

(b) Buffering agents, for example, Citrate, gluconates, lactates.

(c) Preservatives, for example, Sodium benzoate, methyl paraben, propyl parabens.

(d) Anti-oxidants, for example, Butylated hydroxy anisole (BHA), Butylated hydroxy toluene (BHT), ascorbic acid.

(e) Wetting agents, for example, Polysorbate, sorbitan esters.

(f) Anti-foaming agents, for example, Simethicone.

(g) Thickening agents, for example, Methylcellulose or hydroxyethyl cellulose.

(h) Sweetening agents, for example, Sorbitol, saccharin, aspartame, acesulfame.

(i) Flavouring agents, for example, Peppermint, lemon oils, butterscotch, etc.

(j) Humectants, for example, Propylene glycol, glycerol, sorbitol.

(a) Vehicles

1. **Solvents:** In liquid pharmaceutical formulations, vehicles are major components used as a base in which drugs and other excipients are dissolved or dispersed. They function by breaking of bonds and reducing effective charge on ions thus increasing solute-solvent forces of attraction which are eventually greater than solute-solute and solvent-solvent forces of attraction.

   Examples: Water, hydro-alcoholic liquid systems, polyhydric alcohols, acetic acid, ethyl acetate, and buffers. These may be thin liquids, thick syrupy liquids, mucilage or hydrocolloid bases. The oily vehicles include vegetable oils, mineral oils, organic oily bases or emulsified bases etc.

2. **Co-solvent:** Co-solvents are defined as water-miscible organic solvents that are used in liquid drug formulations to increase the solubility of poorly water soluble substances or to enhance the chemical stability of a drug. Co-solvent increases the solubility of a drug. An ideal co-solvent should possess values of dielectric constant between 25 and 80. The most widely used system that will cover this range is a water/ethanol blend. It should not cause toxicity or irritancy when administrated for oral or parental use. Other co-solvents are sorbitol, glycerol, propylene glycol and syrup.

   Examples: Ethanol, sorbitol, glycerine, propylene glycol etc.

   (i) Water: Natural water contains large number of dissolved and suspended particles as impurities. The dissolved impurities include inorganic impurities like salts of sodium, potassium, calcium, magnesium and iron as chlorides, sulfates and bicarbonates. Organic impurities present in purified water are either in soluble or insoluble state. Micro-organisms are the other impurities present in water. Potable water used for drinking contains less than 0.1% of total solid. This water should meet the requirements of IP. IP acceptable drinking water should be clear, odorless, colorless and neutral with slight deviation in pH due to dissolved solids and gasses. Drinking water, due to possible incompatibility of formulation components with dissolved impurities in it, is not used in liquid pharmaceutical formulation. Purified Water IP is commonly used as vehicle or as a component of vehicle for aqueous liquid formulations but not for those intended for parenteral administration. Water used to prepare injectables is obtained by distillation, ion exchange treatment, reverse osmosis or any other suitable process from drinking water.

Difference between Purified Water IP and Water for Injection IP

Specifications	Purified Water IP	WFI IP
Conductivity	< 1.3 µ S/cm at 25°C	<1.3 µ S/cm at 25°C
Total Organic Carbon (TOC)	< 500 ppm	< 500 ppm
Microbial limit	100 cfu/ml	10 cfu/100ml
Endotoxin	NA	< 0.25 EU/ml
Endotoxin	5-7	5 - 7
Production Method	Not Specified	Distillation

(ii) Ethanol: Ethanol, frequently referred to as 'Alcohol', is the most commonly used solvent in liquid pharmaceutical formulations next to water. It is generally used as hydro-alcoholic mixture to dissolve water and alcohol soluble drugs and excipients. Diluted ethanol prepared by mixing equal volumes of Ethanol IP and Purified Water IP is a most useful solvent in various pharmaceutical processes and formulations to dissolve poorly soluble substances. Alcohol is used in the pharmaceutical industry in a variety of manufacturing processes. It has bactericidal activity and is often used as a topical disinfectant, especially in alcohol gel for hands. It is also widely used as a solvent and preservative in liquid pharmaceutical preparations.

(iii) Glycerol: Glycerol also called glycerin is a clear, colorless liquid, with thick, syrupy consistency, oily to the touch, odorless, very sweet and slightly warm to the taste. When exposed to the air, it slowly absorbs moisture. Glycerol is obtained by the decomposition of vegetable or animal fats or fixed oils and containing not less than 95% of absolute glycerin. It is soluble in all proportions, in water or alcohol; also soluble in a mixture of 3 parts of alcohol and 1 part of ether, but insoluble in ether, chloroform, carbon di-sulphide, benzene, benzol, and fixed or volatile oils. Glycerin is used as vehicle in Phosphoric Acid Elixir, Ferric Ammonium Acetate Solution, Tragacanth Mucilage, Boric acid Glycerin, Tannic Acid Glycerin, and in many extracts, syrups and tinctures.

Glycerin is an excellent solvent for substances such as iodine, bromine, alkalies, tannic acid, many neutral salts, alkaloids, salicin etc. and thus is a good vehicle for applying these substances to the skin and to sores. It does not evaporate nor turn rancid. Being it hygroscopic it absorbs moisture and thus commonly used in liquid formulations to maintain skin moist. It also has sweet taste and thus it is an excellent flavouring agent. It is demulcent, and is used as a vehicle for applying substances, such as tannic acid, to the throat. It is rarely administered orally for any medicinal purpose. Although it has been reported to be administered orally for dyspepsia, for diabetes, and as a nutritive agent, the results of treatment are not guaranteed. In oral liquid formulations, glycerin is used as co-solvent to increase solubility of drugs that show low solubility in water. In addition, it is used to improve viscosity, taste and flavour of the products. In dosage forms for external applications it is used as humectant.

(iv) Propylene Glycol: Propylene glycol (PG), also called monopropylene glycol, has a specified purity of not less than 99.8%. PG is an important excipient used in number of preparations for variety of its functionalities. It is colorless and odorless and has a very slight characteristic taste which is not objectionable. These properties make propylene glycol particularly suitable as a solvent for flavourings and dyes in cosmetics, toothpastes, shampoos, and mouth washes. It is solvent for aromatics in the flavour-concentrate industry and also used as wetting agent for natural gums. It is important ingredient in the compounding of citrus and other emulsified flavors. In pharmaceutical preparations such as elixir, lotion, shampoos, creams and other similar products it is used as solvent. It is very effective humectant, preservative and stabilizer and thus used as emulsifier in cosmetic and pharmaceutical creams. Propylene glycol is an excellent solvent for many organic compounds. It is non-allergenic and may be used in cosmetics and other toilet goods specifically formulated for sensitive skin. Propylene glycol is used in liquid orals and, topical and parenteral preparations as an antimicrobial preservative. It has quite less toxicity in comparison to many other co-solvents generally used. The LD_{50} of propylene glycol is 24 g/kg, 8 g/kg and 9.7 g/kg when administered orally, intravenously and intraperitoneally, respectively, to mouse. Its use in large volumes in children is discouraged because it has CNS adverse effects, especially in neonates.

(v) Lipids: A large number of new drugs being developed show low water solubility and are characterized as either Biopharmaceutical Classification System (BCS) Class II or IV. To overcome low solubility and low bioavailability issues of these drugs there has been a growing interest in developing novel oral delivery strategies using lipid-based formulations. While oral liquid emulsions have been used for many years, self-emulsifying drug delivery systems, which utilize a lipid/surfactant-based vehicle, are becoming a more widely used approach to solubilize water-insoluble drugs. Benefits of these types of formulations are that lipids that keep a hydrophobic drug in solution may facilitate the dissolution and absorption of the drug as the lipid vehicle is metabolized in the GI tract. The erratic bioavailability of some drugs may be overcome by formulation into a microemulsion, which includes oil.

(b) Solubilizers

Wetting agents and surfactants

The homogeneous dispersion of solute particles in a liquid vehicle is prime requirement of any dosage form. In such pharmaceutical formulations wetting agents are routinely used. The air adsorbed at solid particles surfaces keep them away from vehicles. Even particles with a high density floats on the surface of the vehicle. The air present at surfaces is needed to be displaced completely to disperse them uniformly in vehicles. Wetting agents help to remove adsorbed air which ultimately promotes penetration of the liquid vehicle into pores and capillaries of the particles. In case of aqueous based formulations generally alcohol, glycerin, and PG are frequently used to facilitate the removal of adsorbed air from the surface of particles. Whereas for non-aqueous vehicle based liquid formulations mineral oils are commonly used as a wetting agents. Generally, hydrophobic drug particles are difficult to wet even after the removal of adsorbed air. In such cases it is necessary to reduce the surface tension between the particles and the liquid vehicles. Surface active agents that work as wetting agents, comprises of branched hydrophobic chains with central hydrophilic groups or short hydrophobic chains with hydrophilic end groups. Sodium lauryl sulfate is one of the most commonly used surface-active agents as a wetting agent. When it is dissolved in water, it lowers the contact angle of water and support in spreading of water on the particles surface to remove the air layer at the surface and replace it with the liquid phase. Wetting agents have a hydrophilic-lipophilic balance (HLB) value between 7 and 9. While selecting wetting agent for any liquid formulation it is important to know minimum surface tension that can be attained, regardless of the amount of agent required. In addition, the information about depression of surface tension achieved with a specified concentration of agent and the time required for an agent to achieve equilibrium are very important issues.

A good wetting agent decreases surface tension in water about 2.5 mN/m within 15 seconds. Wetting agents used for the purpose should not have any unwanted change in the potential activity and bioavailability of the drugs or other excipients. When wetting agents are incorporated in formulations drastic changes in the bactericidal action of certain excipients has been observed due to altered solubilities by surfactants. Increased solubilization sometimes modifies stability of excipients against oxidation and hydrolysis. Some of the non-ionic surfactants at higher concentrations exhibit a characteristic temperature called cloud point. At this point the liquids appear cloudy due to formation of lamellar micelles as result of dehydration of the polyoxyethylene chains. Thus, for such surfactants, it is essential to consider the risk of exceeding this point. The location of the drug or excipient in the micelle structure also influences its stability. For example, at the positive surface of the cationic micelle there would be a relatively higher concentration of $^-$OH from the surrounding solution. In such cases drugs or excipients are prone to hydrolysis but if it is stable under alkaline conditions then there may be least hydrolytic degradation. Therefore, a formulator has to optimize the choice of surfactant to prevent degradation.

The wetting agents used in liquid dosage forms includes lecithin, sodium lauryl sulphate benzalkonium chloride, benzethonium chloride cetylpyridinium chloride, docusate sodium, nonoxynol, octoxynol, poloxamers, polyoxyl 40 hydrogenated castor oil, polyoxyl 10 oleyl ether, polyoxyl 20 cetylstearyl ether, polyoxyl 40 stearate, polysorbate 20, polysorbate 40, polysorbate 60, polysorbate 80, sodium lauryl sulfate, sorbitan monolaurate, sorbitan monooleate, sorbitan monopalmitate, sorbitan monostearate, tyloxapol etc.

(c) pH Modifiers and Buffering Agents

The pH of liquid formulations especially those for oral administration is a crucial point. In maintaining the formulation, the pH helps to prevent unwanted changes during storage. Therefore, buffers being able to prevent changes in pH, are added in to most formulations to control potential changes in the pH. Buffers act by binding hydrogen ions in acids and donating hydrogen ions in bases. The amount of buffer capacity needed is generally between 0.01 and 0.1 M, and a concentration between 0.05 and 0.5 M is usually sufficient. The selection of a suitable buffer should be based on suitability of acid-base form for use in oral liquids, stability of the drug and excipients in the buffer, and compatibility between the buffer and container.

A combination of buffers has also been used to prepare wide range of pH compared to the individual buffers. It is important to note that not all buffers are suitable for use in oral liquids. For example, a boric acid buffer is not used in oral liquids because of its toxicity. Stability of formulation containing non-ionizable drugs depends on pH. However, the buffer may negatively influence the solubility of the drug and other excipients. The effect depends on a combination of the polarity of the solute and of the salt. Non-polar solutes are solubilized by less polar organic salts and are desolubilized by polar salts and vice-versa.

The stabilizing effect of buffers determines the potential reaction between excipients and drug. For example, buffers containing carbonate, citrate, tartarate, and phosphate salts may precipitate with calcium ions by forming sparingly soluble salts. This precipitation is dependent upon the solution pH. The activity of phosphate ions may be lowered due to interactions with other solution components. Other factors that may affect the solution pH include temperature, ionic strength, dilution, and the amount and type of co-solvents present. For example, the pH of acetate buffers is known to increase with temperature, whereas the pH of boric acid buffers decreases with temperature. It is important to know that the drug in solution may itself act as a buffer. If the drug is a weak electrolyte, such as salicylic acid or ephedrine, the addition of base or acid, respectively, will create a system in which the drug can act as a buffer.

Examples: Phosphate buffers, Acetate buffers, Citric acid Phosphate buffers etc.

(d) Suspending and Viscosity Enhancing Agents

Selection of an appropriate suspending agent is one of the most crucial factors in formulating a pharmaceutical suspension. Suspending agents impart viscosity, and thus retard particle settling. Other factors considered in the selection of the appropriate suspending and viscosity enhancing agent include desired rheological property, suspendability in the system, chemical compatibility with other excipients, pH stability, hydration time, reproducibility, and the cost. The examples of suspending agents are cellulose derivatives, clays, natural gums, and synthetic gums. In many formulations these excipients are employed in combination for enhanced effects.

Examples: Sodium alginate, methyl cellulose, hydroxyethyl cellulose, hydroxylpropylcellulose, hydroxypropylmethylcellulose, carboxy methylcellulose, sodium carboxy methylcellulose, microcrystalline cellulose, tragacanth, xanthan gum, bentonite, carrageenan gum, guar gum, colloidal silicon dioxide etc.

(e) Preservatives

Microbiological contamination is major problem encountered by aqueous based liquid dosage forms. Use of preservatives becomes unavoidable in such cases to prevent the growth of micro-organisms during production and over storage time. In fact, it is desirable to develop a preservative-free formulation to avoid unwanted effects of these excipients. Formulations such as syrups, emulsions, solutions etc., require preservative to prevent microbial growth. The majorities of preservatives are of both acid and non-acid types and are bacteriostatic rather than bactericidal. The pH of solution and the pKa of the preservative are important criterion for their selection. In liquid formulation with alkaline pH being insignificant microbial growth use of preservative is not generally recommended. Many preservatives are listed in the FDA inactive ingredient list for liquid dosage forms. Many of them are not recommended for use in liquid orals and hence the choice of an acceptable preservative is limited. In addition, many of them have low aqueous solubility and thus are ineffective for the purpose. Some of them partition between organic and aqueous phases of heterogeneous liquid formulations such as emulsions and their activity is significantly reduced. Substances such as non-ionic surfactants, quaternary ammonium compounds, gelatin, ferric salts, calcium salts and salts of heavy metals prevent microbial growth. Preservatives contain reactive moiety responsible for antimicrobial activity but sometimes lead to undesired reactions. Therefore, while selecting preservatives other parameters need to be evaluated for its compatibility with the drug, other excipients, and the container system.

Examples: benzyl alcohol, thiomersal, bronopol, chlorbutol, chlorocresol, butyl paraben, methyl paraben, propyl paraben, phenol, phenyl ethanol, sodium benzoate, phenol, chloro-cresol, p-hydroxybenzoic acid, benzoic acid, boric acid, and sorbic acid, chlorobutanol, benzyl alcohol, and beta-phenylethyl alcohol and antimicrobial solvents like propylene glycol and chloroform, etc.

(f) Stabilizers

Oxidation, photolysis, solvolysis and dehydration are common transformations taking place in liquid dosage forms. Amongst them for oxidation and photodecomposition of drug are very common pathways of drug decomposition and are very difficult to control due to low activation energies. Trace amounts of impurities, which are invariably present in the drug or excipient initiates the oxidation reaction. Drugs exist in reduced form show increased susceptibility when it is consistently exposed an open environment. The pH of the solution may contribute in the oxidation of drugs because ionized forms of these drugs at particular pH are very prone oxidation. For example, epinephrine is slowly oxidized at pH less than 4 but rapidly degrades in alkaline pH conditions. Antioxidants are the compounds that can reduce oxidation of a drug, or are compounds that are more readily oxidized than the drugs that are to protect. In some cases, antioxidants act as chain terminators where it reacts with free radicals in solution to stop the free-radical propagation cycle. A combination of chelating agents with antioxidants is often used to exert synergistic effect. This is because many of these agents act at differing steps in the oxidative process. Oxidation of formulation component leads to products with an unpleasant odour, taste, appearance, precipitation, discoloration or even a slight loss of activity. The term rancidity refers to auto-oxidation of unsaturated fatty acids that are present in oils and fats, and it affects many oils and fats. The distinct rancid odour may result from short-chain, volatile monomers resulting from the cleavage of the longer chain, less volatile oils and fats.

Some substances prone to oxidation include unsaturated oils/fats, compounds with aldehyde or phenolic groups, colors, flavors, sweeteners, plastics and rubbers, the latter being used in containers for products.

Examples: Tocopherol acetate, acetone sodium bisulfite, acetylcysteine, ascorbic acid, ascorbyl palmitate, butylated hydroxyanisole (BHA), butylated hydroxytoluene (BHT), cysteine, cysteine hydrochloride, d α-tocopherol, natural d-α-tocopherol, synthetic dithiothreitol, monothioglycerol, nordihydroguaiaretic acid, propyl gallate, sodium bisulfite, sodium formaldehyde, sodium metabisulfite, sulfoxylate, sodium sulfite, sodium thiosulfate, thiourea etc.

(g) Emulsifying Agents

Prevent coalescence of the dispersed globules. Forms barriers at interface, and reduces interfacial tension.

Examples: Sodium lauryl sulphate, cetrimide, macrogols, esters, sorbitan esters etc.

(h) Antifoaming Agents

The formation of foams during manufacturing processes or when reconstituting the liquid dosage forms can be undesirable and disruptive. Anti-foaming agents are effective at discouraging the formation of stable foams by lowering surface tension and cohesive binding of the liquid phase.

Examples: Simethicone, organic phosphates, alcohols, paraffin oils, stearate and glycols.

(i) Humectants

Humectants are the hygroscopic substances that help to retard evapouration of aqueous vehicles from dosage forms. These excipients are used at ~5% strength in aqueous suspensions and emulsions for external application. They are also used to prevent drying of the product after application to the skin as well as prevent drying of product from the container upon opening. It also helps to prevent cap-locking caused by condensation onto neck of container-closure at first opening.

Examples: Propylene glycols, glycerol, polyethylene glycol, etc.

(j) Flocculating agents

Flocculating agents prevent caking. Addition of an electrolyte reduces the magnitude of zeta potential of dispersed particles.

Example: Starch, sodium alginate, carbomer etc.

(k) Chelating agents

Chelating agents are substances that form complexes with metal ions inactivating their catalytic activity in oxidation of medicaments. These agents are capable of forming complexes with the drug involving more than one bond it's a complex compound contains one or more ring in its structure. Protect drug from catalysts that accelerate the oxidative reaction.

Examples: Disodium EDTA, dihydroxy ethyl glycine, citric acid and tartaric acid. Ethylene diamine is bidentate and ethylene diamine tetraacetic acid is hexadentate.

(l) Flavouring agents

The flavouring agent in liquid pharmaceutical products is added to the solvent or vehicle component of the formulation in which it is most soluble or miscible. That is, water-soluble flavorants are added to the aqueous component of a formulation and poorly water-soluble flavorants are added to the alcoholic or other non-aqueous solvent component of the formulation. In a hydro-alcoholic or other multi-solvent system, care must be exercised to maintain the flavorants in solution. This is accomplished by maintaining a sufficient level of the flavorants solvent.

Examples: Salty-apricot, butterscotch, liquorice, peach, vanilla; Bitter -anise, chocolate, mint, passion fruit, wild cherry; Sweet - vanilla, fruits, berries; and Sour -citrus fruits, liquorice, raspberry. For extemporaneous preparations flavouring agents used are syrup, orange syrup, raspberry syrup, conc. raspberry juice, concentrated peppermint emulsion, sorbitol, saccharin, sodium cyclamate, anise water, conc. camphor water, liquorice liquid extract, glycerol, peppermint, lemon oils, butterscotch etc.

(m) Sweetening Agents

Sucrose enhances viscosity of liquids and also gives a pleasant texture in the mouth. The term 'sugar free' solutions include sweetening agents such as sorbitol, mannitol, xylitol, saccharin and aspartame as alternatives to sugar such as sucrose, fructose and glucose. In addition to sucrose, a number of artificial sweetening agents have been used in foods and pharmaceuticals over the years. Some of these, including aspartame, saccharin, and cyclamate, have faced challenges over their safety by the FDA and restrictions to their use and sale; in fact, in 1969, FDA banned cyclamates from use in the United States. Sucralose is most popular due to its excellent sweetness, non-cariogenic, low calorie, wide and growing regulatory acceptability but is relatively expensive.

Examples: Saccharin, cyclamate, saccharin, cyclamate, fructose, polyalcohol, sucrose, and aspartame, scesulfame potassium, sevia powder, sucralose.

(n) Colouring Agents

Colouring agents are used in pharmaceutical preparations for aesthetics. A distinction should be made between agents that have inherent colour and those that are employed as colorants. Colours used in liquid dosage form must be certified by FDA as per D&C Act 1940. Certain agents - sulphur (yellow), riboflavin (yellow), cupric sulfate (blue), ferrous sulfate (bluish green), cyanocobalamin (red), and red mercuric iodide (vivid red)—have inherent colour and are not thought of as pharmaceutical colorants in the usual sense of the term. Although most pharmaceutical colorants in use today are synthetic, a few are obtained from natural mineral and plant sources. For example, red ferric oxide is mixed in small proportions with zinc oxide powder to give calamine its characteristic pink colour, which is intended to match the skin tone upon application. The age of the intended patient should also be considered in the selection of the flavouring agent, because certain age groups seem to prefer certain flavours. Children prefer sweet candy-like preparations with fruity flavours, but adults seem to prefer less sweet preparations with a tart rather than a fruit flavour.

Examples: Natural colorants - derived from animals or plants (for example, carotenoids, chlorophylls, caramel, cochineal, saffron and red beetroot extract); Mineral pigments - as iron oxide not used in sols due to their low water solubility and Synthetic organic dyes such as the azo compounds. Amaranth, erythrosine, eosin, tartarazine etc.

MODEL QUESTIONS

1. Give advantages and disadvantages of liquid dosage form.
2. Enlist different excipients used in liquid dosage form. What is selection criteria and function of excipients in liquid dosage form?
3. Explain vehicles and solubilizers used in liquid dosage form.
4. Why pH modifier and buffering agents are used in liquid dosage form?
5. Explain different excipients used in liquid dosage form.

■■■

Chapter **8**...

Monophasic Liquids

LEARNING OBJECTIVES

Although liquid dosage forms are used for multiple reasons, they are especially desirable for the elderly as well as young children who have difficulty swallowing tablets or capsules. Other benefits of these liquid forms is that they may contain flavors that make them palatable and help to disguise the awful taste of the actual medicine, and can have more of a soothing feel on the way down.

The objectives of this chapter includes

- To recognize the route of drug administration through liquid form.
- Types of monophasic liquid dosage forms.
- To understand the principle and procedure of various monophasic liquid formulations.
- To know about storage, packaging, uses and special instructions of commonly used monophasic liquids.
- To formulate and describe various physical properties of monophasic liquid formulations.

8.1 INTRODUCTION

The liquid dosage forms are classified as monophasic liquid dosage forms and polyphasic liquid dosage forms. In pharmaceutical term, solutions are clear liquid preparations containing one or more active ingredients dissolved in a suitable solvent or mixture of mutually miscible solvents.

Monophasic liquid dosage forms are true or colloidal solution. The component of the solution which is present in a large quantity is known as solvent and the component present in a small quantity is termed as solute. Water is commonly used as solvent for majority of monophasic liquid dosage forms. A solution is homogenous because the solute is in an ionic or molecular form of subdivision. In case of colloidal solution, the solute is present as aggregates although they cannot be seen by naked eye or under ordinary microscope.

Monophasic liquid dosage forms are classified as:

(I) Route of administration:

1. Liquid for internal use, for example, syrup, elixirs, linctus, drops and draughts.
2. Liquid for external use.
    (a) Liquid to be applied to the skin, for example, liniments, and lotions
    (b) Liquid meant for body cavities, for example, gargles, throat paints, mouth washes, eye drops, eye lotions, ear drops, nasal drops, sprays and inhalations.

(II) Type of vehicle

1. Aqueous liquid dosage forms.
2. Non-aqueous liquids dosage forms.

8.2 PREPARATIONS OF MONOPHASIC LIQUIDS

8.2.1 Solutions

The solutions are dosage forms prepared by dissolving active ingredients in an aqueous or non-aqueous solvent. Solution is a homogenous mixture of two or more substances. In such a mixture, solute is dissolved in another substance known as solvent. The common example is solid dissolved in liquid such as salt or sugar in water.

The solutions are further classified as:

(i) According to route of administration:

(a) Oral solution – administered through oral cavity, for example, Methylphenidate Hydrochloride Oral Solution (Methylin[®]).

(b) Otic solutions – instilled in the ear, for example, Glycerin and Butylene Glycol Otic Solution (Phyteneo[®]).

(c) Ophthalmic solutions – instilled in the eyes, for example, Tobramycin Ophthalmic Solution (Falcon[®]).

(d) Topical solutions – applied over the skin surface, for example, Clindamycin Topical Solution (Dalacin T[®]).

(ii) According to composition and uses:

(a) Syrup – Aqueous solution containing sugar.

(b) Elixir – Sweeten hydro-alcoholic solution.

(c) Spirit – Solution of aromatic materials in alcohol.

(d) Aromatic water – Solution of aromatic materials in water.

(e) Tincture – Solution prepared by extracting constituents from crude drugs.

(f) Injection – Solution prepared to be sterile and pyrogen free intended for parenteral use.

(iii) According to vehicle:

(a) Aqueous solutions: Solutions that contains water as solvent, for example, sugar in water.

(b) Non-aqueous solutions: Solutions that contain solvent other than water, for example, naphthalene in benzene.

Concentrated and Dilute solution: The solution with greater proportion of solute is called concentrated solution whereas solution with less proportion of solute is called dilute solution.

Saturated solutions: A solution in which no more solute can be dissolved at given temperature is called saturated solution.

Unsaturated solution: A solution in which more solute can be dissolved at given temperature is called unsaturated solution.

A saturated solution at particular temperature can be unsaturated, dissolving more of the solute if temperature is increased. The pharmacist can in certain instances, dissolve greater quantities of solute than be possible using different solubilizing agents or a different chemical salt form of the drug. For example, Iodine topical solution, solubility of iodine crystals in water can be increased by addition of aqueous solution of potassium or sodium iodide.

Advantages of solutions:

1. Solutions being liquids, are easier to swallow therefore easier for children, old age and unconscious people.
2. Solutions are more quickly effective than tablets and capsules. A drug in solution is at molecular level and thus it can be absorbed rapidly.
3. A solution being a homogenous system, the drug is uniformly distributed throughout the preparation and uniform dose can be withdrawn.
4. Some drugs in other state than liquid can irritate the gastric mucosa if localized in one area. Irritation is reduced by administration of a solution of the drug.

Disadvantages of solutions:

1. Liquids are bulky and inconvenient to transport and store.
2. The stability of ingredients in aqueous solution is often poor than in solid dosage form.
3. Solution provide suitable media for the growth of micro-organisms and may require the addition of preservative.
4. Accurate dose measuring depends on the ability of patient to measure the dose (needs an accurate spoon to measure the dose.
5. Nature of the solute and the solvent.
6. The maximum possible concentration to which a pharmacist may prepare a solution varies greatly and depends in part on the chemical constitution of the solute.

Packaging: Plain, amber medicine bottles should be used, with a re-closable child-resistant closure with some exceptions. A 5 mL measuring spoon or an appropriate oral syringe should be supplied with product.

Label: An expiry date should appear on the label for extemporaneously prepared solutions.

8.2.2 Gargles

Gargles are liquid preparations intended to apply locally to the oral and throat cavities. The vehicles used in preparing gargles may be aqueous or hydroalcoholic solutions. Gargling is the human act in which air from the lungs is bubbled through a liquid in the mouth. Vibration caused by the muscles in the throat and back of the mouth cause the liquid to bubble and percolate through the throat and mouth cavity.

Uses: Gargles are used to treat sore throat and throat infections and for soothing and healing.

Contents: They may contain antiseptics, analgesics or weak astringents. Active constituent in gargle is phenol, thymol, potassium chlorate etc. Examples, Phenol Gargle and Potassium Chlorate (also called Golden gargle) and Phenol Gargle BPC. Solid type preparations are dissolved in water before use is also included in the category. Gargles tend to contain higher concentrations of active ingredients than mouthwashes. The liquid is usually not intended for swallowing:

1. Phenol Gargle

Phenol glycerin	50 mL
Amaranth solution	10 mL
Water to make	1000 mL

Phenol gargle is diluted with equal volume of warm water before use. It is used as an antiseptic and soothing effect in throat.

Method of preparation: Mix phenol glycerin and small amount of amaranth solution in a beaker. Add 3/4th quantity of water and mix again. Transfer contents to the measuring cylinder. Wash and adjust to the final volume with water. Transfer to a clean bottle, close the bottle with closure and stick on the label.

Gargles are usually prepared by dissolving drug substances with suitable excipients in a solvent together with suitable excipients and filtering. In the case of solid preparations which are dissolved before use, prepare as directed Tablets or Granules. Herbal gargles may be swallowed to obtain secondary systemic effect. Many gargles must be diluted with water prior to use.

Packaging: Manufactured gargles are usually packed in plain, clear, fluted glass bottle closed with plastic screw cap. It is recommended to use tight containers for preservation. An amber ribbed bottle should be used for extemporaneously prepared solutions. Medicine bottles may be used for products which are intended to be swallowed.

Label: The container should be labelled 'For External Use Only'. Directions for diluting the preparations should be given to the patient. If the preparation is not intended for swallowing, the following label is appropriate: 'Not to be swallowed in large amounts'.

8.2.3 Mouthwashes

The need for mouthwash is a result of a condition called halitosis, or bad breath. It is estimated that over half the population occasionally has foul-smelling breath. Mouth washes are aqueous solutions with pleasant taste and odour used to make clean and deodourize the buccal cavity. Mouthwashes are designed to eliminate bad breath in two ways. First, they relieve it by killing the bacteria responsible for producing the foul odour. The best of these products prevent bad breath for as long as eight hours. The second way that mouthwashes help reduce bad breath is by masking the odour. This is a much less effective method which lasts no more than 30 minutes.

Uses: Mouthwashes are used to make clean and deodourize the buccal cavity. Mouthwashes are used on the mucous membranes of the oral cavity, rather than the throat, to refresh and mechanically clean the mouth.

Contents: The active constituents include antibacterial agents, glycerol, sweetening agent, flavouring agent, soaps, colouring agents and astringent. The primary ingredient in most mouthwashes is deionized water, a diluent, making-up over 50% of the entire formula. Alcohol is another diluent typically used in up to 20% of the formula. Antibacterial agents employed in mouthwash formulations include ingredients like phenols, thymol, salol, tannic acid, hexachlorophene, chlorinated thymols, quaternary ammonium compounds; parachlormetacresol, thymol, hexachlorophene. Flavorants such as peppermint, menthol, methyl salicylate, and eugenol are commonly used. The most commonly used colours are blue and green approved and certified FDA. Some mouthwash formulas also include a synthetic detergent to give extra foaming and cleansing action.

Example: Compound Sodium Chloride Mouth Wash B.P. 1993.

Formula:

Sodium chloride	1.5 g
Sodium bicarbonate	1.0 g
Concentrated Peppermint emulsion	2.5 mL
Chloroform water, double strength	50 mL
Water to produce	100 mL

Method of preparation: Dissolve sodium chloride and sodium bicarbonate in 3/4 volume of water in a beaker. Add the concentrated peppermint emulsion, chloroform water and mix well. Transfer contents to the measuring cylinder and adjust the volume with the remaining amount of water. Transfer contents to a bottle, close and stick on the label.

Packaging: Manufactured mouthwashes are usually packed in plain, clear, flutted glass bottle closed with plastic screw cap. It is recommended to use tight containers for preservation. An amber, ribbed bottle should be used for extemporaneously prepared solutions.

Label: The label should clearly indicate proper direction for diluting the mouthwash before use. 'For External Use Only' and if the preparation is not intended for swallowing 'Not to Be Swallowed in Large Amount' are other labelling instructions.

Future: In the past, mouthwashes were primarily powerful breath fresheners. They eventually evolved into tooth protectors. Today, products are available to not only fight bad breath but whiten teeth and help battle cavity formation and gum recession. For example, mouthwash containing peptide known as p1025 can bond to the teeth and prevent the growth of naturally occurring bacteria preventing cavity-causing bacteria to adhere to the tooth and thus inhibits cavity formation for up to three months.

8.2.4 Throat Paints

Throat paints are viscous liquid preparations used for the mouth and throat infections. Glycerin is commonly used as a base because being viscous, it adheres to mucous membrane for a long period and it possesses a sweet taste. Throat paints must be more viscous because they are designed to prolong contact of the medicament with the affected site.

Examples: Iodine Throat Paint (Lecare®), Iodine Potassium Throat Paint (Gleem®), Tannic Acid Throat Paint (Koral®), Clotrimazole Mouth Paint (Nuforce® and Candid®)

Iodine is a naturally occurring mineral that the body needs to produce hormones and control the body's metabolism. In a liquid form, it is also used as an antibacterial agent and anti-inflammatory. When you apply iodine to an inflamed throat, the treatment eliminates infection, kills fungus and bacteria, and eradicates the underlying cause of a sore throat. It also offers immediate relief as it helps reduce inflammation on contact. Iodine is a nutrient that many people are deficient in, so supplementing iodine can help support immune function and relieve a sore throat.

Uses: Painting the external throat with iodine can reduce pain of the throat, may curb and even eliminate throat infections; boosts overall immune function and help with conditions such as tonsillitis, pharyngitis, laryngitis and more. The action of iodine paint in the case of throat infections has been observed to be much greater when the solution is painted internally on throat tissue. While using this type of preparation we need to be sure that an appropriate formulation is selected. Iodine is considered safe for most people, but some people should avoid it and it should not be taken with certain medications. Anyone with Hashimoto's Autoimmune Thyroid Disease or overactive thyroid should not take Iodine. According to the Merck manual, chronic toxicity may develop when intake of iodine paint is greater than 1.1 mg/day. Also, a precaution needs to be taken by people who may have an allergy to iodine. A simple test is to spread a very small amount on the skin of inner thigh and observe for small blisters to appear within a few hours. If blisters do appear, you may be allergic to or have an allergic reaction to iodine paint. Iodine throat paint is designed to kill germs. It can be used on sore throats and ulcers to ease them.

1. **Compound Iodine Throat Paint**

    Synonym: Mandle's paint

Potassium iodide	24 g
Iodine	12 g
Alcohol (96%)	40 mL
Water	24 mL
Peppermint oil	4 mL
Glycerin...q.s...	1000 mL

Iodine is slightly soluble in water, but it is soluble in presence of potassium iodide and forms polyiodides. These polyiodides are highly soluble in water and hence produce monophasic liquid.

$$I_2 \quad + \quad KI \quad \rightarrow \quad I_2KI$$
Iodine   Potassium iodide   Potassium mono iodide

$$2I_2 \quad + \quad KI \quad \rightarrow \quad 2I_2KI$$
Iodine   Potassium iodide   Potassium di-iodide

$$3I_2 \quad + \quad KI \quad \rightarrow \quad 3I_2KI$$
Iodine   Potassium iodide   Potassium di iodide (Poly iodides)

Alcohol (90%) acts as co solvent, to increase the solubility of iodine. It is also used to dissolve peppermint oil, which acts as flavouring agent. Glycerin is viscous in nature hence Mandle's paint will remain in contact with mucous membrane of throat for longer time; it also acts as humectant and soothing agent.

Method of Preparation:

1. Triturate iodine in glass mortar, to get fine powder and accurately weigh the required amount of iodine.
2. Dissolve potassium iodide in water. To this solution, add iodine powder and dissolve by stirring.
3. Dissolve peppermint oil and half of the portion of glycerin in alcohol.
4. Add this solution to the above iodide and potassium iodide solution, with continuous stirring and adjust the final volume with remaining portion of glycerin.

Label: Apply with camel hairbrush, every four hours. The auxiliary label instructions include 'For External Use Only', 'Store In Cool Place', 'Not To Be Swallowed In Large Quantities', 'Keep The Container Tightly Closed'. Since there are chances of separation of oil globules of peppermint oil during storage 'Shake Well Before Use' is one more important instruction to the patients.

Packaging: Mandes paint contains volatile ingredients like iodine, alcohol (90%) and peppermint oil. Iodine is sensitive to the light, hence transfer the paint to a light resistant, wide mouthed, glass bottle, close it tightly with plastic screw cap, polish and label. Supply with camel hairbrush.

Storage: Store in cool and dark place.

Uses: Mandl's paint is used in the treatment of pharyngitis, laryngitis, tonsillitis and abscilles of throat.

2. **Tannic Acid – Glycerin Throat Paint**

Tannic acid	20 g
Sodium citrate	1 g
Dried sodium sulphide	0.2 g
Glycerin...q.s...	100 mL

Tannic acid is slightly soluble in water (1:0.35), but aqueous solution of tannic acid leads to decomposition during storage. Tannic acid is soluble in glycerin (1:1), hence glycerin is used as a vehicle to dissolve the tannic acid and because of its high viscous nature, it does not flow, quickly and adhere to the mucous membrane of the throat for longer time. In addition, glycerin also acts as sweetening agent. Dried sodium sulphide and sodium citrate acts as stabilizers, which prevents the deterioration of tannic acid.

Method of Preparation:

1. Separately weigh tannic acid, dried sodium sulphide and sodium chloride. Triturate them, to fine powder in a porcelain dish.
2. To this powder, add half of the portion of glycerin and triturate until a smooth mixture is produced, then add the remaining amount of glycerin and mix well.
3. Heat this mixture on a sand bath to a temperature between 115 to 120°C with occasional stirring, until a solution is formed and cool it to room temperature.
4. Throat paints contains glycerin which is hygroscopic in nature, hence it should be protected from moisture. Therefore transfer the paint to a light resistant, wide mouthed glass bottle, close it tightly with plastic screw cap, polish and label. Supply with camel hairbrush.

Label: The label of this paint must contain instructions 'APPLY WITH CAMEL HAIRBRUSH, WHENEVER NECESSARY'. Other auxiliary instructions include 'FOR EXTERNAL USE ONLY', 'NOT TO BE SWALLOWED IN LARGE QUANTITIES', 'KEEP THE CONTAINER TIGHTLY CLOSED'.

STORAGE: Store in dry place.

Uses: It is used as an astringent in the treatment of sore throat and receding gums, because tannic acid precipitates the proteins. It also has a haemostatic property that stops the bleeding in gums.

8.2.5 Ear Drops

Ear drops are solutions of one or more active ingredient which exert a local effect in the ear. They may also be referred to as otic or aural preparations.

Propylene glycol, oils, glycerol (to increase viscosity) and water may be used as vehicles.

Uses: Ear drops are a form of medicine used to treat or prevent ear infections, especially infections of the outer ear and ear canal (otitis external). Bacterial infections are sometimes treated with antibiotics. They may be useful for softening earwax or treating infection or inflammation.

Examples: Polysporin Ear Drop, Murine Ear Drop, Ciprosine Ear Drop, Ciprodex Ear Drops, etc.

Benzocaine Ear Drops

Benzocaine (1 % v/v)	10 mL
Phenazone (antipyrine)	50 g
Glycerol...qs...	1000 mL

Advantages:

1. They are not necessarily sterile.
2. Used for clearing up infections or cleaning out ear wax buildup.
3. They are safer than systemic therapy.
4. They are delivered directly to the infected organ bypassing the systemic circulation.
5. Drugs delivered as ear drops have minimal side effects, local irritation and local allergy.
6. They are usually less expensive than comparable systemic medications.

Disadvantages:

1. They need to be isotonic and non-irritating.
2. If the eardrum of the ear being treated is perforated, there is a slight risk that a permanent reduction in hearing may take place.
3. There is a slight risk of dizziness with long term use.
4. Proper administration skills are required.
5. There may be pain upon use of ear drop.

Packaging: Extemporaneously prepared ear drops should be packed in an amber, ribbed hexagonal glass bottle fitted with a teat and dropper. Manufactured ear drops are usually packed in small glass or plastic containers with a dropper.

Label: Not to share ear drops in order to minimize contamination and infection. Patients should be given advice on how to administer extemporaneously prepared ear drops, accompanied by written information if possible. Extemporaneous preparations should be labelled with the appropriate expiry date following the official monographs. "For External Use Only" is not an appropriate label and so 'Not to be taken" is advised.

8.2.6 Nasal Drops

Nasal drops are the solutions of drugs that are instilled in to the nose with a dropper. Nasal drops are isotonic to nasal secretions and buffered to the normal pH range of nasal fluids (pH 5.5-6.5) to prevent damage to ciliary transport in the nose. These are usually aqueous and not oily drops since the latter inhibits the movements of cilia in the nasal mucosa and if used for the long periods may reach the lungs and cause lipoid pneumonia.

Uses: Nasal drops are used to treat colds and allergies and work on the specific site rather than the whole body. Nasal route is useful for new biologically active peptides and polypeptides which need to avoid the first pass metabolism or GI destruction. The most frequent use of nasal drops is as a decongestant for the common cold or to administer local steroids for the treatment of allergic rhinitis.

Examples: Otrivin Nasal Drops (Xylometazoline HCl), Nozolin Nasal Drops (Sodium chloride), Xylomet Nasal Drops (Xylometazoline HCl) etc.

Xylometazoline Hydrochloride BP

Xylometazoline hydrochloride BP	0.1% w/v
Benzalkonium chloride	0.015% w/v
Disodium edetate...qs...	
Sodium phosphate dihydrate ...qs...	
Sodium acid phosphate ...qs...	
Sodium chloride ...qs...	
Water ...qs...	10 mL

Advantages:

1. Suitable for drugs that easily cross mucous membranes as they are directly absorbed into the blood stream.
2. This direct absorption into the blood stream avoids gastrointestinal destruction and hepatic first pass metabolism.
3. Drugs are rapidly absorbed and predictably bioavailable.
4. The rates of drug absorption and plasma concentrations are comparable to intravenous administration.
5. They are easy, convenient and safe to administer.
6. They may rapidly achieve therapeutic brain and spinal cord (CNS) drug concentrations.
7. They are cheaper than injections.

Disadvantages:

1. Limited medications that can be delivered through nasal drops.
2. Many medications are not adequately concentrated to achieve ideal dosing volumes.
3. Mucosal health impacts absorption.
4. Repeated use can cause permanent damage to the sinus membranes.
5. Most nasal drops have various side effects including fatigue, nosebleeds, throat irritation, and cough.
6. Nasal drops may also exacerbate headaches or even cause strokes in patients taking some antidepressants, diet pills or anti-migraine drugs.

Packaging: Manufactured nasal solutions may be packed in flexible plastic bottles which deliver a fine spray to the nose when squeezed, or in a plain glass bottle with a pump spray or dropper.

Label: Not to share nasal drops in order to minimize contamination and infection. Patients should be given advice on how to administer extemporaneously prepared nasal drops, accompanied by written information if possible. Extemporaneous preparations should be labelled with the appropriate expiry date following the official monographs. "For External Use Only" is not an appropriate label and so 'Not to be taken" is advised.

8.2.7 Enema

Enemas are oily or aqueous solutions that are administered rectally. Enemas are also known as clyster. Microenemas are single-dose, small volume solutions. Large-volume (0.5-1 litre) enemas should be warmed to body temperature before administration. Enemas are usually given at body temperature in quantities of 450 to 900 mL injected slowly with enema syringe. If they are to be retained in the intestine, they should not be used in larger quantities than 180 mL for an adult.

There are two types of enema namely evacuation enema and retention enema.

Example: Hydrocortisone Enema for local action and Aminophylline Enema for systemic effects.

Evacuation Enemas: These are rectal enemas employed to promote evacuation of bowel and to cleanse the colon for retention and for diagnosis. Available in disposable plastic squeeze bottles containing a pre measured amount of enema solution. The agents present are solutions of sodium phosphate, sodium biphosphate, glycerin and docusate potassium and light mineral oil.

Retention Enemas: In this enema, a number of solutions are administered rectally for the local effects of the medication. There are three types of retention enema.

1. Nutritive Enema - supply nutrient to the patient.

2. Medicated Enema - supply medication for systemic effect.

3. Diagnostic Enema – Barium Sulphate ($BaSO_4$) and Fleet Enema.

Uses: Enemas are rectal injections employed to evacuate the bowel, to influence the general system by absorption, affect locally the seat of disease and for diagnostic visualization of GIT. Enemas are used to deliver anti-inflammatory, purgative, anthelmintic, nutritive, sedative or stimulating substances in the bowel. Retention enemas are administered to give either a local action of the drug or for systemic absorption. They may contain radioopaque substances for roentgenographic examination of the lower bowel. They are used after defecation.

Examples:

1. Enema of Soft Soap**:**
    It is prepared by dissolving 50 g of soft soap with purified water to make 1000 mL.
2. Barium Sulfate Enema (for diagnostic visualization of GIT).

Barium sulfate	120 g
Acacia mucilage	100 mL
Starch enema q.s. to make	500 mL

Method of preparation: Prepared by mixing barium sulfate with acacia mucilage and sufficient starch enema to make 500 mL. Starch enema is made by triturating 30 g of powdered starch with 200 mL cold water followed by addition of sufficient quantity of water to make 1000 mL.

Packaging: If extemporaneously produced, enemas are packed in amber fluted glass bottles. Manufactured enemas will usually be packed in disposable polythene or polyvinyl chloride bags with a nozzle for insertion into the rectum.

Label: Patients should be advised on how to use the enema if they are self-administering and the time that the product will take to work. The label 'For rectal use only' should be used.

8.2.8 Syrup

Syrup is a highly concentrated, aqueous solution of sugar or a sugar substitute that traditionally contain a flavouring agent. The strength of sugar in syrup is 66.7%w/w. The syrup used as a vehicle for medicine. It is usually used as a flavoured vehicle for drugs. It also masks the taste of bitter substances of the formulation.

Types of Syrups

(i) **Simple syrup:** Simple Syrup I.P. is 66.7%w/w sucrose solution in water prepared by simple solution method. In simple syrup USP sucrose at the concentration of 85% is dissolved in water. These are sometimes used as a coating on to the surface of the tablets. Syrup, is protected from bacterial contamination by virtue of its high solute concentration. More dilute syrups are good media for microbial growth and require the addition of preservatives. Syrups are saturated solutions of sucrose in water thus exerts high osmotic pressure and no free water is available for microbial growth. Hence preservative is not required to be added in simple syrup.

   Example: Simple Syrup IP, Simple Syrup USP, Simple Syrup BP.

   The USP simple syrup is 85%w/v or an approximately 65% w/w sucrose solution with a specific gravity of 1.313 whereas BP simple syrup is 87.5% w/v or 66.7% w/w of sucrose as the solute in 33.3% w/w of water as the solvent. The USP syrup is 850 g sucrose and enough distilled water to make 1000 mL. The BP syrup is 865 g – 875 g sucrose and enough distilled water to make 1000 mL.

(ii) Medicated syrup: Medicated syrup is nearly saturated solution of sugar in water in which drug or drugs are dissolved. These syrups contain medicinal substances giving them therapeutic value.

Example: Ephedrine Sulfate Syrup (for cough)

Formula:

Ephedrine sulfate	4 g
Citric acid	1 g
Amaranth solution	4 mL
Caramel	0.4 g
Lemon oil	0.125 mL
Orange oil	0.25 mL
Benzaldehyde	0.06 mL
Vanillin	0.016 g
Alcohol	25 mL
Sucrose	800 g
Purified water, q.s. to make	1000 mL

Some syrups are used as cathartic, cholinergic, decongestant, expectorant, fecal softener, sedative and others.

Other examples of medicated syrups

1. Analgesic**:** Meperidine HCl Syrup (Demerol®).
2. *Anticholenergics***:** Dicyclomine HCl Syrup (Bentyl®) and Oxybutynin Chloride (Ditropan®).
3. Antiemetic**:** Chlorpromazine HCl Syrup (Thorazine®), Dimenhydrinate Syrup (Dramamine®).
4. Anticonvulsant**:** Sodium Valproate Syrup (Depakene®).
5. Antipsychotic**:** Lithium Citrate Syrup.
6. Antihistamines**:** Chlorpheniramine Maleate Syrup (Chlor-Trimeton®), Cyproheptadine HCl Syrup (Periactin®), Hydroxyzine HCl Syrup (Atarax®).
7. Sedative**:** Dextromethrophan Hydrobromide Cough Syrup (Chericof®).
8. Asthma and Bronchitis**:** Acebrophylline Sugar Free Syrup (Abpex®).

Uses:

1. Due to sweetness, can mask the taste of salty and bitter drugs and therefore serve as pleasant tasting vehicle.

2. Used as vehicle for pediatric use due to their high viscosity and the "smoothness" and mouth feel qualities.

3. Due to the wide variety of flavours of syrups such as orange, lemon, peppermint, these are widely acceptable.

(iii) Non-medicated or flavoured Syrup: Some syrup does not contain therapeutic agent, instead they consist of various aromatic and pleasantly flavoured substances and is intended as a vehicle or flavour for preparations called non-medicated or flavoured syrups.

Examples: Cherry Syrup, Orange Syrup, Cocoa Syrup etc.

Components of Syrups:

1. Sugar - usually sucrose and other substitutes for sweetness and viscosity.

2. Antimicrobial preservatives.

3. Flavourants.

4. Colorants.

5. Miscellaneous - special solvents, solubilizing agents, thickeners or stabilizers.

The syrup may be prepared from sugars other than sucrose such as glucose, fructose or non-sugar polyols such as sorbitol, glycerine, propylene glycol and mannitol, or other non-nutritive artificial sweeteners such as aspartame, saccharin, when a reduction in calories or glucogenic properties is desired, as with the diabetic patient. The non-nutritive sweeteners do not impart the characteristic viscosity of syrups and require the addition of viscosity adjusting agents such as methylcellulose. The polyols, though less sweet than sucrose, have the advantage of providing favourable viscosity, reducing cap-locking and in some cases acting as co-solvents and preservatives. A 70% sorbitol solution is commercially available for use as a vehicle.

Label and storage: Syrup should be kept in well-closed containers and stored at temperature below 30°C. Generally, syrups are stored at room temperature in tightly closed bottle and well-filled bottles in cool dark place. A low temperature, about 25°C is suitable for preservation.

Preservatives in syrups: The amount of preservatives required in syrup varies with the proportions of water available for microbial growth. Among the preservatives, glycerine, benzoic acid (0.1% to 0.2%), sodium benzoate (0.1 to 0.2%) and combination of methyl, propyl, and butyl parabens totaling 0.1% are most commonly used.

Advantages:

1. Syrups has ability to disguise bad taste of drug and can be administered easily to children.
2. Thick character of syrup has soothing effect on irritated tissues of throat.
3. Contain little or no alcohol.
4. Easy to adjust the dose for a child's weight
5. Resistant to microbial growth.
6. Attractive for youngsters.

Disadvantages:

1. Patients who have to consume food having less calories should be aware of amount of sugar present in syrup.
2. Patient taking syrups regularly are at risk of dental carries.
3. Not suitable for diabetic patients.
4. Crystallization of sugar takes place if is container is left open.

Method of Preparation: Syrups should be carefully prepared in clean equipment to prevent contamination. Preparation of syrup depends on the physical and chemical characteristics of the substance employed for its preparation. Four methods are commonly used for preparation of syrups.

1. **Agitation without Heat:** This method is used for the preparation of syrups to contain volatile and thermally unstable substances and when syrups are to be made rapidly. In this process, active substance is added in solution and agitated in a glass-stoppered bottle. Closing of bottle is necessary to protect the syrup from contamination and loss of solution during the process. For preparation of large quantities, glass lined tank with mechanical agitators is employed. This method is used for the preparation of wide variety of syrups. Cough syrups are commonly prepared by this process, (e.g. Codeine Syrup, Ephedrine Sulfate Syrup etc.)

2. **Solution with heat:** This process is generally preferred as it is simple and less time consuming method, particularly if the constituents are not effected by heat and are non-volatile in nature. In this process sucrose is added in the aqueous solution and heated till the sucrose is dissolved completely. Adding remaining amount of distilled water makes-up volume of the solution. If the syrups contain any substances which are coagulated, it can be separated subsequently by straining. Excessive heating of syrups at the boiling temperature is undesirable because more or less inversion of the sucrose occurs with an increased tendency to ferment. Syrups cannot be sterilized in an autoclave without some caramelization. This is indicated by a yellowish or brownish colour resulting from

the formation of caramel by the action of heat upon sucrose. The concentration of the syrup is measured using saccharometer if the specific gravity of the solution is known. Excessive heating of syrup is not suitable because more inversion of sucrose occurs with the increase in temperature. Syrups cannot be sterilized in autoclave without caramelization. This solution is converted in yellowish to brown colour due to formation of caramel by the effect of heat on sucrose.

3. **Addition of a medicated liquid:** This method is used in those cases in which tinctures, fluid extracts or other medicated substances in liquid form are added to syrup to medicate it. Syrups made in this way usually develop precipitates because alcohol is often an ingredient of the liquids used, and the resinous and oil substances dissolved by the alcohol precipitate when mixed with the syrup, producing unsightly preparations. It is necessary to take care that medicated substance should not get precipitated in this process. A modified process can be used which consist of mixing the fluid extract or tincture with the water, allowing the mixture to stand to permit the separation of insoluble constituents, filtering and then dissolving the sucrose in the filtrate. It is obvious that this procedure is not permissible when the precipitated ingredients are the valuable medicinal agents.

4. **Percolation:** In this process, purified water or an aqueous solution is allowed to pass slowly through a bed of crystalline sucrosein, a cylindrical percolator. A pledget of cotton is put in the neck of the percolator and purified water or aqueous solution is added in the percolator containing sucrose. The flow rate is controlled by the stopcock and maintained such that drops appear in rapid succession. If required, a small portion of liquid is re-passed through the percolator to dissolve the sugar completely in the liquid or aqueous solvent. A coarse granular sugar must be used; otherwise it will coalesce into a compact mass, which the liquid cannot permeate.

5. **Reconstitution:** To improve stability and minimize microbial contamination, dry syrup formulations can be prepared and purified water is added just prior to dispensing or use.

   Although the hot method is quickest, it is not applicable to syrups of thermolabile or volatile ingredients. When using heat, temperature must be carefully controlled to avoid decomposing and darkening the syrup (caramelization). When heat is used in the preparation of syrups, inversion of a slight portion of the sucrose may take place. This reaction is termed inversion because invert sugar (dextrose plus levulose) is formed.

$$C_{12}H_{22}O_{11} + H_2O \rightarrow C_6H_{12}O_6 \qquad + C_6H_{12}O_6$$

Sucrose   Dextrose (glucose)   Levulose (fructose)

The speed of inversion is increased greatly by the presence of acids. The levulose formed during inversion is sweeter than sucrose, and thus the resulting syrup is sweeter than the original syrup. The levulose formed during the hydrolysis also is responsible for the darkening of syrup. If a sugar solution is excessively heated, the sweet taste is destroyed and a dark brown liquid is formed. This process is known as caramelization.

8.2.9 Elixirs

The USP XVII defines elixirs as clear, sweetened hydro-alcoholic liquids intended for oral use containing flavouring substances or active medicinal agents. Their primary solvents are alcohol and water, with glycerin, sorbitol and syrup sometimes as an additional solvent and/or sweetening agents. They are prepared by simple solution or admixture of the several ingredients. They are used either as vehicles or for the therapeutic effect of the medicinal substances that they contain. According to their definition, elixirs are divided into two groups:

1. **Flavored Elixirs:** It is used for flavour and vehicles in prescriptions, for example, Aromatic Elixir USP.
2. **Medicated Elixirs:** It is used for the therapeutic effect or property of the medicinally active agent or as vehicle for other drugs. The examples of medicated elixirs are Dexamethasone Elixir USP, Phenobarbital Elixir USP etc.

Elixirs have low viscosity than syrups thus flow more freely. It contains very less use of agents that increase viscosity like sucrose. There is no clear cut difference between elixirs and syrups, but the amount of alcohol in elixir may vary greatly, for example, Compound Benzaldehyde Elixir (3 to 5%) and Aromatic Elixir USP (21 to 23%). Similarly, distinction between some of the medicated syrups and elixirs is also not much clear however elixir must contain alcohol. Elixirs also may contain glycerin and syrup added to increase the solubility of the medicinal agent, for sweetening purposes or to decrease the pharmacological effects of the alcohol. Some elixirs contain propylene glycol as a satisfactory substitute for both glycerin and alcohol. To call a formulation as elixir, it must be hydroalcoholic solution. Elixir are used as flavours and vehicles for drug substances (e.g. Aromatic Elixir USP). Elixirs are sometimes better choice over solid dosage forms as certain adverse effects such as mucosal erosions may be eliminated or reduced if potassium chloride is administered in elixir than in a solid dosage form.

Elixirs contain alcohol thus incompatible or precipitate tragacanth, acacia, and agar from aqueous solutions, inorganic salts from similar solutions. So such substances should be absent from the aqueous phase or should be present in such concentrations that there is no danger of precipitating on standing. In addition, alcohol increases the saline taste of bromides so the formulator has to seek some other solvent during these conditions. Aqueous solutions added to elixir will cause a partial precipitation of ingredients due to the reduced alcohol content of the final preparation. Usually, however, the alcohol content of the mixture is not sufficiently high to cause separation. As vehicle for tinctures and fluid extracts, the elixirs generally cause a separation of extractive matters from these products due to a reduction of the alcoholic content. Syrup is the best choice when taste is the main concern.

Dry elixirs: Dry elixirs are the formulations in which non-steroidal anti-inflammatory drug (NSAID) and alcohol are encapsulated. Dextrin is used for encapsulation. As a result, the solubility will be enhanced and so the bioavailability of the drug.

Advantages:

1.   Maintain both water-soluble and alcohol-soluble components in solution.
2.   They are more stable.
3.   Easily prepared by simple solution method.
4.   Elixirs have low viscosity than syrups.
5.   They flow more freely as it contains low amount of sucrose which impart viscosity.

Disadvantages:

1.   Less effective than syrups in masking taste of medicated substances.
2.   Contains alcohol, accentuates saline taste of bromides.

Components: Elixir along with drug mainly contain alcohol and water. In addition, glycerine, sorbitol, propylene glycol, preservatives and flavouring agents are also added to enhance drug solubility, product stability, palatability and patient compliance. The solvents are often used to increase the solubility of the drug substance as well as to mask undesired taste in the dosage form. Glycerine is used to enhance the solubility of drug or to make preparation sweet, for example, Phenobarbital Elixir USP.

Method of preparation: Elixirs are prepared more easily than syrups as they contain fewer amounts of ingredients that are to be dissolved. If formulation has water and alcohol soluble ingredients, the following procedure is generally followed.

1.   Add all the water soluble ingredients to water and dissolve them.

2.   Mix sucrose in above solution and allow it dissolve completely.

3.   Dissolve all the alcohol soluble ingredients in alcohol.

4.   Add the first solution to second solution.

5.   To make elixir clear, filter it and make-up the final volume with water.

Sucrose will enhance the viscosity and reduces the solubility of water. To make the elixir clear which is compulsory, talc or siliceous earth are used as adsorbents for unwanted substances to be removed from preparation.

1. Aromatic Elixir, USP

Compound Orange Spirit	12 mL
Syrup	375 mL
Talc	30 g
Alcohol and Purified water, each q.s.t. make	1000 mL

Preparation: Add to the compound orange spirit, sufficient quantity of alcohol to make 250 mL, add to this the syrup in several portions, agitating vigorously after each addition and then add in the same manner, the required quantity of purified water. Mix the talc with the liquid and filter through a filter wetted with diluted alcohol, returning the filtrate until a clear liquid is obtained. Compound Orange Spirit is used to ensure a uniform proportion of the several oils (i.e. orange, lemon, coriander, and anise), in every lot of the elixir. The alcoholic solution also preserves the delicate flavours of orange and lemon for a considerable time.

Uses: Pleasantly flavoured vehicle used in the preparation of many elixirs.

2. Red Aromatic Elixir, NF

Amaranth solution	14 mL
Aromatic Elixir, q.s.t. make	1000 mL

Preparation: Mix the ingredients.

Use: A red-coloured, flavoured vehicle.

3. Compound Benzaldehyde Elixir, NF

Benzaldehyde	0.5 mL
Vanillin	1 g
Orange flower water	150 mL
Alcohol	50 mL
Syrup	400 mL
Purified Water, q.s.t. make	1000 mL

Preparation: Dissolve the benzaldehyde and the vanillin in alcohol; add the syrup, orange flower water and sufficient quantity of purified water in several portions, shaking the mixture thoroughly after each addition, to make 1000 mL. Filter, if necessary, until clear.

Uses: Vehicle for administering bromides and other salts, especially when a low alcoholic content is desired.

4. Three Bromides Elixir, NF

Ammonium bromide	80 g
Potassium bromide	80 g
Sodium bromide	80 g
Amaranth solution	3 mL
Compound benzaldehyde Elixir q.s.	3 mL
Purified water q.s.t. make	1000 mL

Preparation: Dissolve the bromides in 800 mL of Compound Benzaldehyde Elixir, add the amaranth solution and sufficient compound benzaldehyde elixir to make the product measure 1000 mL. Filter, if necessary, until clear.

Use: Sedative action from bromine ion.

8.2.10 Liniments

Liniments are solutions or mixtures of various substances in oil, alcoholic solutions of soap, or emulsions, may contain suitable antimicrobial preservatives and are intended for external application. These preparations may be of liquid or semiliquid type. They were once called embrocation. Liniments usually are applied with friction and rubbing of the skin. Liniments should not be applied to skin that is bruised or broken. The oil or soap base provides ease of application and massage. Alcoholic liniments are used for their rubefacient, counterirritant, mildly astringent and penetrating effect as they penetrate the skin more easily than oil base liniments. The oily liniments are milder in their action but are more useful when massage is required. Depending on ingredients present liniments may function solely as protective coatings, for example, White Liniment BP.

1. White Liniment BP

Oleic acid	85 mL
Turpentine oil	250 mL
Dilute ammonia solution	45 mL
Ammonium chloride	12.5 g
Purified water	625 mL

Liniments for other use contain antipruritics, astringents, emollients, or analgesics and are classified on the basis of their active ingredient. Liniments usually contain methyl salicylate, menthol and camphor in their preparations.

2. **Compound Calamine Liniment**

Calamine	100 g
Zinc oxide	50 g
Wool fat	25 g
Zinc stearate	25 g
Yellow soft paraffin	250 g
Liquid paraffin	550 g

3. **Camphor Liniment, NF, BP**

Camphor	200 g
Cottonseed oil q.s.t.	1000 g

Procedure: Place the cottonseed oil into a suitable dry flask or bottle, heat on a steam bath, add camphor and stopper the container securely. Agitate to dissolve the camphor without further heating. The liniment should never be prepared in an open dish, because much of the camphor will volatilize upon heating.

Uses: Mild counterirritant for inflamed joints, sprains, rheumatism and in other inflammatory conditions such as cold in throat and chest, in infants and children.

4. **Camphor and Soap Liniment, NF**

Camphor, in small pieces	45 g
Soap, dried and granulated	60 g
Rosemary Oil	10 mL
Alcohol	700 mL
Purified Water, q.s.t.	1000 mL

Procedure: Dissolve camphor and rosemary oil in alcohol, add the soap and sufficient quantity of purified water to measure 1000 mL. Agitate to dissolve the soap, set aside in a cool place for 24 hours and filter. The official hard soap should be used; soap made from animal oils will cause felatinization. If soap shaving from bar soap are used, dry thoroughly and then run through a mill or grater.

Uses: Local irritant, mild rubefacient, and weak local anesthetic for sprains, bruises and rheumatism. It also forms the basis for other liniments.

Label: Liniments are applications and therefore labelled clearly as "For External Use Only".

Packaging: Liniments should be kept in well-closed containers and stored at temperature below 30°C. Generally, liniments are stored at room temperature in tightly closed bottle and well-filled bottles in cool dark place.

8.2.11 Lotions

Lotions are usually liquid suspensions or dispersions intended for external application to the body. They may be prepared by following methods.

1. **Trituration:** Triturating the ingredients to a smooth paste and then cautiously adding the remaining liquid phase or in larger quantities by the use of high-speed mixers or homogenizers. Classical example is the Calamine Lotion, which consists of finely powdered insoluble solids held in more or less permanent suspension by the presence of suspending agents and/or surface active agents.

2. **Chemical interaction:** Lotions can be prepared by chemical interaction in the liquid. For example, White Lotion, a freshly prepared formulation that does not contain a suspending agent. The second type of formulation is the o/w type stabilized by a surface active agent, for example, Benzyl Benzoate Lotion.

3. **Solution method:** Some Lotions are clear solutions and the active ingredients are water soluble substances. For example, Dimethisoqun Hydrochloride Lotion.

Lotions are usually applied without friction. The insoluble matter should be finely divided as particles approaching colloidal dimensions are more soothing to inflamed areas and are more effective in contact with infected surfaces. A wide variety of ingredients may be added to the preparation to produce better dispersion or to accentuate the cooling, soothing, drying, or protective properties of the lotion. A good example of suspending agent is bentonite. Methylcellulose or sodium carboxymethylcellulose will localize and hold the active ingredient in contact with affected site. A formulation containing glycerin will keep the skin moist for a considerable period of time. Addition of alcohol to the formula will accentuate the drying and cooling effects.

Uses: Dermatologist frequently prescribe lotions containing anesthetics, antiseptic, astringents, germicides, protective or screening agents, to be used in treating and preventing various types of skin disease and dermatitis. Antihistamines, benzocaine, calamine, resorcin, steroids, sulfur, zinc oxide, and zirconium oxide are common ingredients in unofficial lotions.

Label and Storage: Lotions tend to separate or stratify on long standing, so a "SHAKE WELL" label is required for them. All lotions should be labelled "FOR EXTERNAL USE ONLY".

(a) Benzyl Benzoate Lotion, USP, BP

Benzyl Benzoate	250 mL
Triethanolamine	5 g
Oleic acid	20 g
Water to make	1000 mL

Preparation: Mix together the triethanolamine and oleic acid add the benzyl benzoate and mix well. Transfer the mixture to a suitable container of about 2000 mL capacity, add 250 mL of water and shake thoroughly. Add the remaining 500 mL of water and shake again.

Uses: Scabicide. It is applied with a brush after the entire body has been thoroughly scrubbed with soft soap and hot water. A second coating is applied when the first is dry and the lotion is left on the body for 24 hrs. Then the body is again bathe thoroughly and dressed in clean clothes.

Application: Adults require from 120 – 180 mL. Children require from 60 – 90 mL.

Caution: Do not apply to the face.

(b) Calamine Lotion, USP

Calamine	80 g
Zinc Oxide	80 g
Glycerin	20 mL
Bentonite Magma	20 mL
Calcium Hydroxide Solution to make	1000 mL

Preparation: Dilute the bentonite magma with an equal volume of calcium hydroxide solution. Mix the powders intimately with the glycerin and about 100 mL of the dilute magma, triturating until smooth, uniform paste is formed. Gradually incorporate the remainder of the diluted magma. Finally add enough calcium hydroxide solution to make 1000 mL and shake well.

Uses: Astringent and protective.

Label: Shake lotions thoroughly before dispensing. If a more viscous consistency is desired, the quantity of bentonite magma may be increased to not more than 400 mL.

(c) Phenolated Calamine Lotion, USP

Liquefied Phenol	10 mL
Calamine Lotion to make	1000 mL

Preparation: Mix the ingredients thoroughly.

Uses: Astringent and protective for skin diseases. Shake well before using.

(d) White Lotion, USP

Zinc Sulfate	40 g
Sulfurated Potash	40 g
Purified Water, to make	1000 mL

Preparation: Dissolve the zinc sulfate and the sulfurated potash separately, each in 450 mL of purified water, and filter each solution. Add slowly the sulfurated potash solution to the zinc sulfate solution with constant stirring. Then add sufficient amount of purified water and mix. The lotion is a result of the chemical reaction between zinc sulfate and sulfurated potash and can be illustrated as follows:

$$ZnSO_4 \quad + \quad K_2S_3 \quad + \quad K_2SO_4 \quad + \quad ZnS \quad \rightarrow \quad 2S$$

Zinc Sulfate   Sulfurated Potash   Potassium Sulfate   Zinc Sulfate   Sulfur

The sulfurated potash solution should be added to zinc sulfate solution with constant stirring. This ensures a fine dispersion of the insoluble precipitates, upon long standing tends to become lumpy and yellowish in colour.

Uses: Topically as astringent and protective.

Label: Lotion should be freshly prepared and shaken thoroughly before dispensing.

MODEL QUESTIONS

1. Define Monophasic liquid dosage form. Give its classification.

2. Define gargles. Give formulation of gargles.

3. Give formulation of mouthwashes.

4. Explain formulation of throat paint.

5. Define and give advantages and disadvantages of nasal drops and eardrops.

6. Define and give classification of syrup. Explain method of preparation of syrup.

7. What is the difference between liniment and lotion?

8. Write a note on:

   (i) Enema

   (ii) Invert syrup

   (iii) Elixir

Chapter 9...

Biphasic Liquids : Suspensions

LEARNING OBJECTIVES

A liquid dosage form that consists of a dispersion of tiny undissolved drug particles suspended in the solution. When the solution is shaken, the particles disburse to create a uniform heterogeneous mixture.

The objectives of this chapter includes

- To recognize the route of drug administration through suspensions.
- To know the principle of formulating stable suspension.
- To understand basic formulation considerations and method of preparing suspension.
- To know about storage, packaging, uses and special instructions for suspensions.
- To describe various physical properties of suspensions.

9.1 INTRODUCTION

Drug substances are rarely administered alone. They are given in the form of a formulation in combination with one or more excipients that serve variety of pharmaceutical functions. Proper selection and use of these excipients produces dosage forms of different types. Excipients help to solubilize, suspend, thicken, dilute, emulsify, stabilize, preserve, colour, favour, and fashion drug substances into effective and appealing dosage forms. Every dosage form is unique in its physical and pharmaceutical characteristics. Since decades among all the pharmaceutical products available, oral drug delivery has gained a higher scope and popularity and has been widely employed for the systemic delivery of drugs. The positive aspect regarding the oral dosage form which created its high level of acceptance was its ease of administration, patient compliance and stability of formulation. For drugs that are insoluble in the delivery vehicle, bitter taste, has low drug stability and if required to achieve controlled/sustained release, commonly used solution form is not suitable. In such case drugs are formulated as suspension to overcome aforementioned issues.

Suspensions are important pharmaceutical dosage forms widely in use today. They are dispersions of solids in liquids. Owing to their versatility, they are often used in situations where an 'emergency' formulation is required. A pharmaceutical suspension is a coarse dispersion in which internal phase consists of insoluble solid particles of a specific range of size is dispersed uniformly throughout the external aqueous or organic or oily liquid phase with aid of single or combination of suspending agent. According to BP 'oral suspensions are oral liquids containing one or more active ingredients suspended in a suitable vehicle'.

The internal phase consists of insoluble solid particles of a size 0.5 to 5 microns which is maintained uniformly throughout the suspending vehicle with aid of single or combination of suspending agent. The external phase (suspending medium) is generally aqueous in some instance, may be an organic or oily liquid for non-oral use. However, it is difficult and also impractical to impose a sharp boundary between the suspensions and the dispersions having finer particles. Therefore, in many instances, suspensions may have smaller particles than 0.5 mm and may show some characteristics typical to colloidal dispersions, such as Brownian movement. There are two types of insoluble solids which constitute the internal or dispersed phase.

1. **Diffusible solids:** These are insoluble solids that are light in weight and easily wetted by water. They get mixed readily with aqueous medium, and remain dispersed over long time for an adequate dose to be measured. They sediment slowly to enable satisfactory dose removal after redispersion. Settled solids of this type redisperse easily. Examples include magnesium trisilicate, light magnesium carbonate, bismuth carbonate and light kaolin.

2. **Indiffusible solids:** These are insoluble solids that sediment too rapidly and require the addition of other materials to reduce settling rate to an acceptable level. Most of these solids are not easily wetted, and particles forms large porous aggregates in the liquid, whereas others may remain on the liquid surface. These solids do not remain evenly distributed in the vehicle for long enough to withdraw an adequate dose to be measured. They may not redisperse easily. Examples for internal use includes aspirin, phenol barbital, sulfadirnidine and for external use calamine, hydrocortisone, sulphur and zinc oxide

Basic requirements of suspension

1. The suspended particles should not settle rapidly.
2. The particle should not form a cake on settling
3. The sediment produced must be easily re-suspended by moderate shaking.
4. The viscosity of suspension should be such that the preparation can be easily poured.
5. It should have an elegant smooth appearance.
6. The medicament must stay in suspended for long enough to allow withdrawal of accurate quantity of drug in each dose as measured.
7. It should have constant particle size and size distribution so that the product is free from a gritty texture.
8. It should be chemically and physically stable.
9. It should be free from gritting particles (external use).

Applications of suspension

1. To overcome the instability of certain drug in aqueous solution:
   (a) Insoluble derivative formulated as suspension, for example, Oxytetracycline HCl (unstable) as its calcium salt (stable).
   (b) Reduce the contact time between solid drug particles and dispersion media to increase the stability, for example, Ampicillin powder for reconstitution.
   (c) A drug that degrades in the presence of water can be suspended in non-aqueous vehicles, for example, phenoxymethypencillin in coconut oil and tetracycline HCl in mineral oil.
2. Suspensions can be used to mask the taste of bitter drugs, for example, Paracetamol Suspension, Chloramphenicol Palmitate Suspension.
3. Some materials are needed to be present as finely divided forms to increase the surface area to adsorb some toxins, for example, M-cid$^®$ (Mg carbonate) and Care+$^®$ (Mg trisilicate).
4. Suspension can be used for topical applications wherein after evapouration of dispersing media, the drug will be left as light deposit, for example, Calamine lotion BP.
5. Suspensions can be used for parental administration intramuscular (i.m.) to control arte of absorption, for example, Betamox LA$^®$ (Amoxicillin).
6. In vaccines to absorb antigen, for example, Diphtheria and Tetanus vaccines.
7. As an x-ray contrast media used for cholecystography, bronchography and myelography via oral and rectal administration, for example, Iopanoic acid, Propyliodone, etc.
8. In aerosol systems, suspension of active agents in mixture of propellants, for example, Ventidos$^®$ (Salbutamol).

9.2 FORMS OF SUSPENSIONS

The common pharmaceutical suspension preparations are differentiated into suspensions, gels, magmas and milks, lotions, ear drops, enemas, inhalations, and mixtures for oral use.

(i) **Suspensions:** Simple suspension is the insoluble solid dispersed in a liquid. The stability considerations suggest that the manufacture of drugs in dry form is ideal. They are reconstituted as suspensions using a suitable vehicle before administration, for example, Cephalexin Powder (Keflex$^®$) and Azithromycin Powder (Zmax$^®$)

(ii) **Gels:** Gels are semisolid two-phase systems consisting of small inorganic particles suspended in a liquid medium to form a network of small discrete particles, for example, Aluminium Hydroxide Gel USP.

(iii) **Magmas and Milks:** Magmas and milk are aqueous suspensions of larger insoluble, inorganic drugs. Freshly prepared magmas and milks are thick and viscous and thus require no suspending agents, for example, Bentonite Magma, Milk of Magnesia etc.

(iv) Lotions: Lotions are suspensions which are intended to be applied to the unbroken skin without friction, for example, Calamine Lotion (Lacto®) and Hydrocortisone Lotion USP.

(v) Ear drops: Ear drops suspensions are topical otic (ear) preparations, acidic in nature (pH 5), and may have less side effects, for example, Gentamicin/ Betamethasone/Clotrimazole Ear Drops (Otomax®).

(vi) Enemas: Enema suspensions are fluid preparations containing un-dissolved solids in aqueous medium injected into the lower bowel by way of the rectum for retention or evacuation, for example, Mesalamine Rectal Suspension USP

(vii) Inhalations: Inhalation suspensions are fluid preparations containing sterile undissolved solids in suitable non-aqueous propellant or propellant mixture inhaled via jet nebulizer, for example, Budesonide Suspension (Pulmicort®).

(viii) Mixtures: Mixtures are oral liquids containing one or more active ingredients, dissolved, suspended or dispersed in a suitable vehicle. Suspended solids may separate slowly on standing, but are easily re-dispersed on shaking, for example, Kaolin Mixture with Pectin.

(ix) Injections: Suspensions for injection contain less than 5% of sterile drug in solid form with mean particle diameter within 5-10 μm dispersed in suitable liquid.

Advantages:

1. **Stability:** Suspension can improve chemical stability of insoluble drug, for example, Procaine Penicillin G.

2. **Choice of solvent:** If the drug is insoluble in water and solvents other than water are not acceptable, suspension is the only choice, for example, parenteral corticosteroid.

3. **Prolonged action:** Suspension has a sustaining effect. Because, before absorption solid particles should be dissolved which takes some time, for example, Protamine Zinc Insulin Suspension and Procaine Penicillin G Suspension.

4. **Mask the taste:** Suspension can mask the unpleasant/bitter taste of drug, for example, Chloramphenicol palmitate. Chloramphenicol base is very bitter in taste; hence the insoluble chloramphenicol palmitate is used which does not have the bitter taste.

5. **Palatability and convenience:** Insoluble drugs may be more palatable. Suspended insoluble powders are easy to swallow. Lotions will leave a cooling layer of medicament on the skin. Suspended solids may slowly separate on standing but are easily re-dispersed.

6. **Bioavailability:** Drugs in suspension exhibit a higher bioavailability compared to other dosage forms (except solution) due to its large surface area, higher dissolution rate, for example, antacid suspensions, provides immediate relief from hyperacidity than its tablet chewable tablet form.

Disadvantages:

1. Physical stability, sedimentation and compaction can cause problems.

2. Susceptible to degradation and the possibility of chemical reaction between the ingredients in the solution where there is water as a catalyst.

3. Uniform and accurate dose cannot be achieved unless suspensions are packed in unit dosage form.
4. Suspensions are bulky, difficult to transport and prone to container breakages.
5. Preparation requires shaking before use.
6. Storage conditions can affect disperse system.
7. Suspensions are difficult to formulate.

9.3 CLASSIFICATION OF SUSPENSIONS

(I) Based on therapeutic class:

1. Antacid suspensions, for example, Magaldrate and Simethicone Oral Suspension (Clodrate®).
2. Antibacterial suspensions, for example, Ciprofloxacin Oral Suspension (Cipro®).
3. Analgesic suspensions, for example, Paracetamol oral suspension (Panadol®).
4. Anthelmintic suspensions, for example, Albendazole oral suspension (Wintil®).
5. Anticonvulsant suspensions, for example, Phenytoin oral suspension (Dilantin®).
6. Antifungal suspensions, for example, Posaconazole Oral Suspension (Noxafil®).
7. Dry antibiotic powders for oral suspensions, for example, Doxycycline Oral Suspension (Vibramycin®), Azithromycin Oral Suspension (Zithromax®).
8. Anticancer suspensions for intravenous injection, for example, Paclitaxel for i.v. inj. (Abraxane®).
9. Contraceptive suspensions for intramuscular injection, for example, Medroxyprogesterone Acetate Suspension for i.m. inj. (Depo-Provera®).
10. Antidiarrheal suspensions for Intramuscular injection, for example, Ampicillin Suspension for i.m. inj. (Ampivil®).
11. Topical lotions for various skin conditions, for example, Hydrocortisone Topical Lotions (Cortizone-10®).

(II) Based on particle size:

1. Nano suspension (10 -100 nm), for example, Celecoxib Suspension.
2. Colloidal suspension (1nm- 0.5 mm) for example, Acacia Suspension.
3. Coarse suspension (> 0.5 mm) for example, Calamine Lotion.

(III)Based on the proportion of solids:

1. **Dilute suspensions:** Solid content 2-10% for example, Cortisone Acetate Suspension and Prednesolone Acetate Suspension.
2. **Concentrated suspensions:** Solid content 10-50% for example, Zinc Oxide Suspension for external use, Procaine Penicillin G Injection, Antacid Suspension, etc.

(IV) Based on nature and behaviour of solids:

1. Flocculated suspensions, for example, Cefuroxime Axetil for Oral Suspension.
2. Deflocculated suspensions for example, Paracetamol Oral Suspension Drops (Parald®).

(V) Based on route of administration:

1. Oral Suspension: for example, Calcium Oxytetracycline HCl Suspension.
2. Topical Suspension: for example, Calamine Lotion.
3. Parenteral Suspension: for example, Desoxycorticosterone Pivalate Suspension (Zycortal®).
4. Ophthalmic Suspension: Ciprofloxacin and Dexamethasone Ear Drops (Ciprodex®).
5. Inhalation Suspension: Budesonide Suspension (Pulmicort®).

(VI) Mode of dispensing

1. Extemporaneous suspensions, for example, Rifampin Suspension for i.v. infusion (Rifadin®).
2. Reconstituted suspensions, for example, Tetracycline Suspension (Sumycin®).

9.4 COMPONENTS OF SUSPENSION FORMULATION

The pharmaceutical suspension must be physically and chemically stable over the required time, possess a viscosity that allows it to be used for its intended purpose, be easily reconstituted upon shaking and easy to manufacture and be acceptable in use to the patient. Thus, in order to deal in-depth, with these requirements selection of suitable excipients is of prime importance in preparing good quality suspension.

The main components of any suspension are insoluble solid drug particles and liquid medium. The other includes excipients such as suspending agent, surfactant, viscosity enhancer, preservative, antioxidants (stabilizers) flavouring agent, sweetener, colours, buffers, etc.

(a) Wetting agents:

Wetting agents are added in suspension to reduce interfacial tension between solid particles and dispersion liquid. Hydrophilic solid particles are easily wetted by water while hydrophobic particles are not. However, hydrophobic, particles are easily wetted by non-polar liquids. The extent of wetting by water is dependent on the hydrophilicity of the solid particles. If the particles are more hydrophilic it finds less difficulty in wetting by water. The inability of solids for particle wetting is due to higher interfacial tension exhibited by air (non-polar) at particle surface. Wetting agents work by reducing the contact angle and interfacial tension between the dispersed phase and dispersed medium. A liquid phase containing suitable wetting agent helps to displace air at the surface particles.

Non-ionic surfactants: Polyoxyethylene sorbitan fatty acid esters (Polysorbate, Tween ®), Polyoxyethylene 15 hydroxystearate (Macrogol 15 hydroxystearate, Solutol HS15 ®), Polyoxyethylene castor oil derivatives (Cremophor ® EL, ELP, RH 40), Polyoxyethylene stearates (Myrj®), Sorbitan fatty acid esters (Span ®), Polyoxyethylene alkyl ethers (Brij®), Polyoxyethylene nonylphenol ether (Nonoxynol ®).

Cationic Surfactants: Phosphatidyl choline

Anionic surfactants: Docusate sodium and sodium lauryl sulfate

Amphoteric surfactants: Cocamidopropyl amino betaine

Hygroscopic liquids: Alcohol and glyrecin

Hydrophilic colloids: Acacia, tragacanth, alginates, guar gum, pectin, gelatin, wool fat, egg yolk, bentonite, veegum, methylcellulose etc.

Ionic surfactants are not generally used because they are not compatible with many adjuvant and causes change in pH. Surfactants are used in low strengths because of their inherent solubilization property as well as toxicity at higher concentrations. Hydrophilic colloids are used to coat hydrophobic drug particles in one or more than one layer to provide hydrophilicity to drug particles to facilitate wetting. They cause deflocculation of suspension because force of attraction is declined.

(b) Flocculating Agents:

Flocculating agents are suspending agents which help to entrap particle and reduce sedimentation of particles. Flocculating agents are added to enhance particle redispersability. The best approach to prepare stable suspension is to achieve a controlled flocculation of the particles. Controlled flocculation of particles is achieved by adding flocculating agents such as electrolytes, surfactants and polymers.

Electrolytes: Electrolytes are added to floc the drug particles. Solid particles dispersed in a suspension may have charge in relation to their surrounding vehicle, because of selective adsorption of a particular ionic species present in the vehicle or ionization of functional group of the molecules in the particle. The ions that gave the particle its charge, serve to repel the particles. Electrolytes acts as flocculating agents by reducing the electrical barrier between the particles, thus, decrease the zeta potential. This leads to decrease in repulsion potential and makes the particle come together to form loosely arranged structure (floccules). The flocculating power increases with the valency of the ions. Calcium ions are more powerful than sodium ions because the valency of calcium is two whereas sodium has valency of one. Polymeric flocculating agents are branched-chain molecules that form a gel-like network within the system and become adsorbed on to the surfaces of the dispersed particles, thus holding them in a flocculated state. The examples of most widely used electrolytes include the sodium salts of acetates, phosphates and citrates, bismuth subnitrate, monobasic potassium phosphate and silicates.

Surfactants: Ionic (Tween 80) and non-ionic (sodium lauryl sulfate) surfactants are used to control flocculation. The concentration of surfactants required to achieve flocculation is critical as these substances may also act as wetting agents to achieve dispersion. Optimum concentrations of surfactants bring down the surface free energy by reducing the surface tension between liquid medium and solid particles. The particles possessing less surface free energy are attracted towards each other by Van der Waal forces and forms loose agglomerates.

Polymers: Natural polymers are long chain, high molecular weight compounds containing active groups spaced along their length. These polymers act as flocculating agents. One part of the chain is adsorbed on the particle surface while the other projecting out in the dispersion medium. Bridging between these portions leads to the formation of floccules. Polymers exhibit pseudo-plastic flow in solution promoting the physical stability of suspension.

Natural agents

(i)   Animal source, for example, Gelatine
(ii)   Plant source, for example, Acacia, Tragacanth, Starch, Sea weed (alginates)
(iii) Mineral sources, for example, Bentonite, Kaoline

Semi-synthetic agents

(i)   Hydroxyethyl cellulose
(ii)   Sodium carboxymethylcellulose
(iii) Methylcellulose
(iv)   Microcrystalline cellulose

Synthetic agents

(i)   Carboxypolymethylene (carbopol)
(ii)   Polyvinyl alcohol
(iii) Polyvinyl pyrrolidone iodine complex (PVP-I)

(c) Deflocculating agents:

Flocculating agents (non-ionic wetting agents) decreases the interfacial tension between the particles and liquid medium to achieve deflocculation. These agents are not effective in wetting as they have low capacity to reduce surface tension and contact angle. The ionic surfactant based on the charge at particle can produce both flocculated and deflocculated suspension. Electrolytes generally reduce the zeta potential and increase in flocculation whereas ionic and non-ionic surfactants cause flocculation. Various polymers have been employed to form network to assist in flocculation. Care must be exercised to avoid too high viscosity which is undesirable as it causes difficulty in pouring and administration of suspension. In addition, it may affect drug absorption as they adsorb on to the particle surface which may suppress drug dissolution. Although, these substances added to reduce the sedimentation of particles, not necessarily completely eliminate the particle settling. Sometime deflocculated particles in a structured vehicle may form solid hard cake upon long storage. The caking may be avoided by forming flocculated particles in a structured vehicle.

(d) Solvents and co-solvents:

The most commonly used solvents in suspensions are distilled water or deionized water, Water-alcohol mixture, alcohol, glycerin, polyethylene glycol, polypropylene glycol and non-aqueous vehicles for topical use. The mechanism by which they provide wetting is that they are miscible with water and reduce liquid air interfacial tension. Liquid penetrates in individual particle and facilitates wetting.

Structured vehicles: Structured vehicles are also called as thickening or suspending agents. They are aqueous solutions of natural and synthetic gums. These are used to increase the viscosity of the suspension. Structured vehicles are vehicles containing thixotropic polymers like acacia which are pseudo-plastic or plastic in nature. These polymers form a three-dimensional gel network structure which entrap the particles in order to avoid particle settling. During shaking, the gel network is completely destroyed so that administration is facilitated. Structured vehicles are used only in deflocculated suspensions. For example, methyl cellulose, sodium carboxy methyl cellulose, acacia, gelatin and tragacanth.

Co-solvents: Some solvents which themselves have high viscosity are used as co-solvents to enhance the viscosity of dispersion medium. Glycerin has high viscosity and the preparations are difficult to pour as well as spread on the skin. It also shows undesirable property of stickiness. It is too hygroscopic to use in undiluted form. The solvents that themselves have high viscosity and are used as co-solvents to enhance the viscosity of dispersion medium are glycerol, propylene glycol and sorbitol.

(e) Suspending agents/Thickeners:

Suspensions being heterogeneous system have least physical stability due to sedimentation and cake formation. Viscosity of suspensions is of great importance for stability and pourability of suspensions. When viscosity of the dispersion medium increases, the terminal settling velocity decreases thus the dispersed phase settle at a slower rate and they remain dispersed for longer time with providing a higher stability to the suspension. On the other hand, as the viscosity of the suspension increases, it's pourability decreases and may cause inconvenience to the patients during dose withdrawal.

Use of viscosity enhancer is one of the approaches been suggested to enhance the viscosity of suspensions. Natural gums (acacia, tragacanth), cellulose derivatives (sodium CMC, methyl cellulose), clays (bentonite, veegum), carbomers, colloidal silicon dioxide (Aerosil), and sugars (glucose, fructose) are used to enhance the viscosity of the dispersion medium. They all are known as suspending agents because of their contribution in maintaining the particles in suspended form.

(f) Buffers:

In order to encounter stability problems, all liquid formulation should be formulated to an optimum pH. Buffers are the solutions of substances which resists any change in pH when an acid or base is added. Rheology, viscosity and other properties of suspension are dependent on the pH. Thus, they are used to control the pH of the suspension products. Generally, pH of suspension should be kept between 7-9.5, preferably between 7.4-8.4. Buffers used should be compatible with other additives and simultaneously they should have less toxicity. Most commonly used buffers are salts of weak acids such as carbonates, citrates, gluconates, phosphate and tartrates.

(g) Osmotic agents:

Osmotic agents are added to produce osmotic pressure comparable to biological fluids when suspension is to be intended for ophthalmic or injectable administration. Most commonly used osmotic agents are dextrose, mannitol, sorbitol, sodium chloride, sodium sulfate, glycerol.

(h) Preservatives:

Water is the most commonly used vehicle in the preparation of suspension but is main source of microbial contamination. In addition, natural materials such as acacia and tragacanth used in suspension may be source of microbes and spores as they are highly susceptible to microbial contamination. Thus, preservatives which prevent growth of such micro-organisms are added to suspension products. Preservative action may be affected by its adsorption onto solid particles of drug, or interaction with suspending agents. Other effect of adsorption includes reduction in suspending activity of suspending agents, loss of colour, flavour and odour and change in product elegance. Useful preservatives in extemporaneous preparations include chloroform water, benzoic acid and hydroxybenzoates. For large scale production of suspension propylene glycol (5-10%), disodium EDTA (0.1%), benzalkonium chloride (0.01-0.02%), benzoic acid (0.1%), butyl paraben (0.006-0.05% in oral suspension and 0.02-0.4% in topical formulation), propylene glycol (5-10 %), bisodium edentate (0.1%), cetrimide (0.005%), chlorobutanol (0.5%), phenyl mercuric acetate (0.001-0.002%), potassium sorbate (0.1-0.2%) sodium benzoate (0.02-0.5%), sorbic acid (0.05-0.2%), methyl paraben (0.015-0.2%), etc. are used.

(i) Sweetening Agents:

Sweetening agents are used for taste masking of bitter drug particles. They are employed specifically to increase the palatability of the therapeutic agent. The use of artificial sweetening agents in formulations is increasing and, in many formulations, saccharin sodium is used either as the sole sweetening agent or in combination with sugars or sorbitol to reduce the sugar concentration in the formulation. The use of sugars in oral formulations for children and patients with diabetes mellitus is to be avoided. Following sweetening agents are used in suspension preparations.

Bulk sweeteners	:	**Sugars:** Xylose, ribose, glucose, mannose, galactose, fructose, dextrose, sucrose, maltose Hydrogenated glucose syrup

Sugar alcohols: Sorbitol, xylitol, mannitol, glycerin

Partially hydrolysed starch: Corn syrup

Artificial sweetening agents : Sodium cyclamate, sodium saccharin, aspartame, ammonium glycyrrhizinate.

(j) Flavoring Agents:

Sweetening agent alone is not capable of complete taste masking of unpleasant drugs therefore, a flavouring agent is incorporated to increase patient acceptance. The four basic taste sensations are salty, sweet, bitter and sour. It has been proposed that certain flavours should be used to mask these specific taste sensations. Most widely used flavouring agents are ginger, sarsaparilla syrup, anise oil, glucose, spearmint oil, benzaldehyde, glycerin, thyme oil, fennel oil, peppermint, raspberry, caraway oil, rose oil, cardamom, glycerrhiza, rosemary oil, cherry syrup, honey, cinnamon, lavender oil, citric acid syrup, lemon oil, clove oil, mannitol, vanilla, cocoa, nutmeg oil, tolu balsam syrup, coriander oil, orange oil, wild cherry syrup, ethyl vanillin and orange flower.

(k) Coloring agents

Colours impart preferred colour to the formulation and thus aid in identification of the certain products. The choice of colour should be associated with flavour used to improve the attractiveness by the patient. Only colours approved by regulatory agencies of particular country are used. Natural colours are obtained from mineral, plant and animal sources. Colours when used in combination with flavours, the selected one should 'match' the flavour of the formulation, for example, green with mint-flavored and red for strawberry-flavoured formulations. Mineral colours (also called as pigments) in suspension are used to colour lotions, cosmetic preparation and other external preparations. Plant colours are most widely used for oral suspension. The synthetic dyes should be used within range of 0.0005 % to 0.001 % depending upon the depth of colour required and thickness of column of the container to be viewed in it. Most widely used colours are white (titanium dioxide), blue (brilliant blue, indigo carmine, indigo), red (amaranth, carmine), yellow (tartarazine, sunset yellow, carrots, saffron), yellow to orange (Annatto seeds), green (chlorophyll), brown (caramel), reddish yellow (Madder plant), etc.

(l) Humectants

Humectants absorb moisture and prevent degradation of drugs sensitive to moisture. Total quantity of humectants should be between 0-10 % w/w. Examples of humectants most commonly used in suspensions are propylene glycol, glycerol.

(m) Antioxidant

Antioxidants are used to enhance the stability of drugs susceptible to chemical degradation by oxidation. Antioxidants are molecules (redox systems) that exhibit higher oxidative potential than the drugs. They inhibit free radical-induced drug decomposition. In aqueous solution, antioxidants are oxidized (and hence degraded) in preference to drugs and protect them from decomposition. Both water-soluble and water-insoluble antioxidants are used in suspensions depending upon nature of vehicle used. Typically, antioxidants are employed in low concentrations (0.2% w/w). Examples of antioxidants most commonly used are ascorbic acid, erythorbic acid, Na ascorbate, thioglycerol, cytosine, acetylcysteine, cystine, dithioerythreitol, dithiothreitol, glutathione, tocopherols, propyl gallate, butylated hydroxy anisole (BHA), butylated hydroxy toluene (BHT), sodium sulfate, sodium bisulfite, acetone sodium bisulfite, sodium metabisulfite, sodium sulfite, sodium formaldehyde sulfoxylate, and sodium thiosulfate, Sodium sulfateacetone and nordihydroguaiaretic acid. Antioxidants may also be employed in conjunction with chelating agents such as ethylene diamine tetraacetic acid (EDTA) and citric acid that act to form complexes with heavy-metal ions that are normally involved in oxidative degradation of drugs.

A perfect suspension is one, which provides content uniformity. The formulator must encounter important problems regarding particle size distribution, specific surface area, inhibition of crystal growth and changes in the polymorphic form. The formulator must ensure that these and other properties should not change after long term storage and do not adversely affect the performance of suspension. Choice of pH, particle size, viscosity, flocculation, taste, colour and odour are some of the most important factors that must be controlled at the time of formulation.

9.5 PREPARATION OF SUSPENSIONS

The main objective in the preparation of suspensions is to keep the suspended particles dispersed. Formulation of a pharmaceutical suspension requires knowledge of the properties of both the dispersed phase and the dispersion medium. The excipients used in the preparation of suspensions should be carefully selected. The criteria for excipient selection includes route of administration, intended application, and possible adverse effects. The following main factors required to be given a consideration during preparations of pharmaceutical suspensions.

    (I)   **Nature of suspended solid:** The particles with low interfacial tension are easily wetted by water and therefore can be suspended easily. On the contrary, particles of materials with high interfacial tensions are not easily wetted. In such cases, surfactant which reduces particles, surface tension are employed to increase wettability.

(II) Size of solid particles: The particle size plays a key role in the formulation of suspension. Care must be taken that the particles must be of small size. Preparation for parenteral and ophthalmic use must have particle size < 5µ. Reduction in particle size decreases rate of sedimentation of the suspended particles. Particles size can be reduced by milling, sieving, and grinding. Particle size has effects on rate and extent of drug absorption, dissolution, and distribution of the drug in the body. Size reduction has a limiting value that beyond particular size reduction lead to formation of a compact cake upon sedimentation.

(III) Viscosity of dispersion medium: Dispersion mediums of higher viscosities produce suspensions with slow rate of sedimentation. Higher viscosity however, affects syringability for parenteral suspensions, spreadability for topical suspensions and ease of dose withdrawal for administration in case of oral suspensions. The medium with shear thinning is always desirable so that the suspension remain viscous during storage when no shear while when shaken at the time of dose withdrawal (high shear), it becomes less viscous to facilitate ease of pourability from the container.

Apart from above mentioned factors, Nernst and zeta potential, flocculation and deflocculation, electrokinetic properties and density of the vehicle, selection of right drug and excipient, sequential step to be followed in the manufacture and preservation and storage of the product needs to be given enough consideration while preparing suspensions.

(IV) Methods of Suspension Preparation: The methods of preparing pharmaceutical suspensions are categorized as follows**:**

1. General methods

    (a) Precipitation method

        (i)   Organic solvent precipitation

        (ii)   Precipitation effected by changing the pH of the medium and

        (iii) Double decomposition

    (b) Dispersion method

        (i)   Small scale (Laboratory): using colloid mill

        (ii)   Large scale (Industrial): using mortar and pestle

2. Extemporaneous method

    (i)   From dry powders and granules for reconstitution

    (ii)   From oral solid dosage form

3. Mechanism involved

    (i)   Controlled flocculation

    (ii)   Structured vehicle

(a) Precipitation Methods

(i) Organic solvent precipitation: This method is used for water insoluble drugs. Drugs can be precipitated by dissolving them in water-miscible organic solvents such as alcohol, acetone, propylene glycol, polyethylene glycol etc. The organic phase mixture so obtained is added to distilled water under standard conditions to produce a suspension. Precipitation of components produces solid sizes in particles of the range of 1 to 5 μm. For example, prednesolone is precipitated using methanol to produce a suspension in water. This method is suitable for administration of parenteral suspensions or inhalation therapy where very fine particles are required. The limitations of this method are that harmful organic solvents are difficult to remove from preparation and occurrence of polymorph or hydrate form of crystals.

(ii) The pH change method: Some drugs are readily soluble at certain pH while at another pH, they form precipitate. Such drugs are first dissolved in the medium of favourable pH and then the solution is poured in another medium (buffer) to change the pH. The drug forms precipitate in the medium of the second pH to produce a suspension. For example, estradiol suspension is prepared by changing the pH of its aqueous solution. Estradiol is readily soluble in medium with alkaline pH (potassium or sodium hydroxide solutions). If concentrated solution of estradiol is prepared in alkaline medium and poured in to a solution of weak hydrochloric, citric or acetic acids, with agitation, estradiol gets precipitated as fine particles to produce suspension. Another example of suspension prepared by this method is insulin suspension. Insulin has an isoelectric point of approximately pH 5 and is soluble at this pH. When it is mixed with protamine (basic pH), it is readily precipitated because the pH of this system becomes 6.9 - 7.3. Protamine-Zinc-Insulin (PZI) suspension contains an excess quantity of zinc to retard the rate of absorption. British Pharmacopoeia recommends use of phosphate buffer to maintain pH in the range 6.9 - 7.3 to form the suspension.

(iii) Precipitation with double decomposition: In this method, two water soluble reagent forms a water insoluble product. For example, White Lotion NF is prepared by slowly adding zinc sulfate solution in a solution of sulphurated potash to form a precipitate of zinc polysulphide. Magnesium carbonate suspension is prepared from double decomposition of magnesium sulphate and sodium carbonate. These two substances are dissolved in water separately and the solutions are mixed at 1 : ratio. The solution is boiled to obtain concentrate. The residue of magnesium carbonate is filtered and washed with water till it becomes free of sulphate ions. The residue is dried and dispersed in medium to obtain suspension. Other example of suspension produced by this method is Aluminium Hydroxide Gel.

(b) Dispersion methods

Preparation of suspension using these methods is simple one. The powder form of the drug is directly dispersed in the liquid medium having good wetting power. Generally, dispersion medium used is water. It should be kept in mind that particles must be dispersed well in water. Dispersing powders that are not soluble in water sometimes find difficult to wet due to presence of air, fat and other contaminants on the surface of the powder.

(i) Small scale method

1. **Mortar and pestle:** Although mortar and pestle is a very old technique it is very efficient and commonly used to make suspension in small quantities (1–10 mL). In this method, solid drug is levigated or grounded or triturated gently with wetting agent or surfactant (0.5 and 2% w/v) solution. Drug powder may be treated with a water miscible material such as glycerin to aid in wetting. Upon trituration for few minutes in the mortar, it forms homogeneous paste or viscous flock. Mortar contents are transferred to the measuring device to make-up the volume with remaining suspending/flocculating agent or surfactant. The container needs to be shaken well before use as usually suspensions tend to settle with time. A proper sequence of steps is required to be followed for obtaining good quality suspension.

2. **Homogenizer:** Use of this method is common practice in pharmaceutical industry to prepare suspensions. It involves breaking of particle agglomerates that form during processing. In this method, solid form of drug is transferred to a bottle (or vial) containing cellulose and/or surfactant solution. The contents in the bottle are mixed well by manual shaking or vortexing and finally the whole dispersion is homogenized to obtain suspension.

3. **Probe sonication:** It is considered to be the most effective technique to reduce particle size significantly and produce best suspension. In this method, solid form of drug is weighed into the bottle. A cellulose and/or surfactant containing solution is added to the bottle. The vial is kept under probe sonicator/ultrasonic homogenizer to reduce particle size at known sonication amplitude. Precaution must be taken to prevent decomposition of the active by heat generated during the probe sonication.

4. **Wet ball milling:** A planetary ball mill in its rotating cylinder with steel balls grinds materials to smaller size. The drug solid and grinding balls are placed in a grinding cylinder and clamped. The milling process involves rotation of sun-wheel to clock-wise, while the cylinder shaft rotation to counter clock-wise. The opposite rotation causes the Coriolis force, between grinding balls and the cylinder at high speeds. The high speed impact causes a high energy collision with drug particles. In addition, the centripetal motion of the grinding action causes frictional forces that help in finer grinding process.

(ii) Large scale preparation method: On large scale dispersion method, the solid particles are suspended using ball, pebble and colloid mills. Dough mixers, pony mixers and similar apparatus are also employed.

(II) Extemporaneous Method

(i) From oral solid dosage form: This method involves crushing of tablet or emptying of capsule contents into the mortar and addition of a suspending agent. A paste is formed with the vehicle which is then diluted to a suitable volume, with the addition any other excipients such as preservative or flavour, if needed. The suspension so prepared has a short expiry of no more than 2 weeks.

(ii) From dry powders and granules for reconstitution: Suspensions from dry powders and granules for reconstitution are prepared when drug has physical or chemical instability problems. The powder or granules are placed at the bottom of the container in which they are to be prepared. The specified amount of cold, purified water is added in two or more portions with shaking. Such suspensions are prepared immediately before opening the pack of powder or bulk solids.

Guide to prepare suspension

Step 1 : Wetting and dispersion of the Active Ingredient: Mill dry powders to achieve target particle size and particle size range. Powder should be added to a low viscosity portion of the product, preferably plain water. This allows for most efficient mixing and homogenization. Wetting agent is added to the water to aid in wetting and displacement of air. Drug powder may be treated with a water miscible material such as glycerin to aid in wetting.

Step 2 : Stabilization of the Dispersed Solid: Add electrolytes to produce charges around each particle and allow for electrical repulsion to prohibit particle interactions.

Step 3 : Preparation of the Vehicle: Polymers may form lumps if added to water improperly. It is often practical to disperse them in a water miscible liquid in which they are insoluble. It is better to make a paste of the drug in glycerin and carefully add this paste to water. Allow this mixture to stand for up to 24 hours to ensure complete hydration of the polymer.

Step 4 : Addition and Dispersions in Vehicle: The dispersion of the solid drug is added to the vehicle with low mixing intensity. The mixture is then homogenized to ensure uniform dispersion of the ingredients.

Step 5 : Addition of other excipients such as volatile components, colouring or concentrated flavouring tinctures such as chloroform spirit, liquid liquorice extract and compound tartarazine solution until near the end, followed by final mixing.

9.6 FLOCCULATED SUSPENSIONS

Flocculation is a process of contact and adhesion whereby the particles of dispersion form larger-size clusters. Flocculation is synonymous with agglomeration and coalescence. Insoluble solids in this system are present as individual particles. The aggregation of particles in a flocculated suspension leads to rapid rate of sedimentation as each aggregate is composed of many individual particles. Flocculation promotes agglomeration and assists in the settling of particles. During flocculation, gentle mixing accelerates the rate of particle collision, and the destabilized particles are further aggregated and trapped into larger precipitates. Flocculation is affected by several parameters, including shear speeds, shear intensity, and shear time.

A commonly used method of preventing aggregation of the small particles of a suspension is the intentional formation of a loose aggregation of the particles held together by weak bonds. Such an aggregation of particles as an open network is termed a 'floc' or a 'floccule'. The floccules have fibrous, fluffy, open network and the dispersion medium can flow through them during sedimentation. They can entrap a large amount of the liquid phase. The volume of the final sediment is large and particles in flocs are easily re-dispersed by moderate agitation. The flocs settle more rapidly than individual discrete particles. Since particles flocculated resists to settle completely, they are less prone to compaction and cake formation than unflocculated particles. The flocculated and deflocculated suspensions are shown in the following figure:

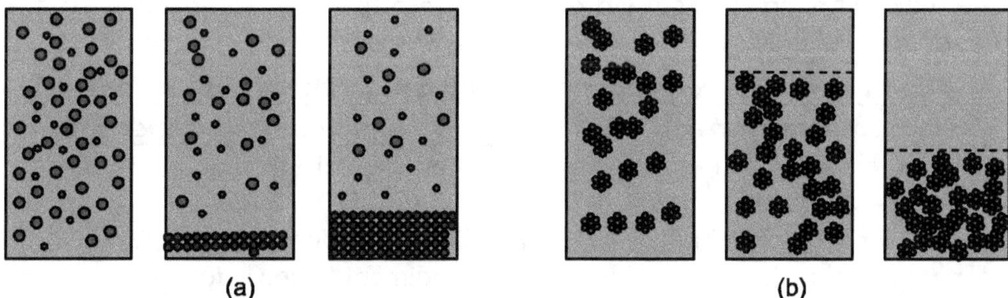

Fig. 9.1: Flocculated and Deflocculated Suspension: (a) Deflocculated and (b) Flocculated

In a flocculated suspension, the supernatant quickly becomes clear, because of the large flocs that settle rapidly. The flocculated suspensions form loose sediments which are easily re-dispersible, but the sedimentation rate is fast and there is a danger of inaccurate dose being administered; also, the product will look inelegant. Ideally, suspension should be prepared with partial flocculation. This is nothing but a compromise between partially flocculated suspension for adequate redispersion upon moderate shaking, and viscosity to control the sedimentation rate at its minimum.

9.7 DEFLOCCULATED SUSPENSION

Deflocculation is the exactly opposite of flocculation. It is defined as "a state or condition of a dispersion of a solid in a liquid in which each solid particle remains independent and unassociated with adjacent particles. In this system, the dispersed particles remain suspended for a long period of time, and only a small portion of the solid is found in the sediment due to the force of gravitation. The supernatant of this suspension remain cloudy for an appreciable time after shaking, due to the very slow settling rate of the smallest particles. During sedimentation, the smaller particles fill the void between the larger ones and thus prevents liquid entrapment within the sediment. The particles in the sediment are gradually pressed together by the weight of the particles above. This closeness of the particles attracts them by a large amount of van der Waals'-London force and forms a compact cake which is very difficult to redisperse. The aggregate formed is a closed one, called coagule. They are tightly packed, produced by surface film bonding. This phenomenon is the most serious of all the physical stability problems encountered in suspension. In cake, particles aggregate themselves by physical bridging. These compact flocs so formed are light, fluffy conglomerate held together by weak van der Waal's forces of attraction. In order to overcome conglomeration of particles systems are provided with addition of a small amount of electrolyte or flocculating agents. A deflocculated system has a zeta potential higher than the critical value when the repulsive forces dominates the attractive forces. In rheological terms, a deflocculated suspension shows zero or very low yield value. Deflocculated suspensions have the advantage of a slow sedimentation rate, thereby enabling a uniform dose to be taken from the container, but when settling does occur, the sediment is compacted and difficult to re-disperse. A comparative study of the properties of flocculated and deflocculated suspensions is shown in table below.

Comparison between flocculated and deflocculated suspensions

Flocculated suspension	Deflocculated suspension
1. Particles forms loose aggregates with network like structure.	1. Particles exist as separate entities.
2. Rate of sedimentation is high.	2. Rate of sedimentation is slow.
3. Sediment is rapidly formed.	3. Sediment is slowly formed.
4. Sediment is scaffold like loosely packed and doesn't form a compact cake.	4. Sediment is very closely packed and a compact cake is formed.
5. Sediment is easy to re-disperse.	5. Sediment is difficult to re-disperse.
6. Suspension is not pleasing in appearance.	6. Suspension is pleasing in appearance.
7. The floccules stick to the bottle wall.	7. They don't stick to the sides of the bottle.
8. Supernatant liquid is generally clear.	8. Supernatant liquid is generally cloudy.
9. Bioavailability is comparatively less due to small specific surface area.	9. Bioavailability is higher due to large specific surface area.

9.8 SUSPENSION STABILITY

(i) Physical Stability

Physical stability of suspension is very important to ensure uniform dosing of drugs they contain. Physical parameters that determine stability of suspensions include physical form and particle size of the dispersed phase, and particle–particle interactions. These properties help to determine whether suspension would form sediment as hard cake or sediment that can be easily dispersed. It is critical to ensure that there are no changes in physical form due to polymorphic changes or increase in particle size due to Ostwald ripening. Other factors that contribute to appreciable appearance, colour, odour and taste of a suspension include specific gravity, sedimentation rate, sedimentation volume, zeta potential, compatibility with packaging components and drug distribution in the system.

Particle size: The particle size plays a key role in the formulation of suspension. Care must be taken that the particles must be of small size. The greater degree of subdivision of a solid by size reduction provides larger the surface area. Increase in surface area increases interface between the solids and liquids leading to an increase in viscosity of a system. This decreases rate of sedimentation. In case suspensions are intended for parenteral and ophthalmic use, particle size > 25μ causes blockage of the needle and hence it is advisable to have particle size < 5μ. Particles with spherical shape are best for suspension as there would be no crystal growth on standing for certain period of time. This is because as the temperature decreases, the solubility decreases that may lead to crystallization. It is better to use uniform sized powder because smaller particles being larger in surface area would become more soluble as their size decreases continuously, whereas the size of larger particles would keep on increasing.

Viscosity: Oral suspensions generally have high viscosity and may contain high amounts of dispersed solid. A parenteral suspension on the other hand usually has low viscosity and contains less than 5% solids. Increasing the viscosity of the continuous phase produces stable suspensions. The rate of sedimentation is low in viscous suspensions. Suspensions can be made viscous by addition of thickening agents to dispersion medium where they usually swell. The rate of drug release from a suspension is dependent of viscosity of a formulation. The more viscous the preparation, the slower is release of a drug. Sometimes this property can be used to deliver drugs by depot preparations.

Temperature: Another factor which negatively affects the stability and usefulness of pharmaceutical suspensions is fluctuation of temperature. Temperature can affect the viscosity of the dispersion medium. Generally, a rise in temperature causes viscosity to go down. The relationship of viscosity to the temperature of a liquid can be shown as:

$$\eta = Ae^{-Ev\,RT}$$

Where, η is the viscosity of the liquid, A is a constant, depends on the molecular weight and molar volume of the liquid and E_v is the energy of activation required to initiate the flow between molecules. Temperature can affect the viscosity of a suspension by modifying interfacial properties and thus inducing or reducing flocculation. Flocculation increases viscosity. Temperature also affects the viscosity of a medium by increasing the Brownian movement. In addition, temperature causes volume expansion in both the dispersion medium and the solid. Temperature fluctuations can lead to caking and claying. During storage or transport, the product may experience a fluctuation of temperature which may lead to crystal growth or physical incompatibilities. For example, crystal growth of sulfathiazole in suspensions is found to accelerate after temperature cycling. The preservative and protective colloid actions may have a profound effect on the physical performance of a suspension under freeze-thaw conditions.

Change in Physical Form: Changes in physical form can result in significant changes in dissolution properties of the drugs, which can lead to changes in exposure. For example, Carbamazepine anhydrates converts to dihydrate when formulated as a suspension. Dihydrate has lower solubility and dissolution which affects the overall exposure. In addition, a number of weakly crystalline compounds and salts of weakly basic compounds can convert into amorphous basic form or crystalline free base in suspension. This could affect the solubility/dissolution rate and the exposure significantly for drugs post oral administration.

(ii) Chemical Stability

Drugs in liquid systems are more prone to chemical reactions than in solid state. Drug in suspended forms with limited solubility are far more stable than the drug in solution. However, chemical stability of drugs in suspension should still be monitored. Often the chemical reactions in suspensions involve hydrolysis, oxidation, complexation etc. Chemical functionalities such as ester and amides are susceptible to hydrolytic degradation and amino functions may undergo oxidative degradation. Chemical changes in formulation components leads to pH change, viscosity change, and degradation of drug and antimicrobial activity of preservatives.

9.9 METHODS TO OVERCOME STABILITY PROBLEMS

Suspension is a liquid preparation of active substance(s) in finely divided form suspended homogeneously in a vehicle. Usually it is prepared using suspending agent or other suitable excipients in purified water or oil and if necessary preservatives, stabilizers, etc. In the case of deterioration, suspensions are prepared by uniformly mixing components just before the use by patient. Unless otherwise specified, suspensions packaged in unit-dose meet the requirements of the test for uniformity of contents in dosage units. Tight containers are used for preservation.

    (i)   **Chemical Stability:** There are various approaches to avoid chemical instability of suspensions. One way is to prepare suspensions of high concentrations (> 100 mg/mL) to minimize the impact of such degradation. If drug is unstable in suspension, which decomposes 2% over the duration of storage, it is recommended to prepare it daily as a fresh formulation prior to dosing. Alternatively, suspension can be stored under refrigerated conditions or freeze and thawed for a few minutes prior to use. Preparing a fresh suspension each time prior to dosing is an option when significant physical or chemical changes occur during storage but is not a convenient method and could potentially result in lot-to-lot variability.

(ii) Packaging and Storage: Suspensions should be packaged in wide mouth containers, having adequate air space above the liquid and should be stored in tight containers, protected from excessive heat and light for sensitive drugs. Some suspensions are stored in cool place but should not be kept in a refrigerator. Generally, they are stored at controlled temperature (20-25°C). Freezing at very low temperatures should be avoided which may lead to aggregation of suspended particles.

(iii) Label: All pharmaceutical suspensions should be properly labelled. In addition to the product name and directions for use, it must have direction *"Shake the Bottle Well Before Use"* as some sedimentation of medicament would normally be expected. Shaking the bottle will re-disperse the drug and ensure that the patient can measure the accurate dose. Other labelling information includes directions to store in a cool place, expiry date etc. In case of dry suspensions powders, the specified amount and quality and state of vehicle to be mixed may be indicated clearly on label.

(iv) Choices of packaging: Packaging of all pharmaceutical suspensions are extremely important aspect of ensuring its stability. Suspensions should be packed in amber coloured bottles- plain for internal use and ribbed for external use. There should be adequate air space above the liquid to allow shaking and easy pouring. A 5 mL medicine spoon or measure or oral syringe should be provided for the suspensions meant for oral administration.

Evaluation of suspension

The following tests are carried out on suspension formulation to assure final quality of suspension:

(a)   Appearance, colour, odour and taste

(b)   Particle size

(c)   Microscopic photography for crystal growth

(d)   Sedimentation rate

(e)   Zeta Potential

(f)   Sedimentation volume

(g) Re-dispersibility

(h) Centrifugation test

(i) Rheological measurement

(j) Stress test

(k) pH

(l) Freeze-Thaw temperature cycling

(m) Compatibility with container and cap liner

MODEL QUESTIONS

1. What are disperse systems?
2. What are various types of disperse systems?
3. What are colloidal and coarse dispersions?
4. What are suspensions? Give classification of suspension.
5. What are advantages/disadvantages of suspensions?
6. Give difference between flocculated and deflocculated suspensions.
7. Explain different components used for preparation of suspension.
8. Give methods of preparation of suspension.
9. What are various stability problems of suspensions?
10. How suspensions are stabilized?
11. Write a note on:
    (i) Stability of suspension.
    (ii) Flocculated and deflocculated suspension.

■■■

Chapter 10...

Biphasic Liquids : Emulsions

LEARNING OBJECTIVES

A liquid dosage form that consists of a dispersion of tiny undissolved drug particles suspended in the solution. When the solution is shaken, the particles disburse to create a uniform heterogeneous mixture.

The objectives of this chapter includes:

- To define and/or identify emulsions and emulsifying agents.
- To identify factors that determines emulsion type and methods of identifying types of emulsions.
- To describe the types of instability and levels to which emulsions know the principle of formulating stable emulsions.
- To understand the mechanisms by which emulsions are stabilized.
- To understand basic formulation considerations and method of preparing emulsions.
- To know about storage, packaging, uses and special instructions for emulsions.
- To know about emulsifying agents by type and their uses, advantages, limitations.
- To know about HLB and methods to calculate for any non-ionic surfactant system.

10.1 INTRODUCTION

Emulsion is two-phase system in which one liquid is dispersed throughout another liquid in the form of small droplets and the system is stabilized by third substance emulsifying agent. Several classes may be distinguished: oil-in-water (o/w), water-in-oil (w/o), and oil-in-oil (o/o). The latter class may be exemplified by an emulsion consisting of a polar oil (for example, propylene glycol) dispersed in a non-polar oil (paraffinic oil) and vice versa. The stabilizing substances called emulsifying agents prevent coalescence, the merging of small droplets into larger droplets and into individual separated phases.

Emulsions being a heterogeneous system are thermodynamically unstable and thus a third substance, the emulsifier is added to stabilize the system. These agents stabilize the system by forming a thin film around the globules of dispersed phase. Either the dispersed phase or the continuous phase may vary in consistency from that of a mobile liquid to semisolid. Thus, pharmaceutical emulsions range from simple emulsion (low viscosity) to creams and ointments (high viscosity). The particle size of the dispersed phase commonly ranges from 0.1 to 100 μm. The pharmaceutical term "emulsion" is most used to indicate preparations prepared for internal use. Emulsions for external use are always given a different title that it's focus may indicate their use. For example, lotion and cream, liniments, vitamin drops.

Advantages:

(i)   Unpalatable oil-soluble drugs can be administered in palatable form.

(ii) Possible to include two incompatible ingredients, one in each phase of the emulsion.

(iii) They can mask the bitter taste and odour of drugs making them more palatable, for example, castor oil, cod-liver oil etc.

(iv) They can be used to prolong the release of the drug providing sustained release action.

(v)   Carbohydrates, fats and vitamins can be emulsified and administered to bed ridden patients as sterile intravenous emulsions.

(vi) Emulsions provide protection to drugs which are susceptible to oxidation or hydrolysis.

(vii) Used to formulate externally used products, for example, lotions, creams, liniments etc.

(viii) The aqueous phase is easily flavoured.

(ix) The rate of drug absorption is increased.

Disadvantages:

(i)   Emulsion needs to be shaken well before use.

(ii) A measuring device is needed for administration of emulsion.

(iii) A degree of technical accuracy is needed to measure a dose.

(iv) Storage conditions may affect emulsion stability.

(v)   They are bulky, difficult to transport and prone to container breakages.

(vi) They are prone to microbial contamination which can lead to cracking.

10.2 CLASSIFICATION OF EMULSIONS

I.   Based on nature of internal and external phase

(i)   o/w type emulsion

(ii) w/o type emulsion

(iii) w/o/w or o/w/o emulsion

II. General types based on type of dosage form

(i)   Lotions

(ii) Liniments

(iii) Creams

(iv) Ointments

(v)   Vitamin drops

III. Based on nature of the emulsifying agents

(i)   Simple molecules and ions, for example, o/w, w/o.

(ii) Non-ionic surfactants.

(iii) Surfactant mixtures, for example, micellar emulsions (microemulsions).

(iv) Ionic surfactants, for example, macroemulsions.

(v)   Non-ionic polymers, for example, bilayer droplets.

(vi) Polyelectrolytes, for example, double and multiple emulsions.

(vii) Mixed polymers and surfactants, for example, mixed emulsions.

(viii) Liquid crystalline phases.

(ix) Solid particles.

IV. Based on structure of the System

(i)   O/w and w/o macroemulsions: Usual size range 0.1–5 μm; average size 1–2 μm.

(ii)   Nanoemulsion: Size range of 20–100 nm.

(iii)   Micellar emulsions or microemulsions: Size ranges 5–50 nm.

(iv)   Double and multiple emulsions: w/o/w, o/w/o emulsions.

(v)   Mixed emulsions: Consisting of two different dispersed droplets that do not mix in a continuous medium, for example, macroemulsions.

(i) Oil in water emulsion

Pharmaceutical emulsions usually consist of mixtures of aqueous phase with various oils and waxes. If the oil droplets are dispersed throughout the aqueous phase, the emulsion is termed oil-in-water (o/w) is as shown in Fig. 10.1. Fats or oils for oral administration, either as medicaments in their own right, or as vehicles for oil soluble drugs, are always formulated as oil in water (o/w) emulsions. They are non-greasy and are easily removable from the skin surface and they are used externally to provide cooling effect and internally to also mask the bitter taste of oil. Water soluble drugs are more quickly released from o/w emulsion. The o/w emulsion is given a positive conductivity test as water, the external phase, is a good conductor of electricity.

(ii) Water in oil emulsion

A system in which the water is dispersed as globules in the oil in a continuous phase is termed water-in-oil emulsion (w/o). Water-in-oil emulsions will have an occlusive effect by hydrating the stratum corneum and inhibiting evapouration of eccrine secretions. It has an effect on the absorption of drugs from w/o emulsions. The w/o type of emulsions are useful to clean the skin consisting oil soluble dirt. The greasy texture is not always cosmetically acceptable. They are greasy and not water washable and are used externally to prevent evaporation of the moisture from the surface of the skin for example, cold cream. Oil soluble drugs are more quickly released from w/o emulsion. They are preferred for formulation meant for external use like cream. w/o emulsion is not given a positive conductivity tests, because oil is the external phase which is a poor conductor of electricity.

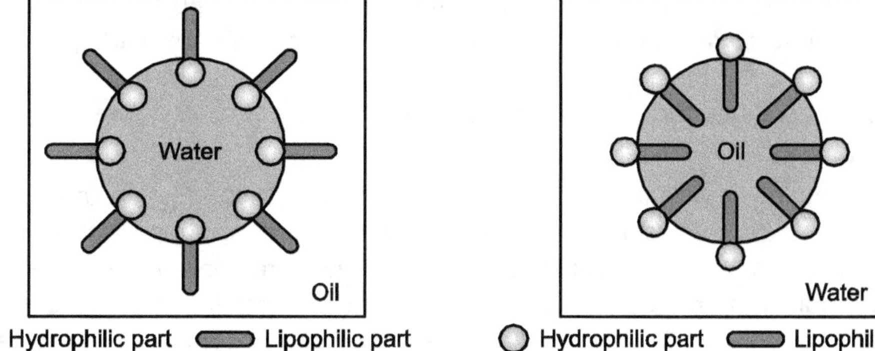

Fig. 10.1: Types of Emulsions

Difference between O/W and W/O emulsions

o/w Emulsion	w/o Emulsion
(i) Dispersion medium is water and dispersed phase is oil.	(i) Dispersion medium is oil while dispersed phase is water.
(ii) Being non-greasy, easily removable from the skin.	(ii) Being greasy, difficult to remove if washed with water.
(iii) Applied externally to provide cooling effect (for example, Vanishing cream).	(iii) Applied externally to maintain skin moist and soft (for example, Cold cream).
(iv) Preferred for internal use to mask bitter taste of oils.	(iv) Preferred for external use (e.g. creams).
(v) Preferred for water soluble drugs to release quickly from emulsion.	(v) Preferred for oil soluble drugs to release quickly from emulsion.

(iii) Multiple emulsions

Multiple emulsions are complex systems. It is a complex type of emulsion system in which the oil-in-water or water-in-oil emulsions are dispersed in another liquid medium. In other words, it can be described as the emulsion system in which the dispersed phase contains smaller droplets that have the same composition as the external phase. In this way, an oil-in-water-in-oil (o/w/o) emulsion consists of very small droplets of oil dispersed in the water globules of a water-in-oil emulsion and a water-in-oil-in-water (w/o/w) emulsion consists of droplets of water dispersed in the oil phase of an oil-in-water emulsion. Their pharmaceutical applications include taste masking, adjuvant vaccines, an immobilization of enzymes and sorbent reservoir of overdose treatments, and sometimes for the augmentation of external skin or dermal absorption. Multiple emulsions have been formulated as cosmetics, such as skin moisturizer. Prolonged release can also be obtained by means of multiple emulsions. These systems have some advantages, such as the protection of the entangled substances and the possibilities of incorporating several drugs in the different compartments. Regardless of their importance, multiple emulsions have limitations because of thermodynamic instability and their complex structure.

(iv) Pickering emulsion

The solid particles in the colloidal size may be used as emulsion stabilizers. These particles are referred to as Pickering emulsion. The solid particles are made partially wetted by the oil phase and by the aqueous phase. Pickering emulsions are recently employed in many areas like cosmetics, food, pharmaceuticals, oil recovery and waste water treatment.

(v) Microemulsions

It may be defined as dispersion of insoluble liquids in a second liquid that appear clear and homogeneous to the naked eyes. Microemulsions are frequently called solubilized systems because on a macroscopic basis, they seem to behave as true solutions. Microemulsions are systems consisting of water, oil and surfactant, which constitute a single optically isotropic and thermodynamically stable liquid solution. There are three basic types of microemulsions namely; Direct, Reversed and Bicontinuous microemulsions.

The term microemulsion was first used by Jack H. Shulman, a Professor of Chemistry at Columbia University, in 1959. They are also termed as, transparent emulsion, swollen micelle, micelles solutions and solubilized oil. A simple method to formulate a microemulsion is suggested by Hoar and Schulman. For preparation of o/w microemulsion, first w/o emulsion is prepared using a low hydrophilic lipophilic balance (HLB) number surfactant. To this emulsion, an aqueous solution of high HLB number surfactant is added with stirring at a certain amount of addition. A 'gel' phase produced to which when surfactant solution is added, an inversion takes place to form o/w emulsion.

Careful examination of these complex systems has shown that clear emulsions can exist in several differentiable forms. Microemulsions should not be confused with solutions formed by co-solvency for example, clear system consisting of water, benzene and ethanol. A drawback of microemulsion is the possibility of disruption of the crystalline structure of stratum corneum which may lead to facilitated transdermal transport and skin irritation.

(vi) Non-aqueous emulsions

Non-aqueous systems are well known as solvents for drugs, suspension vehicles and oleogels. The majority of pharmaceutical emulsions have water as one phase. There has been interest in emulsions as delivery vehicles other than water for topical delivery, for example, Cyclosporine Microemulsion, Propofol i.v. Microemulsion; wherein no aqueous phase is used as drug reservoirs as well as templates for the preparation of microspheres and nanoparticles.

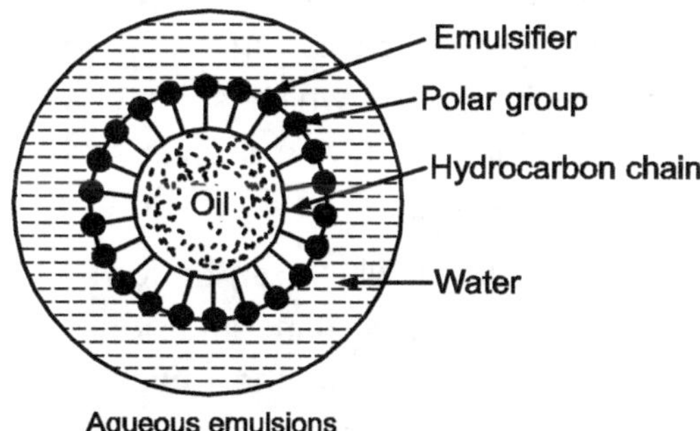

Fig. 10.2: Non-aqueous Emulsions

(vii) Liposome emulsions

Liposomes (liposome-lipid based vesicles) are microscopic vesicles, which can be artificially prepared as globular carriers into which active molecules can be encapsulated. Liposome emulsions are those in which o/w emulsions are produced by using liposomes as the emulsifying agent for stabilizing the oil.

There are two alternative mechanisms involved in preparation of liposomes emulsion. First rapid (or slow) release of liposomes containing encapsulated antigen and lipid for interaction with the immune system at a distant site. And second, retention of liposomes in the o/w emulsion as a depot at the site of injection, resulting in gradual ingestion of the liposomes by phagocytic cells attracted to the site by local inflammation.

Liposomes vesicles with diameters between 25 and 5000 nm are often used as drug carriers for topical purposes in the pharmaceutical and cosmetic industry, such as drug delivery, gene therapy, and immunization. Example: Lubrizol liposome emulsion.

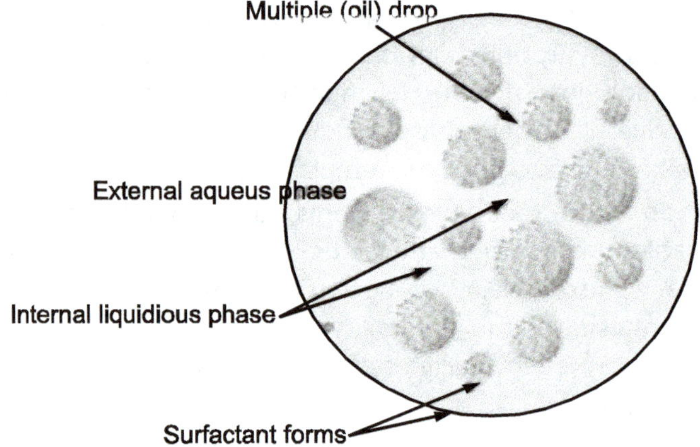

Fig. 10.3: Liposome Emulsions

(vii) Nanoemulsions

Nanoemulsions are a submicron size colloidal particulate carrier system for drug molecules. Their size varies from 10 to 1,000 nm. These carriers are solid spheres and their surface is amorphous and lipophilic with a negative charge. They are used to enhance the therapeutic efficacy of the drug and minimize adverse effect and toxic reactions. The term 'nanoemulsion' also refers to a mini emulsion which is fine o/w or w/o dispersion stabilized by an interfacial film of surfactant molecule having droplet size range 20–600 nm. The small size of nanoemulsions makes them transparent.

There are three types of nanoemulsion which can be formed: (a) o/w nanoemulsion, (b) w/o nanoemulsion, and (c) bi-continuous nanoemulsion. The major applications of nanoemulsion are treatment of infection of the reticuloendothelial system, enzyme replacement therapy in the liver, treatment of cancer, and vaccination.

Advantages:

(a) It is non-toxic and non-irritant in nature.

(b) Used in taste masking.

(c) Small-sized droplets provide greater surface area for increased drug absorption.

(d) It can be formulated as foams, creams, liquids, and sprays.

(e) It helps to solubilize lipophilic drug.

(f) Less amount of energy is required.

(g) It has improved physical stability.

(h) It may be used as substitute for liposomes and vesicles.

10.3 EMULSIFYING AGENT

The choice of the emulsifier is crucial in the formation of the emulsion and its long-term stability. Emulsions may be classified according to the nature of the emulsifier or the structure of the system. It is a substance which stabilizes an emulsion.

I. Ideal properties of emulsifying agents

(i)　Pharmaceutically acceptable emulsifiers must also be stable.

(ii)　It should be compatible with other ingredients.

(iii)　It should be non-toxic.

(iv)　It should possess little or no odour, taste, or colour.

(v)　It should not interfere with the stability of efficacy of the active agent

II. Classification of emulsifying agents

(i) Nature of material

(a) Carbohydrate materials: Acacia, tragacanth, agar, pectin for example, o/w emulsion.

(b) Protein Substances: Gelatin, egg yolk, for example, Caesin o/w emulsion.

(c) High molecular weight alcohols: Stearyl alcohol, cetyl alcohol, glyceryl monostearate for example, o/w emulsion, cholesterol w/o emulsion.

(d) Wetting agents: Anionic, cationic, non-ionic, for example, o/w emulsion, w/o emulsion.

(e) Finely divided solids: Bentonite, magnesium hydroxide, aluminum hydroxide, for example, o/w emulsion.

(ii) Based on HLB values

(a) Lipophilic emulsifying agents: Oleic acid (1.6), Sorbitan tristearate (2.1), ethylene glycol monostearate (2.9), glyceryl monostearate (3.8), sorbitan monostearate (4.7), sorbitan monopalmitate (6.7), PEG-4 dilaurate (6.0).

(b) Hydrophilic emulsifying agents: Sucrose dipalmitate (7.4), PEG-4 monooleate (8.0), PEG-4 monolaurate (9.8), polysorbate 85 (11.0), PEG-8 monooleate (11.4).

(iii) Based on functions

(a) Antifoaming agents: Oleic acid, sorbitan tristearate, Ethylene glycol monostearate.

(b) W/O emulsifier: Glyceryl monostearate, sorbitan monostearate, Sorbitan monopalmitate, PEG-4 dilaurate, sucrose dipalmitate, PEG-4 monooleate.

(c) O/W emulsifier: PEG-4 monolaurate, solysorbate 85, PEG-8 monooleate.

(iv) Based on presence of charged groups in their heads

(a) Anionic (The charge is negative; based on sulfate, sulfonate or carboxylate anions)**:** Perfluorooctanoate, perfluorooctane sulfonate, sodium dodecyl sulfate, ammonium lauryl sulfate, sodium laureth sulfate, alkyl benzene sulfonate.

(b) Cationic (The charge is positive; based on quaternary ammonium cations)**:** Cetyl trimethylamine bromide, cetylpyridinium chloride, polyethoxylated tallow amine, benzalkonium chloride, benzethonium chloride.

(c) Zwitterionic (Two oppositely charged groups; amphoteric)**:** Dodecyl betaine, Cocamidopropyl betaine, Coco amphoglycinate.

(d) Non-ionic (No charge groups)**:** Alkyl poly (ethylene oxide), alkyl phenolpoly (ethylene oxide), poly (ethylene oxide), poly (propylene oxide), octyl glucoside, decyl maltoside, cetyl alcohol, oleyl alcohol, Tween 20 and Tween 80.

III. Mechanism of Emulsifying Agent

Mechanism of action of emulsifying agents depends upon the formation of film at the interface of two phases. There are three types of films formed by emulsifying agents.

(i) **Monomolecular films:** Emulsifying agents with stabilizing action form monolayer at the oil-water interface. The film formed is one molecule thick and thus referred to as a monolayer. This monolayer prevents coalescence of droplets.

(ii) **Multimolecular films:** Multimolecular films around the droplets of dispersed phase are formed by hydrophilic colloids. They act as layer around the droplets making them highly resistant to coalescence. They have the ability of swelling to increase the viscosity of the system so that droplets are less likely to merge to form a separate phase.

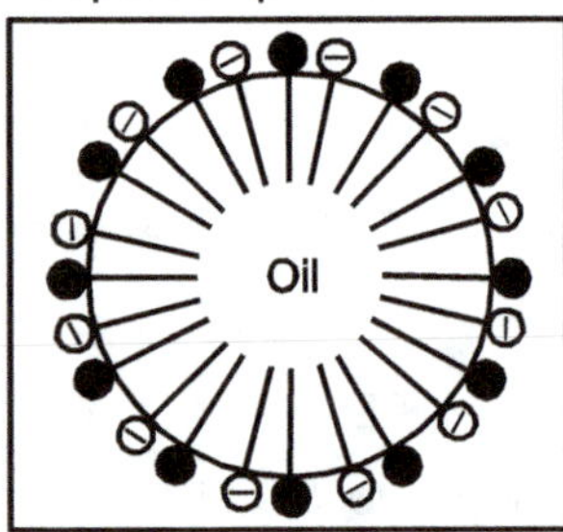

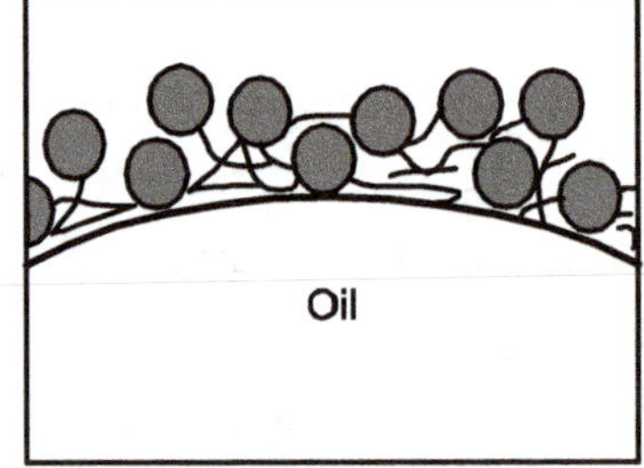

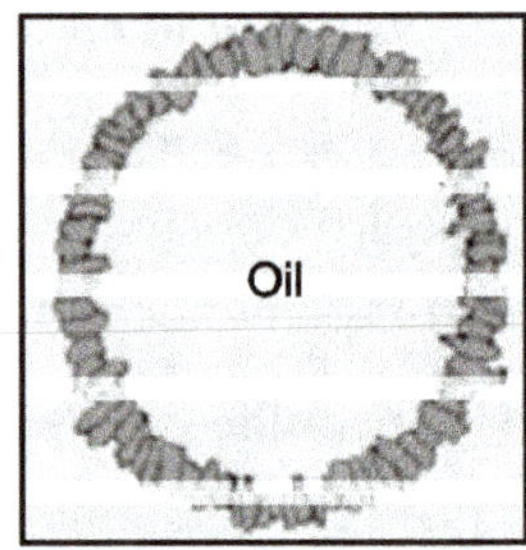

| Monomolecular films | Multimolecular films | Solid particle films |

Fig. 10.4: Types of Films Formed by Emulsifying Agents

(iii) Solid particle films: Small solid particles like bentonite, veegum, hectorite, magnesium hydroxide, aluminum hydroxide and magnesium trisilicate, which are wetted to some degree by both oil and water, can act as emulsifying agents. These solid particles are concentrated at the interface and form a particulate film around the dispersed droplets to avoid coalescence.

(iv) Emulsifying agents as stabilizers: Amongst surfactants, non-ionic surfactants are the most effective emulsifiers that can be used for emulsification of o/w or w/o emulsions. They can stabilize the emulsion against flocculation and coalescence. Ionic surfactants are used for o/w emulsion as emulsifiers but the system produced may sometimes be sensitive to the presence of electrolytes. Emulsifiers alone are less effective and thus their mixtures, for example, ionic and non-ionic, or mixtures of non-ionic surfactants are practically more effective in emulsification and stabilization. Non-ionic polymers such as pluronics are more effective in stabilization of the emulsion when high energy is applied for the process. Mixtures of polymers and surfactants are ideal and most commonly used in achieving ease of emulsification and stabilization. Lamellar liquid crystalline phases produced using surfactant mixtures are very effective in emulsion stabilizers. Solid particles that can accumulate at the o/w interface are effective emulsion stabilizers.

(v) Theories of Emulsification: Theories of emulsification explain the action of emulsifying agents in stabilizing emulsions. The surface or more accurately the interface between the two immiscible liquids plays the important role in producing stable emulsion. Emulsifying agents acts at interface in such a way that they reduce interfacial tension between two phases to obtain stable emulsions. There are three major theories proposed to explain the action of emulsifying agents in stabilizing emulsions.

(i) Surface tension theory: Molecules in a bulk of liquid are attracted equally on all sides by the surrounding similar type molecules through cohesive force; however, at the surface, there is inward attraction of molecules due to the imbalance attractive forces between molecules of oil and water phases. Due to this, tension is exerted at interface known as interfacial tension. The emulsifying agents reduce interfacial tension between the two immiscible liquids. This leads to reduction in the repulsive force between these liquids which ultimately decrease the attraction of liquid's own molecules. Thus surfactants help to convert large globules into small ones and avoid small globules to form coalescence as large molecules.

(ii) The oriented Wedge theory: In this theory, the oil-like or non-polar ends of the emulsifying agents turn towards the oil and the polar ends towards the polar liquid. The oriented Wedge theory of emulsions indicates that if the non-polar end of the emulsifying agent is smaller, the emulsion will be oil-in-water and if the polar end is smaller, the emulsion will be water-in-oil.

(iii) The interfacial film theory: The interfacial film theory suggests that the emulsifying agents make an interface between the two immiscible phases of the emulsion. They surround the droplets of the internal phase as a thin film. This film prevents the coalescence of the dispersed phase.

10.4 EMULSION TEST FOR IDENTIFICATION

Several tests have been proposed for identifying the emulsion type. Although, these tests may be applied rapidly, the results must be interpreted with caution because the tests can not indicate whether a multiple emulsion has been produced or not. In such cases, microscopic examination is a very useful tool to exactly identify type of emulsion produced.

(i)   **Dilution test/miscibility test:** In this test, the emulsion is diluted either with oil or water. If the emulsion is o/w type and it is diluted with water, it will remain stable as water is the dispersion medium. If emulsion is diluted with oil, the emulsion will break as oil and water are not miscible with each other. Oil in water (o/w) emulsion can easily be diluted with an aqueous solvent whereas water in oil (w/o) emulsion can be diluted with an oily liquid.

(ii) **Electrical conductivity test:** The basic principle of this test is that water is a good conductor of electricity. Electric current is conducted by o/w emulsions, owing to the presence of ionic species in water. Thus, an emulsion with water in a continuous phase will readily conduct electricity, while that with oil in a continuous phase will not. In this test, an assembly is used in which a pair of electrodes connected to an electric bulb is dipped into an emulsion. If the emulsion is o/w type, the electric bulb glows. This test fails in non-ionic o/w emulsions.

(iii) **Staining test/dye-solubility test:** In this test, an emulsion is mixed with a water soluble dye (amaranth or methylene blue or brilliant blue) and observed under the microscope. If the continuous phase appears red, it means that the emulsion is o/w type as water is in the continuous or external phase and the dye will dissolve in it to give colour. If the scattered globules appear red and in a continuous phase becomes colourless, then it is w/o type. Similarly, if an oil soluble dye (Scarlet red C or Sudan III) is added to an emulsion and if in the continuous phase appears red, then it is w/o emulsion.

(iv) **Cobalt Chloride Test (Filter paper test):** When a filter paper soaked in cobalt chloride ($COCl_2$) solution is dipped in to an emulsion and dried, it turns from blue to pink, indicating that the emulsion is o/w type. This test may fail if emulsion is unstable or breaks in presence of electrolyte.

(v)   **Fluorescence Test:** Oils fluoresce under UV-light. If an emulsion on exposure to ultra-violet radiations shows continuous fluorescence under microscope, then it is w/o type. If it shows only spotty fluorescence, then it is o/w type.

(vi) **Refractive index measurement:** Refractive index (RI) measurement is a unique way of identifying emulsions. Consider a beam of light is transmitted through w/o emulsion. Because oil has a high optical density than water, the speed of light reduces as the light enters the oil. The beam of light changes direction abruptly as it enters the oil because of the change in speed. This bending of the light ray is called optical refraction. The ratio of the speed of light in water to its speed in oil is called the refractive index. RI is a constant for particular liquid and therefore can be used to identify emulsion type. When oil phase and water phase have equal RI values, light will not bend as it strikes obliquely at the emulsion interface. Instead, light is transmitted through the emulsion without refraction, which produces clarity. This test is most commonly used to identify micro or nano emulsions.

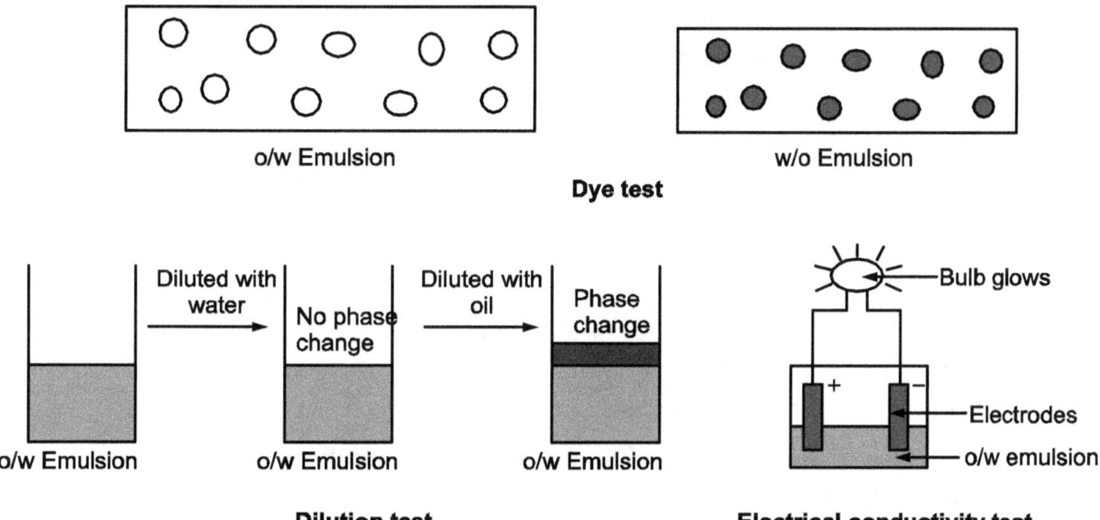

Fig. 10.5: Schematic Presentation of Tests for Emulsion Type Identification

10.5 METHODS OF PREPARATION

We know milk is a natural emulsion, consists of fatty globules surrounded by a layer of casein, suspended in water. The theory of emulsification is based on the nature of milk. When a pharmaceutical emulsion is to be prepared, the principal consideration is the same as that of milk.

(i)   **General method:** Generally, an o/w emulsion is prepared by dividing the oil phase completely into minute globules. Each oil globule is enveloped by emulsifying agent and is suspended in the aqueous phase. Conversely, the w/o type of emulsions are prepared by sub-dividing aqueous phase completely into minute globules. Each water globule is enveloped by emulsifying agent and finally globules are suspended in the oil phase.

(ii) **Phase inversion method:** In this method, the aqueous phase is first added to the oil phase so as to form a w/o emulsion. At the inversion point, addition of more amount of water results in the inversion of emulsion which gives rise to an o/w emulsion. Vice a versa w/o type of emulsions are prepared.

(iii) **Dry gum method or Continental method:** Usually emulsions are made by dry gum method. This method is used to prepare the initial or primary emulsion from oil, water, and a hydrocolloid or "gum" type emulsifier (usually acacia). The primary emulsion, or emulsion nucleus, is formed from 4 parts oil, 2 parts water, and 1-part emulsifier. The 4 parts oil and 1-part emulsifier represent their total amounts for the final emulsion. In a mortar, the 1-part gum is levigated with the 4 parts oil until the powder is thoroughly wetted; then the 2 parts water are added all at once, and the mixture is vigorously and continually triturated until the primary emulsion formed is creamy white and produces a "crackling" sound as it is triturated (usually 3-4 minutes). Additional water or aqueous solutions may be incorporated after the primary emulsion is formed. Solid substances (e.g., drug and excipients) are generally dissolved in water and added as a solution to the primary emulsion. Oil soluble substance, in small amounts, may be incorporated directly into the primary emulsion. Any substance which might reduce the physical stability of the emulsion, such as alcohol (which may precipitate the gum) should be added as near to the end of the process as possible to avoid breaking the emulsion. When all agents have been incorporated, the emulsion should be transferred to a calibrated vessel, brought to final volume with water, then homogenized or blended to ensure uniform distribution of ingredients.

Calculation of the amount of emulsifying agent to be used in the preparation of an emulsion

The amount of emulsifying agent used is dependent on the amount and type of oil to be emulsified. Oils can be divided into three categories: fixed oils, mineral oils and volatile oils.

Fixed oils

Oil	:	4 parts by volume
Aqueous phase	:	2 parts by volume
Gum	:	1 part by weight

Mineral oils

Oil	:	3 parts by volume
Aqueous phase	:	2 parts by volume
Gum	:	1 part by weight

Volatile (aromatic) oils

Oil	:	2 parts by volume
Aqueous phase	:	2 parts by volume
Gum	:	1 part by weight

These proportions are important when making the primary emulsion, to prevent the emulsion from breaking down on dilution or storage.

(iv) Wet gum method or English method: The proportions of oil, water and emulsifying agent for the preparation of the primary emulsion are the same as those used in the dry gum method. The only difference is the method of preparation. In this method, the acacia powder is added to the mortar followed by addition of water and triturated until the gum is dissolved to form mucilage. The oil is then added to the mucilage drop-by-drop with continuous trituration. When nearly all the oil is added, the resulting mixture may appear a little poor. In such case little more water is added to emulsion and trituration is continued until all the oil is added. An extra small amount of water is added if necessary. When all the oil is added, triturate until a smooth primary emulsion is obtained. There is less chance of failure with this method if the oil is added very slowly and in small amounts. But this method is the last choice as it takes more time than the dry gum method.

(v) Bottle (Forbes) Method: This method may be used to prepare emulsions of volatile oils, or oleaginous substances of very low viscosities. It is not suitable for very viscous oils since they cannot be sufficiently agitated in a bottle. This method is a variation of the dry gum method. One part of powdered acacia (or other gum) is placed in a dry bottle and four parts of oil are added. The bottle is capped and thoroughly shaken. To this, the required volume of water is added all at once, and the mixture is shaken thoroughly until the primary emulsion forms. It is important to minimize the initial amount of time when the gum and oil are mixed. The gum will tend to imbibe the oil, and will become more waterproof. It is also effective in preparing an olive oil and lime water emulsion, which is self-emulsifying. In the case of lime water and olive oil, equal parts of lime water and olive oil are added to the bottle and shaken. No emulsifying agent is used, but one is formed "in-situ" following a chemical interaction between the components.

(vi) Beaker Method: When synthetic or non-gum emulsifiers are used, the proportions given in the previous methods become meaningless. The most appropriate method for preparing emulsions from surfactants or other non-gum emulsifiers is to begin by dividing components into water soluble and oil soluble components. All oil soluble components are dissolved in the oily phase in one beaker and all water soluble components are dissolved in the water in a separate beaker. Oleaginous components are melted and both phases are heated to approximately 70°C over a water bath. The internal phase is then added to the external phase with stirring until the product reaches room temperature. The mixing of such emulsions can be carried out in a beaker, mortar, or blender; or, in the case of creams and ointments, in the jar in which they will be dispensed.

(vii) Membrane emulsification method: This method is based on a novel concept of generating droplets as "drop-by-drop" addition to produce emulsion. Here, a pressure is applied direct to the dispersed phase which seeps through a porous membrane into the continuous phase and in this way, the droplets formed are then detached from the membrane surface due to the relative shear motion between the continuous phase and membrane surface.

(viii) Auxiliary Methods: Instead of, or in addition to, any of the preceding methods, the pharmacist can usually prepare an excellent emulsion using an electric mixer or blender. An emulsion prepared by other methods can also usually be improved by passing it through a hand homogenizer, which forces the emulsion through a very small orifice, reducing the dispersed droplet size to about 5 microns or less.

10.6 STABILITY PROBLEMS IN EMULSIONS

I.   Physical Instability

Pharmaceutical emulsion stability is characterized by the absence of coalescence of dispersed phase, absence of creaming and retaining its physical characters like elegance, odour, colour and appearance. The physical instability of emulsion may be classified into four phenomena namely; flocculation, creaming, coalescence and breaking.

(i)   **Creaming:** Creaming is the phenomenon in which the dispersed phase separates out, forming a layer on the top of the continuous phase. This process results from external forces, usually, centrifugal. When such forces exceed the thermal motion (Brownian motion) of the droplets, a concentration gradient builds-up in the system with the larger droplets moving faster to the top, if their density is lower than that of the medium, of the container. It is notable that in creaming, the dispersed phase remains in globules state so that it can be re-dispersed on shaking. Creaming can be minimized if the viscosity of the continuous phase is increased. The o/w emulsions generally face upward creaming when the globules of the dispersed phase are less dense than the continuous phase. In the limiting cases, the droplets may form a close-packed array at the top of the system with the remainder of the volume occupied by the continuous liquid phase.

(ii) **Sedimentation:** This process results from external forces, usually, gravitational. When such forces exceed the thermal motion (Brownian motion) of the droplets, a concentration gradient builds up in the system with the larger droplets moving faster to the bottom, if their density is larger than that of the medium, of the container. In the limiting cases, the droplets may form a close-packed (random or ordered) array at the bottom of the system with the remainder of the volume occupied by the continuous liquid phase. The w/o type of emulsions face downward sedimentation if dispersed phase globules are denser than the continuous phase.

(iii) **Flocculation:** Flocculation refers to the association of small emulsion droplets (without any change in primary droplet size) to form large aggregate which is re-dispersible upon shaking. It is a reversible process in which the droplets remain intact. It is the result of the van der Waals attraction that is universal with all disperse systems. Flocculation occurs when there is insufficient repulsion between droplets to keep them apart to distances where the van der Waals attraction is weak. The presence of excess surfactant in the continuous phase of an emulsion can lead to flocculation of emulsion droplets. The flocculation of emulsion droplets by excess surfactant is also called "depletion effect". The depletion mechanism in system containing excess surfactant in the form of micelles can be explained as, when the dispersed emulsion droplets approach each other to distances closer than the diameter of the surfactant micelles, segregation of micelles from the inter-particle space occurs. This is net result of the loss in configurational entropy of the micelles. In this phenomenon attractive force between the droplets increases due to the lowering of osmotic pressure in the region between the droplets, and flocculation of droplets occurs. Flocculation may be "strong" or "weak," depending on the magnitude of the attractive force involved.

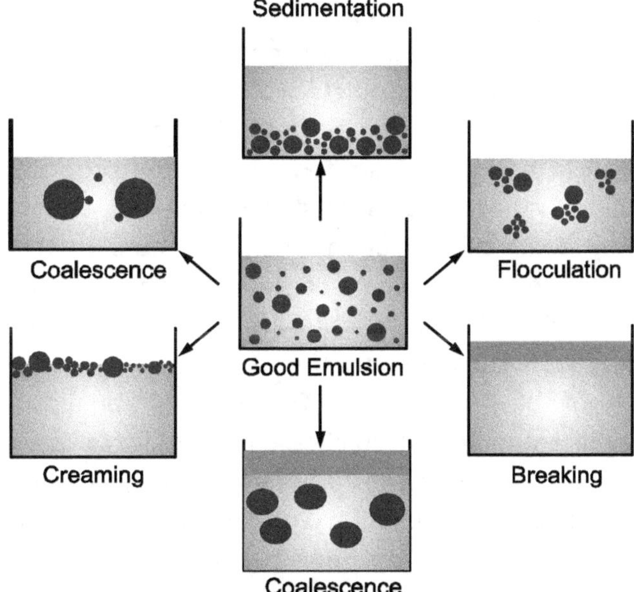

Fig. 10.6: Types of Emulsion Instability

There may be fast or slow. The fast flocculation occurs when the smaller droplets disappear more rapidly than the larger ones as a result of the different rates of movement under gravity or in forced convection, leading to an increased collision rate. The slow flocculation occurs when the build-up of large metastable structures slows due to energy barrier between droplets and the formation of droplet-free spaces between aggregates and the heavier aqueous phase of o/w emulsions; the consequence is called hindered creaming.

(iv) Phase Inversion: Phase inversion means the change of one type of emulsion into the other type that is oil in water (o/w) emulsion changes into water in oil (w/o) type and vice versa. The temperature at which the inversion occurs depends on the emulsifier concentration and is called Phase Inversion Temperature (PIT). This refers to the process whereby there will be an exchange between the disperse phase and the medium. Inversion often can be seen when an emulsion, prepared by heating and mixing the two phases, is being cooled. This takes place presumably because of the temperature dependent changes in the solubilities of the emulsifying agents. It may also be due to addition of an electrolyte, change in the phase-volume ratio, or changing emulsifying agent.

(v) Coalescence (breaking or cracking): The coalescence is most common type of emulsion instability. The coalescence is the complete separation of the emulsion into two distinct liquid phases. The w/o type of emulsions are formed when the film of emulsifying agent at the interface is uncharged and rigid. Coalescence occurs when the mechanical or electrical barrier is insufficient to prevent the formation of progressively larger droplets. This refers to the process of thinning and disruption of the liquid film between the droplets with the result of fusion of two or more droplets into larger ones. The driving force for coalescence is the surface or film fluctuations which results in close approach of the droplets. A surface potential higher than 25 mV is not sufficient to stabilize the droplets of dispersed phase with a radius $\geq$ 1 μ against flocculation. This is because of the high sedimentation velocities. Stabilization against coalescence may be achieved by the addition of high boiling point or high molecular weight components to the continuous phase.

(vi) Ostwald Ripening (Disproportionation): This type of instability results from the finite solubility of the liquid phases. The phases of emulsion that are immiscible often have significant mutual solubilities. Emulsions, which are usually polydispersed systems, the smaller droplets will have larger solubility when compared with the larger ones due to curvature effects. With time, the smaller droplets disappear and their molecules diffuse to the bulk and become deposited on the larger droplets. Finally, on standing for long time, the droplet size distribution shifts to larger values

(vii) Process Variables: The preparation of stable w/o emulsion is critical for the manufacturing of good dosage form.

    (a) Effect of emulsifier concentration: The amount of emulsifier has great impact on emulsion stability. These agents when employed in specific concentration produce stable emulsion. But if used in concentrations outside the range, the emulsion stability quickly declines. At low emulsifier concentration, the emulsion is unstable because of agglomeration of the oil droplets. At high emulsifier concentration, emulsion instability occurs because of rapid coalescence.

(b) Effect of stirring intensity: Emulsification is usually achieved by applying mechanical energy. Stirring intensity is one of the important parameter that can affect emulsion stability. The interfacial areas between phases are increased by increase in rotational speed and diameter of the stirrer and by keeping the diameter of vessel low. In such a process, initially, the interface between the two phases is deformed to extents that large droplets are formed which are subsequently broken into small particles. Stirring is applied to form stable and homogeneous emulsion by converting large globules into small ones. It is clearly indicating that a more stable emulsion can be prepared with a higher stirring speed (< 2500 r.p.m.) but very high speed (> 2500 r.p.m.) will lead the emulsifier to break away from the oil-water interface.

(c) Effect of mixing temperature: Emulsions prepared at low temperature are stable; however, more stable emulsions can be prepared at a temperature of about 30°C. Process temperature indirectly changes in interfacial tension, absorption of emulsifying agent and viscosity. The surface tension of most liquids decreases with the increase of temperature. Due to this high kinetic energy, the surface molecules tend to overcome the attractive force of bulk liquid. Furthermore, at critical temperature value, the cohesive forces between the liquid molecules become zero; therefore, the surface tension will fade-off at critical temperature value. Generally higher temperatures are good for emulsification. However, minute decrease in temperature may cause coagulation of globules that result in destabilization of the emulsion.

(d) Effect of mixing time: In formulation of emulsion, mixing time has great significance. The radius of the droplet of the dispersed phase decrease with the increase of stirring speed and mixing time. Longer mixing times increases performance of emulsifying agents. However, too a long mixing time may cause decrease in its effectiveness. This is because severe stirring causes the emulsifier to separate out from liquids interface.

II. Chemical Instability

Chemical instability of an emulsion causes coalescence of particles of emulsion. It is necessary to ensure that any emulgent system use is not only physically but also chemically compatible with the active agent and with the other emulsion ingredients. Anionic and cationic emulgents are thus mutually incompatible. It has already been demonstrated that the presence of electrolyte can influence the stability of an emulsion either by reducing the energy of interaction between adjacent globules or by a salting out effect, by which high concentration of electrolyte can strip emulsifying agents of their hydrated layers and so cause their precipitation.

Change in pH may also lead to the breaking of emulsion. Soap stabilized emulsions are therefore usually formulated at an alkaline pH. Environmental conditions, such as the presence of light, air, contaminating microbes adversely affect the stability of an emulsion. For light sensitive emulsion, light resistance container is used. For emulsion susceptible to oxidative decomposition, anti-oxidants may be included in the formulation and adequate label warning is provided to ensure that the container is tightly closed to air after each use. Many molds, yeasts, and bacteria can decompose the emulsifying agent, disrupting the system. Even if the emulsifier is not affected by the microbes, the product can be rendered unsightly by their presence and growth and will not off course be efficacious from a pharmaceutical or therapeutic point. Because fungi (molds and yeasts) are more likely to contaminate emulsion than are bacteria, fungi static preservatives, commonly combinations of methyl paraben and propyl paraben are generally included in the aqueous phase of an o/w emulsion. Alcohol in the amount of 12 % to 15 % based on the external phase volume is frequently added to oral o/w emulsion for preservation.

Chemical instability is of three types namely**:**

(i)   Oxidation
(ii) Microbial contamination
(iii) Adverse storage condition

(i) Oxidation

Many of the oils and fats used in emulsion formulation are of animal or vegetable origin and can be susceptible to oxidation by atmospheric oxygen or by the action of micro-organisms. Oxidation of microbiological origin is controlled by the use of anti-microbial preservatives and atmospheric oxidation by the use of reducing agents or more usually, anti-oxidants like butylated hydroxy anisole (BHA) is widely used in the protection of fixed oil sand fats at concentration of up to 0.02 % and for some essential oils up to 0.1 %. The efficiency of an anti-oxidant in a product will depend on many factors, including**:**

(a) Its compatibility with other ingredients
(b) Its o/w partition coefficient
(c) The extent of its solubilization within micelles of the emulgent
(d) Its sorption onto the containers and its closure.

(ii) Microbial contamination

Microbial contamination of emulsion occurs by micro-organisms, they can adversely affect the physicochemical properties of the product, causing such problem as gas production, colour and odour changes, hydrolysis of fat sand oils, pH changes in the aqueous phase and breaking of the emulsion. An emulsion can contain many bacteria and if these include pathogens, may constitute a serious health hazard and most fungi and many bacteria will multiply readily in the aqueous phase of an emulsion at room temperature. Many moulds will also tolerate a wide pH range. Species of the genus Pseudomonas can utilize polysorbates, aliphatic hydro carbons and compounds. Some fixed oils such as arachis oil, can be used by some *aspergillus* and *rhizopus* species, and liquid paraffin by some species of *penicillium*. Water in oil (w/o) product have less chances of microbial spoilage as compared to oil in water (o/w), emulsion, as in the latter case the continuous oil phase act as a barrier to the spread of microorganisms throughout the product, and less water, there is present, the less growth there is likely to be. It is necessary to include an anti-microbial agent to prevent the growth of any microorganisms that might contaminate the product. Example, because fungi are more likely to contaminate emulsion then are bacteria, fungi static preservatives, commonly contamination of methyl paraben and propyl paraben are generally included in the aqueous phase of an oil in water emulsion.

(ii) Adverse storage condition

Adverse storage conditions may also cause emulsion instability by increase in temperature that cause increasing rate of creaming, owing to a fall in apparent viscosity of the continuous phase. Increase in temperature cause an increased kinetic motion, both of the dispersed droplet and of the emulsifying agent at the oil in water (o/w) interface. Increased motion of the emulgent will result in a more expended monolayer and so coalescence is more likely. Certain macro molecules emulsifying agents may also be coagulated by an increase in temperature. Freezing of the aqueous phase will produce ice crystals that may exert a pressure on the disposed globules and their absorbed layer of emulgent. In addition, dissolved electrolyte may concentrate in the unfrozen water, thus affecting the charge density on the globules. Certain emulgents may also precipitate at low temperature. The growth of micro-organisms within the emulsion can cause deterioration and it is therefore essential that these products are protected as far as possible from the ingress of micro-organisms during manufacture, storage and use.

III. Assessment of Emulsion Stability

A very important parameter for emulsion products is their stability. However, the evaluation of emulsion stability is not easy. Emulsion stability is regarded in terms of physical stability of emulsion system and the physical and chemical stability of the emulsion components.

    (i) Macroscopic examination (Phase separation): Testing of physical stability of an emulsion is examined by degree of creaming or coalescence (Phase separation) occurring over a period of time. The rate and extent of phase separation after aging of an emulsion may be observed visually or by measuring the volume of separated phase. A simple means of determining phase separation due to creaming or coalescence involves withdrawing a sample of the emulsion from the top and the bottom of the preparation after some period of storage and comparing the composition of the two samples by appropriate analysis of water content, oil content, or any suitable constituent.

(ii) Globule size analysis: Determination of changes in the average particle size is one of the parameters used for assessing emulsion stability. The coalescence of globules in emulsion results in increased mean globule size. The coalescence rates of a variety of emulsion formulations can be assessed by this size analysis. Optical microscopy, Andresen apparatus, coulter counter or laser diffraction sizing techniques are widely used for this purpose.

(iii) Determination of viscosity: A change in the globule size or number or migration of emulsifying agent during storage can be detected by a change in apparent viscosity of emulsion. Majority of emulsions follow non-Newtonian flow characteristics. The flocculation in o/w emulsions leads to an increase in viscosity. Viscosity can be measured by standard capillary tube and rotational viscometers.

(iv) Determination of electrophoretic properties: Presence of electric charges on the particles affects the rate of flocculation. The strength of charge is determined from the zeta potential of emulsion for assessing its stability. Electrostatically emulsion stabilization is net result of mutual repulsion between electrical double layers of oil and water phases. Electrophoretic stability is very sensitive to the ionic strength of solution. As the concentration of electrolyte increases, the electrical double layers of both the phases are compressed and the distance of electrostatic repulsion is reduced resulting in flocculation.

General emulsion properties and test methods used for assessing stability

Property	Test Method
pH	pH meter
Viscosity	Rotational viscometer
Flow behaviour	Oscillatory shear viscosity with a cone/plate rheometer
Tack/Texture	Extensional and compressional deformation
Colour	Visual or colourimeter
Odour	Organoleptic
Specific gravity	Pycnometer
Separation	Creaming value - visual or instrumental
Conductivity	Conductivity meter
Droplet size distribution	Microscopic examination (image analysis) and instrumental
Preservation	Microbial challenge and/or assay
Vibration	Shipping test or shaker table
Active ingredient(s)	Chemical or bio-assay

10.7 REMEDY FOR EMULSION INSTABILITY

(i) Flocculation: The presence of high charged density on the dispersed droplets will ensure the presence of a high energy barrier and these reduce the incidence of flocculation.

(ii) Creaming

(a) Reduction of the globules size by using an efficient homogenizer.

(b) Increasing the viscosity of the continuous phase by using viscosity imparting agent.

(c) By reducing the density difference between two phases.

(d) By controlling the dispersed phase concentration.

(e) By storing in a cool place or low temperature.

(iii) Coalescence

(a) By adding sufficient amount of emulsifying agent and passing the product through the proper emulsifying machinery.

(b) During preparation, the addition of emulsifying agent should be appropriate because the use of wrong emulsifying agent loses its activity within a short period of time.

(iv) Breaking or Cracking

(a) By incorporating more emulsifying agent.
(b) By controlling the temperature at which emulsion is kept.
(c) By controlling disperse phase concentration.
(d) By adding correct emulsifying agent.

(iv) Phase inversion

The phase inversion can be minimized by keeping the concentration of dispersed phase between 30 to 60 %, storing the emulsion in a cool place and by using proper emulsifying agent in adequate concentration.

(v) Microbial contamination

Add chemical agent that will act specially as preservative. Combination of para-hydroxy benzoates 0.1% to 2% of methyl ester and 0.02% to 0.05% of propyl ester are frequently used for this purpose. Preservative should be adequately soluble in both phases. If not more than one type of preservatives should be used, one for oil phase and other for aqueous phase. The emulsifying agent and other ingredients of the formulation should not form complex with the preservatives.

(vi) Miscellaneous:

Care must be taken to protect emulsion against deterioration caused by light, temperature in box freezing and thawing.

MODEL QUESTIONS

1. Define and classify emulsion.
2. What is emulsifying agents? Give mechanism of emulsifying agents.
3. Give theories of emulsification.
4. Explain different identification tests for emulsion.
5. Explain different methods of preparation of emulsion.
6. Elaborate different stability problems in emulsion.
7. How emulsion stability is assessed? Explain different remedies for instability of emulsion.
8. Write a note on:
   (i)   Multiple emulsion
   (ii) Nano-emulsion
   (iii) Emulsifying agents

■■■

Chapter 11...

Suppositories

LEARNING OBJECTIVES

Suppositories are medicated solid dosage forms intended for insertion into body cavities other than mouth where they melt, soften, or dissolve and exert localized or systemic effects.

The objectives of this chapter includes:

- Define and understand the basic concept, need, types and uses of suppositories.
- Recognize route of drug administration through suppositories with examples.
- To understand general considerations for bases and other excipients, calculation of displacement value and methods of manufacturing and packaging and storage of suppositories.
- To know testing of finished suppositories for its quality.

11.1 INTRODUCTION

Suppositories are medicated solid dosage forms intended for insertion into body cavities other than mouth where they melt, soften, or dissolve and exert localized or systemic effects. The term suppositories have its origin in Latin '*Suppositorium*' and it means, 'to place under'. It is a contemplation that suppositories were first used in nursing facilities to be administered to geriatric patients, who were not able to take medicines through more traditional delivery systems. Suppositories usually melt, soften or dissolve at body temperature. Suppositories act as protectant or palliative to local tissue at the point of introduction or act as carrier of medicaments to systemic circulation or local effect.

Suppositories generally consist of an active drug incorporated into an inert matrix, which may be either a rigid or semi-rigid base. This mixture of drug and inert matrix should not have any interactions. Suppository base disperse or dilute, carry, protect and deliver active drug into patient. Once administered; suppositories melt due to body temperature and release drug by dissolving in mucosal fluids where active drug shows its local effect and after transport to systemic circulation, it shows systemic effect. The physicochemical properties of both the drug and suppository base are important determinants of the clinical and non-clinical performance of suppositories.

Suppositories are available in various sizes, shapes, volume and consistency which facilitate their insertion and retention in the cavity. If it is meant for insertion into rectum, then it is called as suppository. If special form meant for insertion into vagina, then it is called as 'pessaries' and if it is meant for insertion into other body cavities such as urethra and nasal then it is called as 'urethral bougies' and 'nasal bougies' respectively.

Suppositories have been used for the last 200 years but their utility as a medication increased from around 1840 for constipation, haemorrhoids, and pessaries for vaginal infections and bougies for infections of the urethra, prostate, bladder or nose.

Indications of suppositories

The use of suppositories is indicated under the following circumstances:

(i)   To empty the bowel before certain types of surgery.

(ii) To empty the bowel to relieve acute constipation or when other treatments for constipation have failed.

(iii) To empty the bowel before endoscopic examination.

(iv) To introduce medication into the system.

(v)   To soothe and treat hemorrhoids or anal pruritus.

Contraindications of suppositories

The use of suppositories is contraindicated when one or more of the following concern:

(i)   Chronic constipation, which would require repetitive use.

(ii) Paralytic ileus.

(iii) Colonic obstruction.

(iv) Following gastrointestinal or gynaecological operations, unless on the specific instructions of the doctor.

11.2 TYPES OF SUPPOSITORIES

1.   Rectal Suppositories
2.   Vaginal Suppositories/Pessaries
3.   Urethral suppositories
4.   Nasal suppositories
5.   Ear cones
6.   Special Types/Recently developed suppositories

1.   Rectal Suppositories

Rectal suppositories are meant for introduction into rectum (anus) for their local and systemic effect. Rectal suppositories are tapered at one end; to aid insertion and are frequently wider in the middle before tapering towards the other end; thereby aiding retention in the rectum and enabling the suppository to be pressed forward by the anal sphincter. They are also cone shaped with rounded apex. Its weight for children is about 1 g and for adults 2 g, torpedo shape.

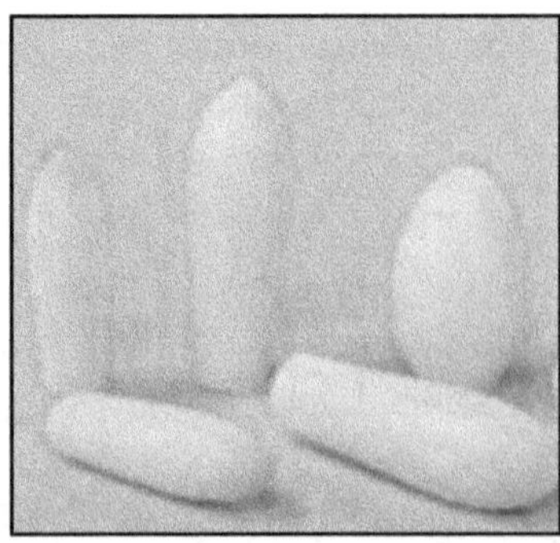

Fig. 11.1: Rectal Suppositories

Use

First wash hands. Read the medication label and remove a suppository from the packet. Moisten the suppository with water or water – based lubricating jelly. Then lie on side with knees pulled up towards chest. Gently insert the suppository into the rectum (back passage) with finger as far as it will go, tapered end first. Lower legs, squeeze buttocks together and lie still for a few minutes. Patients may feel the urge to force the suppository out again. This urge should pass once the suppository has melted which should only take a few minutes. After lying still for a few minutes, then wash hands again. Avoid going to the toilet for at least one hour (unless the suppository is a laxative).

Examples:

1. Suppol® Baby / Child / 250 (Meridian): Paracetamol I.P. 80 mg or 170 mg or 250mg: Antipyretic
2. GV-SOFT (Bliss): Glycerin USP 90% w/w: Laxative
3. Mesacol® Suppositories (Sun Pharma): Mesalamine 500 mg: To treat ulcerative proctitis, a type of bowel disease.

2. Vaginal Suppositories/Pessaries:

Pessaries are solid medicated preparations made for insertion into vagina for local and/or systemic action. Weight of pessaries ranges from 3 g to 5 g and more, hence it requires larger size mould than rectal suppositories. They are available in globular, oviform shaped, rod shaped, wedge shaped or compressed on a tablet press into conical shapes (vaginal tablets) and also available in the form of capsule (vaginal capsule). Pessaries can be inserted using fingers into vagina but for special shaped pessaries, applicators are provided to facilitate insertion into vagina. Pessaries are exclusively used for its local action in vagina except few medications such as prostaglandin, which exert a systemic effect. Commonly used drugs for inclusion into pessaries are antiseptics, contraceptive agents, local anaesthetics, various therapeutic agents to treat trichomonal, bacterial and monilial infections.

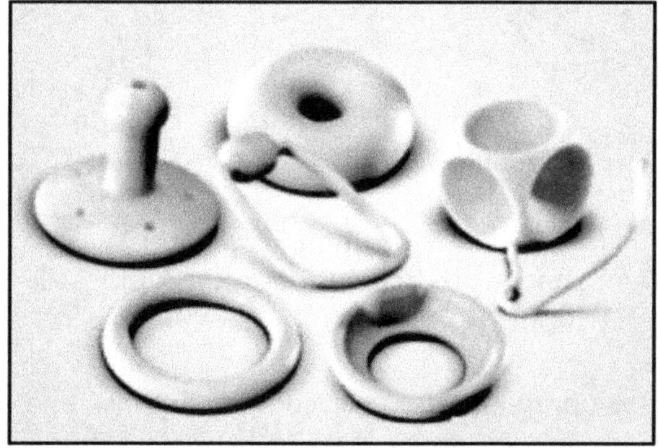

Fig. 11.2: Vaginal Suppositories and Application

Uses of vaginal suppositories / Pessaries

First wash hands and read the medication label before using pessaries. Remove any foil or plastic wrapping from the pessary and applicator (if supplied). If an applicator is supplied, push the pessary into the hole at the end of the applicator. Sit or lie down with knees bent and legs apart. Gently insert the pessary into the vagina as far as is comfortably possible using either fingers or the applicator. If applicator is used, depress the plunger to release the pessary then remove the applicator from vagina. Wash hands again.

Examples:

1. Candid CL® Vaginal Pessary (Glenmark): Clotrimazole-200 mg, Clindamycin-100 mg: Antifungal.
2. TODAY® Vaginal Contraceptive (Bliss GVS): Nonoxynol -9 USP- 5 %w/w: Vaginal Contraceptive.
3. Vagifem® Estradiol Vaginal Tablets (Novo Nordisk): Estradiol 10 mcg: Used to treat menopausal changes in and around the vagina.

3. Urethral Suppositories

Urethral suppositories are meant for insertion into urethra. They are also known as 'urethral bougies'. They are available in long, thin, cylindrical form or pencil shaped. Those intended for males weigh 4 g each and are 100-150 mm long while those for females are 2 g each and 60-75 mm in length. Urethral suppositories are very rarely used.

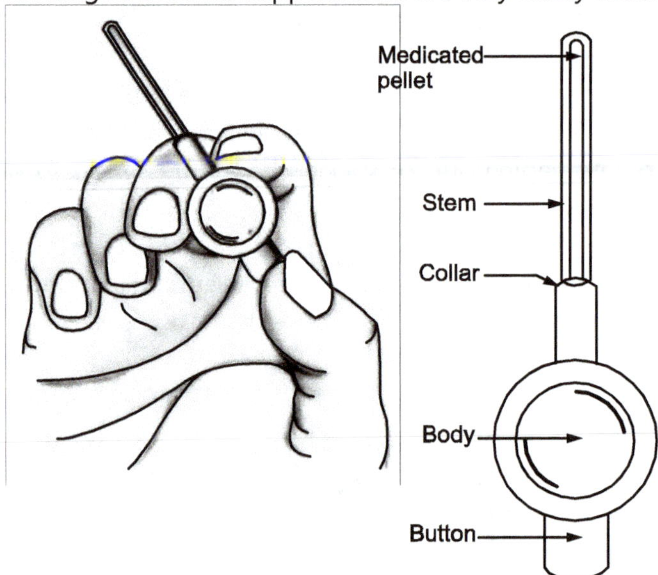

Fig. 11.3: Urethral Suppository

Example: MUSE® (Alprostadil) urethral suppository: Alprostadil 125 mcg: used for the treatment of erectile dysfunction.

4. Nasal Suppositories

Nasal Suppositories are prepared using glycerogelatin base and are meant for insertion into nasal cavity. They are also called as 'nasal bougies' or 'buginaria'. They have similar shape as that of urethral suppositories having weight 1 g and length 1-2 cm.

5. Ear Suppositories

Ear Suppositories are prepared using theobroma oil as a base and are meant for insertion into ear. They are also called as 'aurinaria'. They are prepared using urethral suppository mould and then cut into required size. Ear suppositories are rarely used.

6. Recent development as special suppositories

(a) Tablet suppositories: Rectal suppositories and pessaries are compressed into tablet and are called as tablet suppositories. Such tablet suppositories are not necessary to keep at lower temperature as it is prepared using superdisintegrants and it gets disintegrated in presence of low fluids in body cavity. Tablet suppositories are generally coated with polyethylene glycol (PEG) for protection and also to facilitate its insertion into rectum.

(b) Capsule suppositories: They are same as soft gelatin capsules. Liquid or semisolid content of drug is filled into soft gelatin capsule of various size and shape so that it can be inserted into rectum or vagina.

(c) Layered suppositories: In this type of suppositories, different drugs having incompatibility with each other or are having different melting points can be incorporated in single suppository. It can be prepared by partial filling of mould with matrix of one drug and base, once it gets solidified or congealed, fill mould with matrix of another drug and base as a separate layer.

(d) Packaging in disposable moulds: Now-a-day's, suppositories are directly made into disposable plastic or tin foil's mould instead of metallic mould where latter is necessary to be packed into individual wrapper and supplied in boxes. Advantage of such type of suppository is; if the content melts due to any reason during transportation or storage, it will remain in mould itself and can be used after cooling in refrigerator.

(e) Hollow-Type Suppositories: It has a hollow cavity to hold drugs in various forms such as a powder and solution. It is considered better than conventional suppository as it is not affected by properties of base, as in conventional suppository. From hollow suppositories, drug gets released faster than from conventional suppositories.

(f) Hydrogel Suppositories: Hydrogel means the macromolecular network that swells but does not dissolve in water and is used as base in this type of suppositories. The rate and extent of drug release from this hydrogel matrix depends upon the water migration into the matrix and rate of drug diffusion out of the swollen matrix.

(g) Sectile or Bisected Suppositories: This type of suppository has bisected or beveled edge at middle. The purpose of having bisect at middle is that, for child; half part of suppository can be used after cutting and for adult, whole suppository can be used.

(h) Thermo-Reversible-Liquid Suppository: These liquid suppositories form gel at body temperature. It has suitable gel strength so that it will not leak out from anus after administration. Such a gel has suitable mucoadhesive force hence it will not reach to end of the colon.

(i) Effervescent Suppository: In this type of suppository, composition of citric acid or tartaric acid and sodium bicarbonate is incorporated into suppository base. After administration uptake of fluid causes effervescence which break suppository and release medication.

(j) Sustained Release Suppositories: In order to maintain desired concentration of drug for longer period of time, sustained release suppositories are prepared either by modification of suppository base or by using special additives or sustained release polymers or polymer coated drug particles. These types of suppositories are prepared to retard release of drug from base for longer period of time so as to avoid multiple administrations and also to maintain therapeutic effect.

11.3 ADVANTAGES AND DISADVANTAGES

Advantages:

1. Self-administration is possible with suppository.
2. It can be used for systemic absorption of drugs and avoid first-pass metabolism.
3. It can exert local effect on rectal mucosa.
4. It protects drug from harsh conditions in stomach.
5. It avoids gastrointestinal irritation of drug if any.
6. Drug causes nausea and vomiting which can be administered using suppositories.
7. Suppository is convenient to use when oral intake is restricted before surgery.
8. It is convenient to use for the post-operative people who cannot be administered oral medication.
9. It can be used for patient suffering from severe vomiting and for unconscious patients (for example, during fitting).
10. It has high drug loading capacity.
11. Lymphatic delivery is possible using suppository.
12. It provides constant and static environment for drug absorption.
13. It shows rapid onset of action than that of after oral administration as drug is directly absorbed from the mucosa into the venous circulation.
14. It can be used for site targeted delivery system.

Disadvantages

1. Un-comfort: As administration of rectal suppository requires privacy; it has problem of patent acceptability.
2. Difficult to self-administer by arthritic or physically compromised patients.

3. Leakage: Melted suppository may leak from body cavities especially in vaginal and rectal products.
4. Unpredictable and variable absorption of drug may be found in suppository.
5. Irritation of mucous may be caused by some drugs or bases due to repeated administration of suppository.

Factors affecting absorption of drug from suppository

(a) Physiological factors

(i)   Quantity of fluid available: The quantity of fluid available for drug dissolution is very small (approximately 3 mL). Thus the dissolution of slightly soluble substances is the slowest step in the absorption process.

(ii) The properties of rectal fluid: The rectal fluid is neutral in pH (7 – 8) and has no buffer capacity.

(iii) Contents of the rectum: When systemic effects are desired, greater absorption may be expected from an empty rectum as the drug will be in good contact with the absorbing surface of the rectum.

(iv) Circulation route: The lower hemorrhoidal veins surrounding the colon receive the absorbed drug and initiate its circulation throughout the body, bypassing the liver. Lymphatic circulation also assists in the absorption.

(b) Physicochemical properties of Drug and suppository base

Physicochemical properties of drug such as relative solubility of the drug in lipid and in water and the particle size, pKa, dose etc. and that of suppository base include its ability to melt, soften, or dissolve at body temperature, its ability to release the drug substance, and its hydrophilic or hydrophobic characters affect absorption of drug through suppository.

(i)   Drug solubility in vehicle: The rate at which a drug is released from a suppository and absorbed by the rectal mucous membrane is directly related to its solubility in the vehicle or, in other words, to the partition coefficient of the drug between the vehicle and the rectal liquids. When drugs are highly soluble in the vehicle, the tendency to leave the vehicle will be small and so the release rate into the rectal fluid will be low.

(ii) Particle Size: For drugs present in a suppository in the undissolved state, the size of the drug particle will influence its rate of dissolution and its availability for absorption. The smaller the particles size, the more readily the dissolution of the particle and greater the chance for rapid absorption.

(iii) Nature of the base: The base must be capable of melting, softening, or dissolving to release its drug components for absorption. If the base interacts with the drug inhibiting its release, drug absorption will be impaired or even prevented. If the base is irritating to the mucous membrane of the rectum, it may initiate a colonic response and a bowel movement, which incomplete drug release and absorption.

(iv) Spreading Capacity: The rapidity and intensity of the therapeutic effects of suppositories are related to the surface area of the rectal mucous membrane covered by the melted base: drug mixture (the spreading capacity of the suppositories). This spreading capacity may be related to the presence of surfactants in the base.

Applications of suppository:

Suppositories are mainly used for their mechanical, local and systemic action.

(i)   Mechanical action: Suppositories are used to get mechanical action to facilitate evacuation of bowel in the treatment of hemorrhoids, anal irritation and in constipation by irritating the mucous membrane of rectum or by lubricating action.

(ii) Local action: Suppository can be used for local action for drug such as emollient, astringent, antiseptic, local anesthetic, antibacterial etc.

(iii) Systemic action: For drugs such as analgesic, antispasmodic, sedative, hypnotics, tranquilizer, vasodilator, hormone etc.

11.4 FORMULATION OF SUPPOSITORY

For formulation of suppository following components are required:

(I)   Drug (active pharmaceutical ingredient)
(II)   Suppository base
(III) Additives
(IV) Packaging material

I. Drug

Drug which has stability problem in GIT or drug which irritate gastric mucosa can be used for preparation of suppository. Drugs which are used for treatment of disorders of lowest bowel can be used in formulation of suppository. Drugs which are required to be administered in unconscious and pediatric patients as well as for the treatment of pregnancy, chemotherapy and allergy induced emesis can be manufactured in the form of suppository. Drug for which sustained-release is required for long-term treatment of chronic diseases like essential hypertension, asthma, diabetes, AIDS, anemia etc are used for preparation of suppositories. Drug to be incorporated into suppository should require minimum base so as to produce smaller weight suppository. Drug should be soluble in base so as to get homogeneity but should not lower melting point of base. It should be stable and compatible with base and other additives of suppository during its processing and use.

II. Suppository Base

Suppository base are substances used to carry drug, dilute drug to non-irritating level, control release of drug from suppository and represent drug in acceptable usable form. Suppository base must melt, soften or dissolve in order to facilitate or promote the release of drug in such a way that it is readily available for absorption. Physico-chemical interactions between drug and suppository base may affect stability and bioavailability of drug hence such possible interactions must be checked in preformulation studies. If suppository base irritates mucous membrane, it will initiate a colonic response and hence promote unwanted bowel moment which may cause expulsion of dosage form and affect absorption of drug.

Ideal characteristics of suppository base

(i)   It should be non-toxic, non-irritant and non-sensitive to inflamed tissue.

(ii)   It should melt at rectal cavity temperature (36°C) or other body cavities temperature.

(iii)   It should be compatible with drug and additives and has no meta-stable form.

(iv)   It should have enough volume contraction on cooling for easy release from moulds.

(v)   It should be able to incorporate more amount of water in it (should have high 'water number').

(vi)   It should have wetting and emulsifying properties.

(vii)   It should be chemically and physically stable over the period of storage (shelf-life).

(viii) Acid value should be less than 0.2, saponification value ranges from 200 to 245 and iodine value should be less than 7.

(ix)   Solid fat index (SFI) should be sharp i.e. the interval between melting point and solidification point should be small.

(x)   Suppository base should have a high viscosity at negligible shear (during shelf storage), and should have a low viscosity at high shearing rate (agitation pouring and spreading). Thus thixotropic as well as pseudoplastic bases are useful as they form a gel on standing and become fluid when disturbed.

(xi)   Easily available and economic.

As suppository must retain its shape, solidity and firmness during storage and administration but should melt in the body cavity, it should possess all above ideal properties. But it is difficult to get all ideal properties from single base hence many times combination of different suppository base is used to get desired properties of suppository.

Types of suppository base

Suppository bases can be classified according to their composition and physical properties as Oleaginous (fatty) bases that melt at body temperature and water soluble or water miscible bases that dissolve or disperse in rectal secretion. It is broadly classified into four types:

1.   Oily base/Oleaginous or fatty bases
2.   Hydrophilic base:
3.   Water dispersible base:
4.   Emulsifying base:

1. Oily (oleaginous or fatty) base

(a) Cocoa butter/ Theobroma oil

Cocoa butter is fat obtained from roasted seed of *Theobroma cocoa* belonging to family Sterculiaceae. It is a yellowish white solid which becomes white on storage. It has butter like consistency and chocolate like odour. It is a mixture of liquid triglycerides entrapped in a network of crystalline, solid triglycerides. Palmitic acid and stearic acid make-up about half of the saturated fatty acids and oleic acid constitutes the only unsaturated fatty acid.

Cocoa butter is widely used rectal suppository base because it is solid at room temperatures but melts readily on contact with the skin. Its melting range is 30-36°C. Cocoa butter satisfies many requirements for an ideal base, since it is innocuous, bland, non-reactive, melts at body temperature and miscible with many ingredients. But it is not suitable for pessaries, nasal and urethral bougies as it leaks out after melting and immiscible with mucous secretions.

Advantages:

(i) Solid at room temperature but melts in the body.
(ii) Readily melted on warming, rapid setting on cooling.
(iii) Miscible with many ingredients.
(iv) Non-irritating.

Disadvantages:

(i) **Polymorphism:** As Cocoa butter contain high proportion of unsaturated triglycerides; it is existing in four crystalline form such as α, β, β', and γ and all these polymorphic form have different melting point. Hence knowledge of this polymorphic form is necessary to control release of drug from cocoa butter.

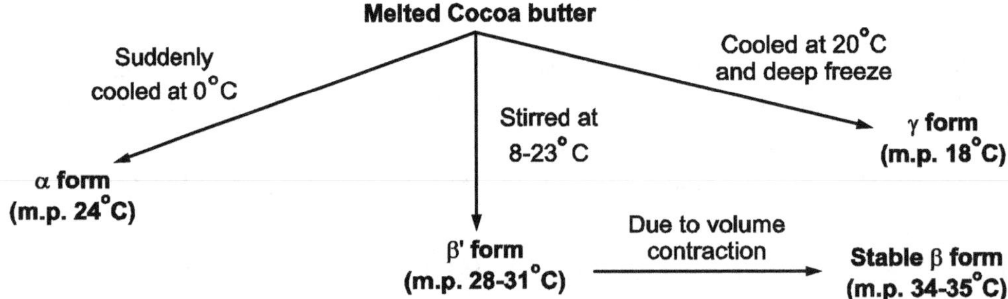

Fig. 11.4: Different polymorphic form of cocoa butter

The formation of unstable form can be avoided by preventing overheating of Cocoa butter: If mass is not completely melted the remaining crystals prevent formation of unstable form. Seeding, i.e. addition of some crystals of stable form of cocoa butter, accelerates conversion of unstable to stable form. One can store solidified melt of cocoa butter at 28-32°C temperature for few days which converts unstable form to stable form.)

(ii) Cocoa butter has tendency to adhere to side of mould when solidified. This problem can be avoided by using suitable mould lubricant/releaser before pouring molten mass into suppository moulds.

(iii) Leakage occurs when it melts.

(iv) Rancidity on storage due to oxidation of unsaturated glycerides.

(v) Poor water-absorbing ability: Improved by the addition of emulsifying agents such as 5-10 % of Tween 61.

(vi) Immiscible with body fluid hence failure to release medicaments.

(vii) Liquefy when mixed with certain medicaments.

(viii) Melts in warm weather.

(ix) Expensive.

(b) Emulsified Theobroma Oil

When large quantity of aqueous solutions is to be incorporated into suppository and to promote the diffusion of the active medicinal agent to the surrounding tissue and its subsequent absorption, this emulsified theobroma oil is used as base. It is prepared by emulsifying theobroma oil with different emulsifying agents. e.g. incorporation of 5% glyceryl monostearate will produce product with 35°C melting point and can be used as base for preparation of suppository either by hot or the cold method. 2% lecithin and 98% theobroma oil forms an oil-in-water emulsified base. 2% cholesterol with theobroma oil will produce water-in-oil emulsion. Other additives used to prepare emulsified theobroma oil are 10% lanette wax, 2-3% cetyl alcohol, 4% bees wax and up to 12% spermaceti wax etc.

(c) Shea Butter

Shea butter has been extracted from the seeds of the shea tree, *Butyrospermum parkii*, belonging to family Sapotaceae. It contains 36-44% of glycerides of stearic acid and 46-59% of oleic acid. It has melting point 37.8°C and compatible with many drugs. It has good water absorption capacity. It can be used along with beeswax and polysorbate 80 to improve physicochemical and drug release properties.

(d) Synthetic Hydrogenated Oils/Hard Fats

Synthetic hydrogenated oils or hard fats are prepared by hydrolyzing different vegetable oils then hydrogenating resulting fatty acids and finally re-emulsifying the acids by heating with glycerol. Different oils used to prepare synthetic hydrogenated hard fat are edible oil, coconut oil, palm kernel oil, pea oil, stearin and mixture of oleic acid and stearic acid. These are recommended as substitute for theobroma oil.

Example: Fattibase®:

It is triglycerides from palm, palm kernel, and coconut oils with self-emulsifying glyceryl monostearate and polyoxyl stearate. It is a pre-blended suppository base that offers the advantages of a cocoa butter base with few of the drawbacks. This base is stable with a low irritation profile, needs no special storage conditions, is uniform in composition, and has controlled melting range. It exhibits excellent mold release characteristics and does not require mold lubrication. Fattibase is a solid with a melting point of 35°C to 37°C, has a specific gravity of 0.890 at 37°C, is opaque white, and is free of suspended matter.

Advantages over theobroma oil:

(i)   Synthetic hydrogenated oils/ hard fats produce white, clean, attractive, polished and odourless suppositories.

(ii)   Solidifying point is unaffected by overheating.

(iii) As difference between melting and setting points is small; they set quickly hence the risk of sedimentation of suspended ingredients is low.

(iv)   As their unsaturated fatty acids have been reduced; they have good resistance to oxidation.

(v)   Good water absorbing capacity.

(vi)   As they contract on cooling, it does not require mould lubricants.

Disadvantages:

(i)   Molten hydrogenated oils/ hard fats are less viscous than theobroma oil hence suspended or added substances get settled down. But this problem can be overcome by addition of thickening agent such as bentonite, magnesium stearate or colloidal silicon dioxide.

(ii)   It becomes brittle after rapid cooling in refrigerator. (avoid refrigeration during preparation).

2. Hydrophilic base

(a) Glycero-gelatin base

Glycero-gelatin base is mixture of glycerin and water which is made thick/a stiff jelly by addition of gelatin. As it is hydrophilic in nature, suppositories prepared using glycerol-gelatin base slowly dissolve in the aqueous secretions and provide a slow, continuous release of medication. It may be used to prepare all types of suppositories and it is particularly useful in vaginal suppositories. It is well adapted for the incorporation of solid extracts such as belladonna. It may also be used for suppositories containing boric acid; bromides, chloral hydrate, iodide, iodoform, opium and other drugs. Glycero-gelatin base is also recommended for their effective use as antiseptics such as hexyl resorcinol, nitromersol, and phemerol in suppository form. The composition for glycero-gelatin base as per different Pharmacopoeia is as follows:

Ingredient	BP and EP	USP	BPC
Gelatin	14 g	20 g	25 g
Glycerin	70 g	70 g	40 g
Water to	100 g	100 g	100 g
	For solid drugs and liquids < 20%		For liquid> 20%

Two types of gelatin are used for preparation of glycero-gelatin base. Type A gelatin (Trade name: Pharmagel-A) which is acidic in nature and used for acidic drugs and Type B gelatin (Trade name: Pharmagel-B) which is alkaline in nature and used for alkaline drugs.

The base does not melt at body temperature, but rather dissolves in the secretions of the cavity in which they are inserted. Solution time is regulated by the proportion of gelatin, glycerin, water used, the nature of gelatin used, and the chemical reaction of the drug with gelatin.

Disadvantages:

(i)   They have a physiological action (Glycerol suppository BP is a laxative)

(ii)   Unpredictable solution time. This varies with the batch of gelatin and the age of the base.

(iii)   Difficult to prepare and handle.

(iv)   Hygroscopic: The base requires protection from heat and moisture and also has a dehydrating effect on the rectal or vaginal mucosa leading to irritation.

(v)   Microbial contamination. The base may require preservatives such as methyl and propyl paraben which may lead to problems of incompatibility.

(vi)   Suppository prepared are difficult to remove from moulds hence lubrication of the moulds is required.

(vii) Gelatin is incompatible with protein precipitants such as tannic acid, ferric chloride, gallic acid etc.

(b) Soap glycerin

It is same as that of glycero-gelatin base; here gelatin is replaced by soap as hardening agent. Soap is produced by interaction between stearic acid and sodium carbonate. Advantages of Soap glycerin base over glycero-gelatin base are larger quantity of glycerin can be incorporated actually up to 95% of the mass which can assist action glycerin. It makes glycerin sufficiently harder than gelatin. Disadvantage of soap glycerin suppository is that it is very hygroscopic, and required to be wrapped in waxed paper or pure tin foil, and protected from the atmosphere.

(c) Polyethylene glycol/ Macrogols

Macrogol is the International Non-proprietary Name (INN) for Polyethylene glycol (PEG). They are polymers of ethylene oxide and water and their ethers. It is also called as 'carbowaxes' and 'polyglycols'. PEG having molecular weight 200 to 1000 are liquid and those having molecular weight more than 1000 are wax like consistency. Their water solubility, hygroscopicity and vapor pressure decreases with increasing molecular weight. Suppositories of different melting point can be prepared using combination of different molecular weight PEG. Following compositions are generally used for preparation of suppository:

Composition of PEG	Use
PEG 1000 - 96 % PEG 4000 - 04 %	This base is soft and used for fast release of drug
PEG 1000 - 75 % PEG 4000 - 25 %	It is used for slow release of drug
PEG 1540 - 70 % PEG 6000 - 30 %	It is used for drug having lower melting point
PEG 1540 - 30 % PEG 6000 - 50 % Water - 20 %	As it contains water, it is used for water soluble drugs

Advantages:

(i)   Physiologically inert (no laxative effect) and chemically stable.
(ii)   As base contracts slightly; there is no requirement of lubricant during moulding.
(iii)   Microbial contamination is less.
(iv)   Can be used for prolonged and immediate action.
(v)   As melting point is above body temperature (42°C); cool storage is not required.
(vi)   It has good solvent property.
(vii)   Produce suppository with clean smooth appearance.
(viii) Because of their high molecular weight, solutions of high viscosity are produced when they disperse in the body and leakage is not a serious problem.

Disadvantages:

(i)   Hygroscopic; hence require special storage condition and it may cause irritation and dehydration of the rectum.
(ii)   Incompatibilities; Polyethylene glycol bases are incompatible with some medicaments, for example, phenols and tannins, and reduce the activity of some antibacterial agent such as quaternary ammonium compounds and hydroxyl benzoate. They also interact with some plastics, hence limits the choice of container.

(iii)   Reduced therapeutic effect: good solvent properties can cause drug retention in the liquefied base with reduced therapeutics effect.

(iv)   It may produce brittle suppository.

3. Water dispersible base

Many non-ionic surfactants chemically related with PEG have been used as suppository base. Most commonly used are the polyoxyethylene sorbitan fatty acid esters (Tweens), the polyoxyethylene stearates (Myrj), and the sorbitan fatty acid esters (Spans).These surfactants may be used alone, blended or in combination with other suppository vehicle materials to yield a wide range of melting points and consistencies.

Surface-active agents are extensively used in combination with other suppository bases. Inclusion of surfactants in the formulation may improve the wetting and water-absorption properties of the suppository. In addition, emulsifying surfactants help to keep insoluble substances suspended in a fatty base suppository. The inclusion of a surfactant in the suppository formulation may enhance the rectal absorption of drugs. Many of these bases can be used for suppository of water soluble and oil soluble medicaments. Checking compatibility of medicament with surfactant must be checked while using this type of suppository base.

4. Emulsifying base

(a) Massa estrinum

It is also called as *Adeps solidus.* It is a mixture of the monoglycerides, diglycerides, and triglycerides of the saturated fatty acids having the formula $C_{11}H_{23}COOH$ to $C_{17}H_{35}COOH$. Several grades of Mass estrinum such as Massaestrinum A, AB, AS, B, BB, BC, BD and C are available. It is white, brittle, almost odourless and tasteless solid. They possess a melting range of 33 to 38°C.

(b) Massupol

It consists of glyceryl esters, mainly of lauric acid, to which a very small amount of glyceryl monostearate has been added to increase water absorbing capacity. It has melting range of 34 to 37°C, and is suitable for mass production.

(c) Witepsol

It is a white and odourless base consist of triglycerides of saturated vegetable acids with varying proportions of partial esters. The bees wax is also added for use in hot condition. Nine grades are available of which Witepsol H_{12}, H_{15}, W_{35}, S_{55}, E_{75} and E_{55} are in common uses. They are suitable for formulation of eutectic mixtures and tropical suppositories. Suppositories prepared with witepsol should not be ice-cooled or should not cool rapidly because it may become brittle and fractured. Also mould must not be lubricated while using this base. It has no polymorphisms when heated and cooled.

(d) Wecobee bases

It is derived from triglycerides of higher melting fractions of coconut oil and palm kernal oil and may contain 0.25% of lecithin. Addition of glyceryl monosterate and propylene glycol monostearate makes them emulsifiable.

(e) Dehydarz bases

Three grades of this base are available to prepare suppository as base I, II and G. Grade I and II contain hardened fatty alcohols and fats and grade G contain saturated fatty alcohol. So as to increase melting point of grade I and II; waxes or high melting alcohols may be added. It does not exhibit polymorphism.

Advantages:

(i) Emulsifying bases will not alter its physical characteristics after over heating.
(ii) As they do not stick to the mould; pre-lubrication of mould is not required.
(iii) They can absorb large amount of aqueous liquid as it contains emulsifying agents.
(iv) They solidify rapidly.
(v) Less liable to get rancid.

Disadvantages:

(i) They are not too viscous; hence added medicaments may settle down.
(ii) They become brittle on refrigeration or after rapid cooling.

III. Additives

Plasticizers such as cetyl alcohol, propylene glycol are used to impart softness and resilience to suppositories. Absorption promoting agents are also used in suppository as additive so as to increase absorptions of drug with low bioavailability like antibiotic and having high molecular weights. Other additives include antioxidants (e.g. BHA, BHT) which are used as per requirement and after checking its compatibility with drug and suppository base.

IV. Packaging material

(i) **Blister packing:** The packing material normally used is PVC film, aluminium foil is also used as per requirements. Normally the blister pack contains 5 suppositories and such blisters are further packed into a carton which contains 2 blisters each.

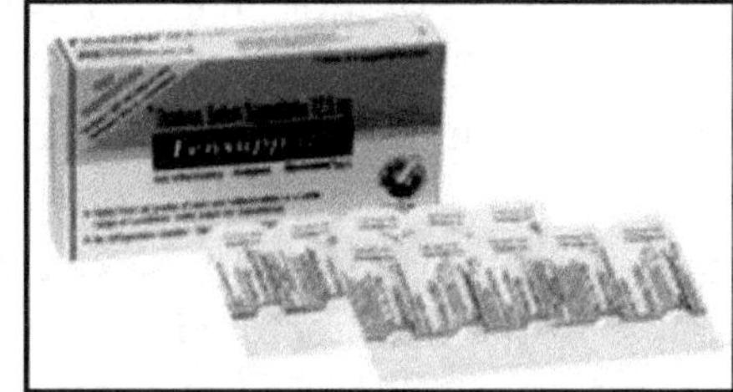

Fig. 11.5: Suppositories in blister packing

(ii) Strip Packing: Pouch type strip packing which contains 5 suppositories each, these strips are of 4 ply material [poly + aluminum + poly + paper (inner layer-poly and extreme outer layer-paper)]. Such strips are further packed into a carton which contains 2 strips each.

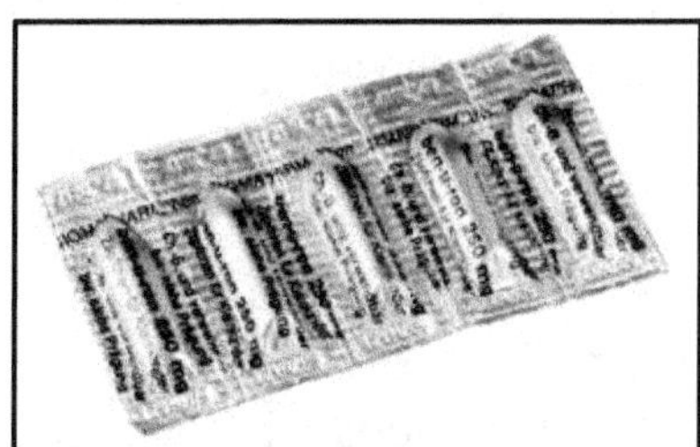

Fig. 11.6: Suppositories in strip packing

(iii) Bottle packing: Plastic bottles sealed with aluminium taggers. Such bottles are further packed in an e-flute carton which contains bottles. Such e-flute cartons are then finally packed into a master corrugated shipper.

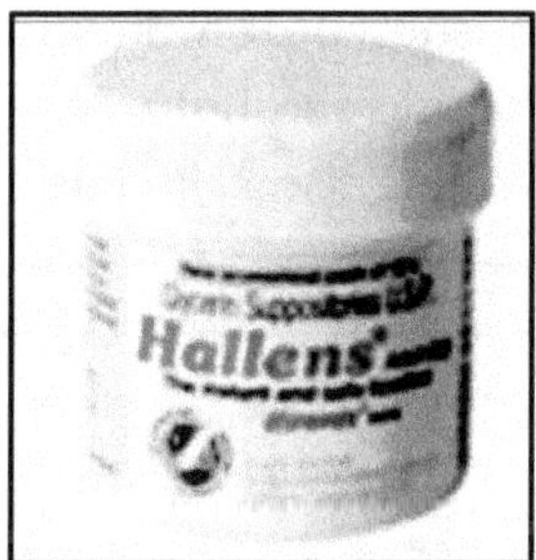

Fig. 11.7: Suppositories in bottle packing

(iv) Plastic disposable moulds: Now-a-days, suppositories are packed into plastic disposable mould. Advantage of such packaging material is that, if suppository gets liquefied during transportation or storage, content will remain in the plastic disposable mould and can be used after refrigeration.

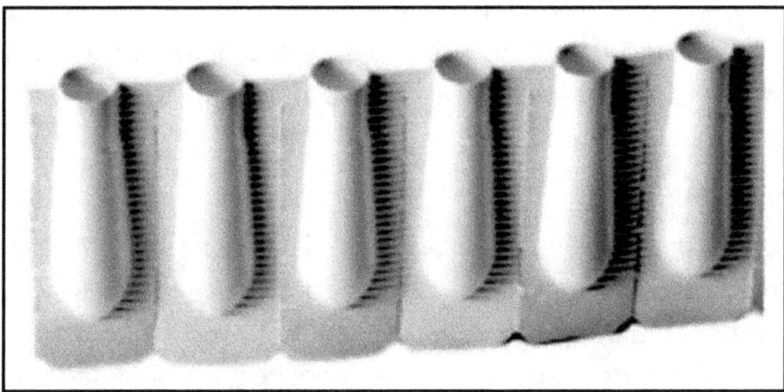

Fig. 11.8: Suppositories in plastic disposable mould

11.5 METHODS OF PREPARATION OF SUPPOSITORY

1. Hand molding

It is one of the oldest and simplest methods of preparation of suppository by which only small number of suppositories are prepared using cocoa butter as a suppository base. In this method, finely divided drug is first blended with wool fat and then this mixture is triturated with suitable base in mortar so as to form plastic - like consistency mass. This mass is formed into ball in palm and then made cylindrical by rolling in the palm. Then this cylindrical rod is cut into suitable length and weight. One end is made tapered by using finger. Talcum powder and starch is used on the rolling surface and on palm so as to avoid adherence of material. This method avoids heating of suppository base. Effective hand rolling requires skill and practice.

2. Compression moulding

In this method, drug is first mixed with suppository base and then the remaining quantity of base is added and blended thoroughly so as to form a mass. This mass is placed into cylinder. Hand turned wheel pushes piston against suppository mass contained in a cylinder so that mass is forced into mould through a narrow opening. As it does not require fusion or heating of suppository base, it is also called as cold compression method.

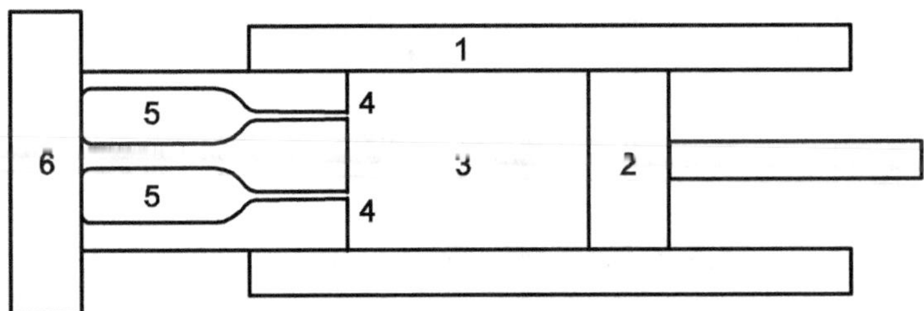

Fig. 11.9: Cold compression machine for suppository: 1- Cylinder, 2- Piston, 3- Prepared mass to be compressed, 4- Narrow opening, 5- Mould, 6- Retaining stop plate

This method is used for insoluble and thermal sensitive medicaments. It is not suitable for suppositories in which glycerogelatin base is used. This method produces more elegant suppository than hand moulding method. It also avoids problem of sedimentation of drug in the base. Disadvantage of this method is air entrapment into the mass and it is a very slow method for production of large number of suppositories.

3. Fusion/Pour molding

It is a hot process in which suppository base is first melted on water bath to avoid overheating and medicaments are either emulsified or suspended in it. This mass is then transferred to pre-lubricated suppository mould and allowed to cool at room temperature. It is a widely used method for preparation of suppository in both laboratory and industry. It has the following requirements and steps.

(a) Suppository mould: It is made-up of stainless steel, nickel-copper alloy, brass or aluminium. It has six to twelve cavities with desired shape and size. For large scale production, mould with 500 cavities can be used.

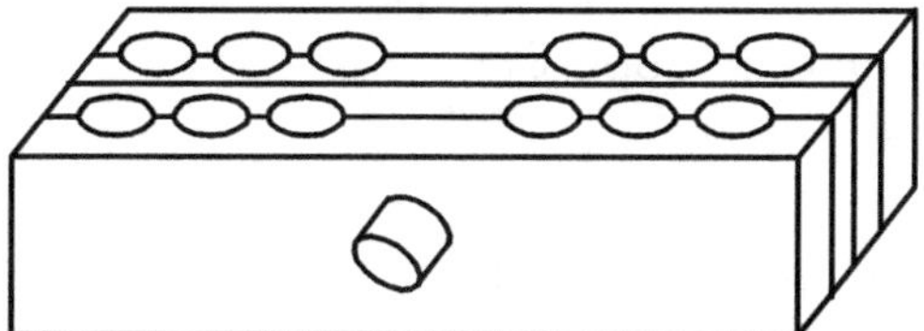

Fig. 11.10: Suppository mould

(b) Lubrication of mould: Suppository mould should be pre-lubricated before filling molten mass into the cavities. Lubricant used should be from different category than that of suppository mould otherwise, it will be absorbed by base and no separating film will be formed between solidified suppository and inner metal surface of mould. Hence oily lubricants for cocoa butter and aqueous lubricants for glycerogelatin base should be avoided. When emulsified or PEG base are used, there is no requirement of pre-lubrication of mould.

Calibration of suppository mould

A suppository mould is filled by volume, but the suppository is formulated by weight. Hence volume of suppository prepared from a particular mould is uniform but its weight can vary when a drug is present due to difference in densities between the drugs and base. Hence it is necessary to calibrate mould by considering displacement value of medicament.

11.6 DISPLACEMENT VALUE

The quantity of drug which displaces one part of base is known as 'displacement value'.

Calculation of displacement of value

If the displacement value of a particular drug is not known, it can be calculated by the following method:

1. Prepare and weigh 10 suppositories using the base alone. Let the weight of these be 'A' gram.
2. Prepare and weigh 10 suppositories containing a known percentage of a drug (medicated suppository). Let the weight of these be 'B' gram.
3. Calculate the amount of base present in the medicated suppositories. Let the weight be 'C' gram.
4. Calculate the amount of medicament present in the suppositories. Let the weight be 'D' gram.
5. Therefore, (A-C) will be the weight of the base displaced by the medicament.
6. Displacement value of the medicament for a particular base will be:

    Displacement value = D/ (A − C) ... (11.1)

Example 11.1: Calculate actual weight of cocoa butter required to prepare 10 suppositories, each containing 0.2 g of drug of displacement value 4.

Solution: Since 1 g weight suppository mould is used. Total weight of cocoa butter alone required for preparation of 10 suppositories is:

$$1 \times 10 = 10 \text{ g}$$

As each suppository should contain 0.2 g of drug, hence total weight of drug required to prepare 10 suppositories is:

$$0.2 \times 10 = 2 \text{ g}$$

As per definition of displacement value; 4 g of drug will displace 1 g of cocoa butter, therefore 2 g of drug will displace:

$$2 \times \frac{1}{4} = 0.5 \text{ g of cocoa butter}$$

Hence actual quantity of cocoa butter required to prepare 10 suppositories will be:

$$10 - 0.5 = 9.5 \text{ g}$$

Therefore, total weight of 10 suppositories will:

9.5 g (cocoa butter) + 2 g (drug) = 11.5 g i.e. 1.15 g for each suppository.

It indicates that; although suppositories are prepared in 1 g mould their volume remains same but weight is higher than 1 g.

Displacement value of few drugs with reference to cocoa butter as a suppository base

Name of drug	Displacement value	Name of drug	Displacement value
Alum	2.0	Ichthammol	1.0
Aminophylline	1.5	Iodoform	4.0
Aspirin	1.1	Boric acid	1.5
Bismuth subgallate	3.0	Phenobarbitone	1.0
Hydrocortisone acetate	1.5	Resorcinol	1.0
Castor oil	1.0	Tannic acid	1.0
Chloral hydrate	1.5	Zinc oxide	5.0
Cocaine hydrochloride	1.5	Zinc sulphate	2.0

Example 11.2: Determine displacement value of drug in cocoa butter suppository containing 40 % of drug prepared in 1 g mould. Weight of 10 suppositories is 14.72 g.

Solution: Weight of 10 suppositories containing cocoa butter alone prepared in 1 g capacity mould:

$$1 \times 10 = 10 \text{ g}$$

Weight of 10 suppositories containing 40 % of drug is given = 14.72 g

Amount of cocoa butter present in medicated suppository (containing 40 % of drug):

$$14.72 \text{ g} \longrightarrow 100 \text{ %}$$
$$X \text{ g} \longleftarrow 60 \text{ %}$$

$$X = 14.72 \times \frac{60}{100} = 8.83 \text{ g}$$

Amount of drug present in medicated suppository (containing 40 % of drug):

$$14.72 \text{ g} \longrightarrow 100 \text{ %}$$
$$X \text{ g} \longleftarrow 40 \text{ %}$$

$$X = 14.72 \times \frac{40}{100} = 5.89 \text{ g}$$

Amount of cocoa butter displaced by 6.184 g of drug:

$$= 10 - 8.83 = 1.17 \text{ g}$$

Therefore, displacement value:

$$\text{Displacement value} = \frac{5.89}{1.17} = 5.03 \approx 5$$

Method of preparation

While preparing suppository by fusion method; always take weight of extra 2 suppositories by considering wastage during transfer of material. For example, if you want to prepare 8 suppositories then take amount of drug and base for 10 suppositories.

Clean and lubricate the mould properly with suitable lubricant as discussed above. Keep mould in inverted position on ice bath so as to remove excess lubricants from mould cavity. Melt suppository base in porcelain dish on water bath and add drug into molten base with continuous stirring. Transfer this content in mould cavity in excess amount and place mould on ice bath. After solidification, scrap excess mount and open mould. Remove suppository and wrap with tin foil or waxed paper and pack into suitable container.

Automatic moulding machine

Various moulding operations such as pouring, cooling and removal are performed on automatic rotary moulding machine. Ejection of solidified suppositories and cleaning of mould are fully automated. On large scale production, about 3500 to 6000 suppositories per hour can be manufactured on rotary machine.

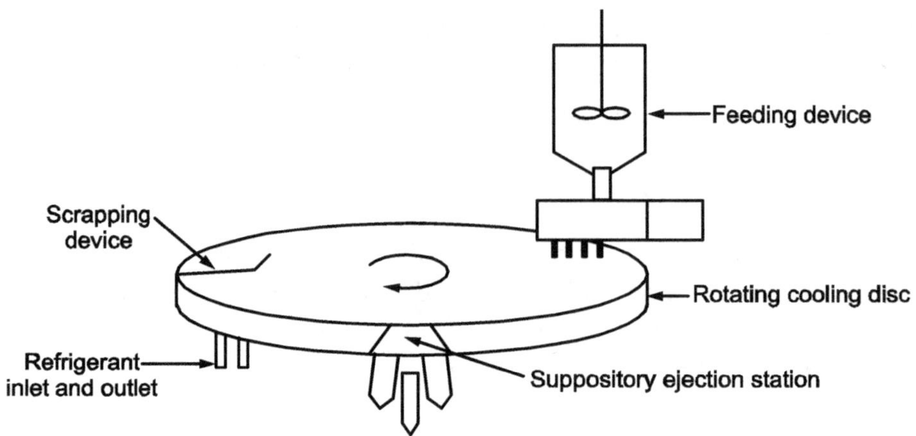

Fig. 11.11: Rotary suppository moulding machine

Problems associated with preparation of suppositories

   (i)   Water in suppositories

   (ii) Hygroscopicity

   (iii) Incompatibilities

   (iv) Viscosity

   (v) Density

   (vi) Volume contraction

   (vii) Brittleness

   (viii) Lubricant or mould release agent

   (ix) Weight and volume control

   (x)   Rancidity

Some marketed formulations of suppositories

   (i)   Dulcolax® Suppositories (Bisacodyl 10 mg).

      Use: Constipation, either chronic or of recent onset, whenever a stimulant laxative is required.

   (ii) Tyridol® Suppositories (Tramadol hydrochloride 100 mg).

      Use: Anti-inflammatory.

   (iii) Galipar® 125 (Children), Galipar® 500 (Adult) Suppositories (Acetaminophen 125 mg for children and 500 mg for adult).

      Use: Antipyretic.

   (iv) Hallens® Adult/Child Suppositories (Glycerin 75% w/w).

      Use: Laxative.

   (v) Proctosedyl® Suppositories (Hydrocortisone 5 mg and cinchocaine 5 mg).

      Use: To treat hemorrhoids and itching/swelling in the rectum and anus.

11.7 EVALUATION OF SUPPOSITORIES

Prepared suppositories are evaluated for following quality control test:

(i) **Visual inspection:** It is necessary to check suppository for the absence of fissuring, pitting, fat blooming, exudation, sedimentation, and the migration of drug. Suppositories are observed as an intact unit and also by splitting them longitudinally. In this test, shape of suppositories, homogeneity of the color and surface condition i.e. brilliance, dullness, mottling, cracks, dark regions, axial cavities, bursts, air bubbles, holes, etc are checked visually.

(ii) **Odour:** Verification of odour can prevent confusion when similar suppositories are being processed. A change in the odour may also be indicative of a degradation process.

(iii) **Weight variation test:** Weigh individually twenty suppositories and determine average weight. Compare the individual weights with the average weight. No suppository should deviate from average weight by more than 5% except two that may deviate by not more than 10%. Weight variation in suppositories could occur due to some mold cavities being under-filled or over-filled, air entrapment or due to inappropriate scrapping.

(iv) **Melting point determination:** A number of different techniques are used to study melting behaviour, including the open capillary tube, the U-tube, and the drop point methods. The use of a U-shaped capillary tube to determine melting point provides precise information for excipient control and consistency in production for those suppositories containing soluble active principles. This method is not suitable for suppositories containing high powder content, which prevents the fat from sliding inside the capillary tube to give the end-point determination.

Melting point can also be determined by placing a small-diameter wire into the mold containing the suppository melt before the form solidifies. The form is then immersed in water, held by the wire, and the temperature of the liquid is raised slowly (about 1°C every 2–3 minutes) until the suppository slips-off the wire; this is the melting point of the suppository.

(v) **Melting range test:** Melting range test is carried out to check physical and absorption characteristics of suppository. This test is also called as macromelting range test. It is time taken for entire suppository to melt when immersed in a constant temperature i.e. 37°C. For this test, USP tablet disintegration test apparatus is used. Suppository under test is completely immersed in the constant water bath and the time for whole suppository to melt or disperse in surrounding water is measured.

                    11.24

(vi) **Liquification or softening time test:** Liquefaction testing provides information on the behaviour of a suppository when subjected to a maximum temperature of 37°C. Krowczynski's method is used to determine Liquification or softening time of suppository, which measures the time required for a suppository to liquefy under pressures similar to those found in the rectum (approximately 30 g) in the presence of water at 37°C. In general, liquefaction should take no longer than about 30 minutes.

(vii) **Mechanical strength/crushing test:** This is the determination of the mechanical force necessary to break a suppository and indicates whether a suppository is brittle or elastic. The Erweka method is used for this test. The mechanical strength should not be less than 1.8 to 2 Kg as measured by Erweka method. The purpose of the test is to verify that the suppository can be transported under normal conditions, and administered to the patient.

(viii) **Deformation Time:** This is the length of time during which a suppository will be able to maintain its original shape under a specific pressure. This can be determined by placing a known weight on a suppository inside a known pH medium at a given temperature not more than 37°C. The time taken for the suppository to lose its shape is the deformation time for the suppository.

(ix) **Content uniformity:** The dose to dose variation can be accomplished by content uniformity in which suppositories are randomly chosen to check drug content uniformity as per specifications given in respective pharmacopoeia. According to Pharmaceutical Codex 1993, preparation of suppositories with an active ingredient less than 2g or less than 2% of the total masses must comply with the test for content uniformity. In this test, active ingredient content of each of randomly selected suppositories should be determined using a suitable assay method.

Acceptance value calculations are not required for suppositories. Assay 10 units individually as directed in the Assay in the individual monograph, unless otherwise specified in the Procedure for content uniformity. The USP 30 "Criteria" for suppositories states the following limits for content uniformity:

Limit A: (if the average of the limits specified in the potency definition in the individual monograph is 100.0% or less). Unless otherwise specified in the individual monograph, the requirements for dosage uniformity are met if the amount of the drug substance in each of the 10 dosage units as determined from the Content Uniformity method lies within the range of 85% to 115% of the label claim, and the relative standard deviation is less than or equal to 6%.

If 1 unit is outside the range of 85% to 115% of label claim, and no unit is outside the range of 75% to 125% of label claim, or if the relative standard deviation is greater than 6.0%, or if both conditions prevail, test 20 additional units. The requirements are met if not more than 1 unit of the 30 is outside the range of 85% to 115% of label claim, and no unit is outside the range of 75% to 125% of label claim and the relative standard deviation of the 30 dosage units does not exceed 7.8%.

Limit B: (if the average of the limits specified in the potency definition in the individual monograph is greater than 100.0 percent). If the average value of the dosage units tested is 100.0 percent or less, the requirements are as in Limit A. If the average value of the dosage units tested is greater than or equal to the average of the limits specified in the potency definition in the individual monograph, the requirements are as specified under Limit A, except that the words "label claim" are replaced by the words "label claim multiplied by the average of the limits specified in the potency definition in the monograph divided by 100.

If the average value of the dosage units tested is between 100 percent and the average of the limits specified in the potency definition in the individual monograph, the requirements are as specified under Limit A, except that the words "label claim" are replaced by the words "label claim multiplied by the average value of the dosage units tested (expressed as a percent of label claim) divided by 100.

(x)   **Dissolution study:** It is one of the most important quality control tools available for *in-vitro* assessment. Under FDA guidelines, dissolution testing is also a requirement for suppository to test for hardening and polymorphic transitions of active ingredients and suppository bases. The methods used in dissolution testing of suppositories includes Basket method, Paddle method, Beaker method, Diffusion method, Dialysis method and Continuous flow method. However, unlike for tablets and capsule dosage forms, there are not enough dissolution testing methods or validations for suppositories. This may be due to the immiscibility of some of the suppository vehicles in water. After thorough discussion US FDA concluded that hydrophilic suppositories that release the drug by dissolving in the rectal fluids can be evaluated by the basket, paddle, or flow-through cell methods. Lipophilic suppositories, on the other hand, release the drug after melting in the rectal cavity and are significantly affected by rectal temperature. Hence recommended equipment for lipophilic suppositories, therefore, includes a modified basket method, a paddle method with a wired screen and a sinker, and a modified flow-through cell with a specific dual-chamber suppository cell.

(xi)   **Stability Studies:** USP defines stability of pharmaceutical product as, "extent to which a product retains with in specified limits and throughout its period of storage and use (i.e. shelf life). In stability study; suppositories in container are placed at respective temperature and relative humidity conditions and should be evaluated for appearance, color, assay, degradation products, particle size, softening range, disintegration and dissolution (at 37°C) and microbial limits.

MODEL QUESTIONS

1. Define suppository. Give advantages and disadvantages of suppository.
2. Explain different types of suppositories.
3. Which are different factors affecting absorption of drug from suppository?
4. What are suppository bases? Give ideal properties of suppository base.
5. Explain different types of suppository base.
6. Define displacement value? Why and how it is calculated?
7. Explain different methods for preparation of suppository.
8. Explain evaluation/quality control tests of suppository.
9. Write a note on:
    (i)   Calibration of suppository mould
    (ii) Cocoa butter as a suppository base
    (iii) Recent development in suppository
    (iv) Packaging of suppositories

■■■

Chapter 12...

Pharmaceutical Incompatibilities

LEARNING OBJECTIVES

A drug incompatibility occurs when drugs are compounded together at the time of administration. In simple terms, it is defined as when two or more ingredients of a prescription are mixed together, the undesired change that may take place in the physical, chemical or therapeutic properties of the medicament is termed as incompatibility.

The objectives of this chapter includes:

- Understand the basics of pharmaceutical incompatibilities
- To know various types of pharmaceutical incompatibilities, reasons and remedies to eliminate them with examples.

12.1 DEFINITION

People take drugs to improve a person's condition, which may not work in the manner intended. Drugs are essentially poison when the dose taken is not stable due to a variety of reasons. The outcome may be contrary to what was expected. It may even cause harm to the patient. Therefore, it is important to know the symptoms that indicate a drug is doing its job properly or not. This is due to a reason called incompatibility. Incompatibility is an undesirable reaction that occurs between the drug and container or another drug or excipient. Therefore, such drugs should not be administered. A drug incompatibility may also occur when drugs are compounded together at the time of administration. Actually, drug incompatibility is a drug interaction that describes the alteration of a drug effect due to the influence of another substance (i.e. drug, chemical substance, nutrition) resulting in a product that is no longer optimal for the patient after the substances are mixed. In simple terms, it is defined as when two or more ingredients of a prescription are mixed together, the undesired change that may take place in the physical, chemical or therapeutic properties of the medicament is termed as incompatibility.

12.2 CLASSIFICATION OF INCOMPATIBILITY

There are three classes of drug incompatibilities:

(i) Physical incompatibility.

(ii) Chemical incompatibility.

(iii) Therapeutic incompatibility.

Reasons of incompatibilities:

The following are the several reasons of incompatibility taking place between or among drugs.

Physical incompatibilities:

(i)   Insolubility of prescribed drug in vehicle.

(ii) Immiscibility of two or more liquids.

(iii) Precipitation due to change in solvent that results in decreased solubility, (called salting out).

(iv) Liquification of solids mixed in a dry state (called eutexia).

(v)   Cementation of insoluble ingredients in liquid mixtures.

Chemical incompatibilities

(i)   Evolution in color.

(ii) Reduction or explosive reaction (called oxidation).

(iii) Precipitation due to chemical reaction.

Therapeutic incompatibilities

(i)   Inactivation of sulfa drugs by procaine HCl.

(ii) Over dose or under dose etc.

12.3 PHYSICAL INCOMPATIBILITIES

Physical incompatibilities are often called pharmaceutical incompatibilities and are evidenced by the failure of the drugs to combine properly. A physical incompatibility involves interaction between two or more substances which lead to change in color, odour, taste, viscosity and morphology. It may cause unsightly, non-uniform products from which removal of an accurate dose is very difficult. Ingredients such as oil and water (which are physically repellant to each other) and substances that are insoluble in the prescribed vehicle are primary examples of physical incompatibilities. This incompatibility depends primarily on the relative solubility, which is evidenced by the failure of the ingredients to combine in such a way as to make a satisfactory product.

Examples of physical incompatibility

(a) Insolubility: The change in pH, milling, surfactant, chemical reaction, complex formation and co-solvent are the factors that affect the solubility of prescribed agent in vehicle and may render it less soluble.

In this case, the pharmacist should protect medicine against these factors.

(i)   If mucilage of acacia and alcohol are put together, the preparation appears to be disagreeable due to the precipitation of acacia by the alcohol. In order to avoid such incompatibility, acacia if left out will produce a nice preparation.

(ii) In liquid preparations containing diffusible solids, suspension produced is settled quickly, from which uniform doses cannot be poured out. In such cases, a thickening agent is added to increase the viscosity and reduce the rate of settling of particles.

(iii) In liquid preparations containing indiffusible solids, suspension produced is settled quickly, from which uniform doses cannot be poured out. For example, chalk, aromatic chalk powder, succinyl sulfathiazole and sulphadimidine (in mixture) and calamine and zinc-oxide (in lotion). Remedy for this is to add thickening agents such as gum acacia, gum tragacanth, methylcellulose etc. to increase the viscosity and reduce the rate of settling of particles.

(b) Precipitation: Precipitation of mucilaginous and albuminous substances and some metallic salts from aqueous solution upon addition of alcohol takes place. For example, precipitation of camphor in camphor water occurs when metallic salts are added. Precipitation of volatile oils in aromatic waters occurs when metallic salts are dissolved in the liquid. Boric acid is precipitated from saturated solution when tragacanth is dissolved in the liquid. Colloidal solutions frequently show precipitation on addition of electrolytes. Phenyl salicylate and acetyl salicylic acid are incompatible when mixed together and produce either a wet mass or a liquid. Thus, phenyl salicylate may be dispensed in a separate capsule.

(c) Separation of immiscible liquids: Oils dissolved in alcohol usually separate on addition of water. For example, Oils are immiscible with water and thus they are emulsified or solubilized.

(i)   Spirit of ethyl nitrite separates and floats as a layer when a substantial proportion of potassium citrate is present in the prescription.

(ii) Mixing of highly alcoholic cannabis tincture with low alcoholic auranti aurora tincture results in the precipitation of the resinous matter of cannabis. In such case, the addition of an equal volume of honey to the highly alcoholic liquid before mixing with lower alcoholic or even aqueous liquid will help in satisfactory suspension of the resin.

(iii) In preparation of castor oil emulsion, the oil is not soluble in water. Hence, gum acacia is added to prepare a stable emulsion.

(iv) In the preparation of cresol soap solution, soap in high concentration in water forms micelles. The overall preparation is transparent.

(v)   Oil-soluble vitamins A, D are solubilized by polysorbates (non-ionic surfactants).

(vi) In the preparation of concentrated hydro-alcoholic solutions of volatile oils, such as spirits (for example, lemon spirits) and concentrated aromatic water (for example, concentrated cinnamon water), when used as flavouring agents in aqueous preparations, large globules of oils separate out. The hydro-alcoholic solution should be gradually diluted with the vehicle before mixing with the remaining ingredients. The hydro-alcoholic solution should be poured slowly into the vehicle with constant stirring.

(vii) Addition of high concentrations of electrolytes (for example, salts) in which the vehicle is a saturated aqueous solution of a volatile oil. The oil separates and collects as an unsightly (looking bad) surface layer, for example, *Potassium Citrate Mixture B.P.C.* When the lemon spirit, used for flavouring, is added the lemon oil is thrown out of the solution, partly by the change of solvent and partly by the salting out effect of the high concentration of soluble salt (potassium citrate). To prevent separation of this oil as surface layer quillaia tincture is included as an emulsifier.

(d) Liquefaction of solid ingredients: This is due in most cases to the formation of eutectic mixture in which the fusing point of the mixed ingredients is lowered more than that of any single one and also lowers than the room temperature. The liquefaction may also be due to liberation of water crystallization, or due to the presence of deliquescent substances. A good example is the mixture of salol and menthol.

(i)   For example, if 2 parts of salol and 1 part of menthol are mixed, it will form a syrupy liquid, while one part of salol and 1-part menthol forms a damp powder. But one-part salol and 2 parts menthol forms a dry mixture.

(ii)   Compounds like acetanilid, antipyrin, betanaphthol, resorcinol, thymol, phenol, etc. may also liquefy when rubbed together.

(iii) If menthol and thymol are required to be dispensed as powder, they are triturated in a mortar to form the liquid mixture. The liquid is triturated with enough adsorbent powder for example, light kaolin or light magnesium carbonate to give a free flowing product. Another method can be used if the final bulk volume of powder is very small. The menthol and thymol are triturated separately with small amount of adsorbent powder. Then both the powders are combined lightly and resultant powder is packed in capsules. The absorbent powders coat the particles and prevent contact between the medicaments and absorb any liquid that may be produced while triturating.

(e) Wrong form of the ingredients prescribed: Sometimes alkaloidal salts are to be dissolved in liquid petrolatum, resulting in failure to dissolve, but by substituting the alkaloid for the alkaloidal salt, complete solution takes place. (Free alkaloids are soluble in liquid petrolatum while alkaloidal salts are insoluble).

(f) Gelatinization: Solution of acacia is gelatinized by the addition of ferric salts. Collodion is also gelatinized by the addition of phenol.

Remedies for physical incompatibilities

1.   Omission of an unimportant ingredient of little therapeutic value.
2.   Addition of an inert ingredient to correct the difficulty.
3.   Alteration in the solvents used (substituting alcohol or glycerin for water or vice versa).
4.   Changing the order of mixing the ingredients.
5.   Dispensing the ingredients separately.
6.   Changing the bulk of the preparation.
8.   Use of a different form of the same ingredient.
9.   Addition of stiffening agents.
10. Addition of an ingredient which promotes solubility.

12.4 CHEMICAL INCOMPATIBILITY

Chemical incompatibility takes place when ingredients in the prescription undergo chemical reaction and the original composition of the formulation is altered. The chemical changes are generally indicated by a change in the physical appearance such as precipitation, a change in color, an explosion or simply effervescence. Sometimes the chemical change improves the product, in this case it is not considered as an incompatibility. For example, a prescription is not considered an incompatibility although potassium-mercuric iodide is formed, because it improves the product. In the modern concept, a chemical reaction is considered to take place between two soluble bodies when one or more products of the reaction are insoluble or gaseous. Thus, if sodium chloride and potassium bromide are mixed in solution although there is formation of potassium chloride and sodium bromide, no chemical reaction is considered to take place because both substances formed are soluble. On the other hand, if sodium chloride and silver nitrate solutions are mixed, there is the precipitation of silver chloride, hence, a chemical reaction is said to take place and thus it is a chemical incompatibility.

It is important to have a general consideration of the solubilities of the reaction products. For example, silver bromide requires 1-2 million times its weight of water to dissolve whereas potassium iodide only requires 7/10 its own weight of water. So substances like silver bromide are generally termed as insoluble.

Chemical incompatibilities are generally caused by pH change, a double decomposition reaction or complex formation. Various types of chemical changes that occur in this type of incompatibility include; oxidation, hydrolysis, polymerization, isomerization, decarboxylation, absorption of CO_2, combination and formation of insoluble complexes.

Examples of chemical incompatibility

(a) **Formation of precipitate:** Precipitate formation is among the more important cases of incompatibilities.

(i) Formation of an insoluble salt.

(ii) Formation of special insoluble organic salts such as tannates of iron, Meconate of lead, when opium preparations are combined with lead solutions; and the production of the insoluble blood-red iron salicylates, when iron preparations are combined with salicylates.

(iii) Precipitation of alkaloids by alkaloidal reagents like the precipitation of cinchona alkaloids when preparations of this drug are combined with potassium iodide and mercuric chloride.

(iv) Formation of insoluble bodies when synthetic organic chemicals are combined with certain reagents. An example of this is the formation of green crystals of iso-nitroso-antipyrine, when antipyrine is treated with spirit of nitrous ether.

(b) Evolution of gas: Mixing of an acid and a carbonate or bicarbonate (should be compounded in open containers to avoid explosion).

(c) Color changes: Color changes brought about by the chemical reaction or formation of a new substance.

(d) Production of an explosion: Explosion occurs when strong oxidizing agent is mixed by trituration with reducing substances or organic materials. Explosions are produced by a sudden evolution of gases, and all substances liable to produce such gaseous evolution on trituration must be handled with utmost caution.

(e) Cementation of ingredients : In some cases, all or part of the ingredients of a prescription may set into a mass cement-like hardness. Separation of an immiscible liquid when organic chemical is decomposed by certain reagent such as the decomposition of chloral, by the action of an alkali into chloroform.

(f) pH effect: Modern drugs are often salts of weak acids and weak bases. These salts are usually soluble in water while free bases are practically insoluble. Consequently, if a solution of a salt of weak acid is acidified, the free weak acid may precipitate out. Similarly, if a solution of a salt of weak base is made alkaline, the free weak base may precipitate out. Precipitation occurs or not depends on the solubility of the unionized acid or base or the pH of the solution or the dissociation constant (K_a) of the acid or base.

(g) Double decomposition: Alkaloidal salts such as emetine hydrochloride react with soluble potassium iodide to produce insoluble iodide salts of alkaloids as a precipitate. The solubility of emetine-HI is less hence may precipitate. For example, potassium iodide is used as expectorant in some alkaloid containing cough mixtures. If the alkaloid concentration is very low then precipitation does not occur. Another example of this type is incompatibility of alkaloidal salts with tannins. Alkaloidal salts react with tannins to form precipitate of alkaloidal tannates. The advantage of this reaction is that in case of alkaloidal poisoning, strong tea (or tannic acid solution) is used to precipitate the alkaloids. The remedy is to suspend precipitate with the help of tragacanth mucilage.

Remedies for chemical incompatibilities

1. Prevent the precipitation by the addition of glycerin, syrup or honey to the incompatible ingredients before mixing, as in the following prescription.

2. Codeine sulfate solution when prepared, slight turbidity is developed due partly to the separation of the resinous matter from the aromatic syrup, when the acid-reacting codeine salt is dissolved therein, and also due to the formation of codeine tannate. However, clear solution is obtained when the codeine salt is triturated with a vehicle made-up of an equal volume of glycerin and aromatic syrup of eriodictyon.

3. If iodine is added directly to the oil of turpentine, a violent reaction takes place, much heat is evolved that the mixture may even catch fire. However, if the iodine is first diluted by dissolving in alcohol and then added gradually to the oil of turpentine, the reaction will be very much moderated although some heat may be developed. The mixing is preferably done in an open container.

4. If the quinine sulfate is dissolved by the use of sulfuric acid and mixed with the solution of sodium acetate, a bulky white precipitate of quinine acetate is formed. The sodium acetate is partly converted to sodium sulfate and acetic acid. However, if the acid is omitted, a fine suspension of quinine sulfate is produced, this should be provided with a "shake well" label.

5. Zinc sulfate solution when first compounded is clear, but sooner or later, there may occur a precipitation of the slightly soluble basic zinc borate, which is objectionable for eye application. By replacing sodium borate with boric acid, precipitation can be avoided.

12.5 THERAPEUTIC INCOMPATIBILITY

Therapeutic incompatibility is the modification of the therapeutic effect of one drug by the prior concomitant administration of another. It is also called drug interactions. It arises when one or more drugs produce response or intensity different from that intended in the patients. This occurs when drugs and/or excipients, which are antagonistic to one another, are prescribed together. Such circumstances seldom occur in hospitals. The drugs may have been used together for one drug to modify the activity of other drug.

Mechanisms of therapeutic incompatibility: There are two types of mechanisms involved:

1. **Pharmacokinetics:** This mechanism is related with the effect of one drug on another drug that affects its absorption, distribution, metabolism and excretion.

2. **Pharmacodynamics:** This mechanism is related to the pharmacological activity of the interacting drugs such as synergism, antagonism, altered cellular transport and effect on the receptor site.

Reasons for Therapeutic Incompatibility:

I. Pharmacokinetic Interactions

1. **Altered GIT absorption:** In this type altered pH, altered bacterial flora, formation of drug chelates or complexes and drug induced mucosal damage and altered GIT motility is involved in the incompatibility of drugs.

    (a) Altered pH: The non-ionized form of a drug is more lipid soluble and more readily absorbed from GIT than the ionized form drug. For example, antacids and H_2 antagonist increases stomach pH that may decrease dissolution of acid soluble drugs such as ketoconazole tablets. In such situations, these drugs must be administered by difference of at least 2h interval in the time of administration of both.

(b) Altered intestinal bacterial flora: Patient taking antibiotics for some reason suffers from gastric disturbances as intestinal flora is damaged. In more than 10% of patients who are under treatment of digoxin, 40% or more of the administered dose is metabolized by the intestinal flora. Thus if intestinal flora is damaged, the concentration of digoxin increases which may be toxic.

(c) Complexation or chelation: Tetracycline interacts with calcium (present in milk) or iron (Hematinic preparations) to form chelates that are not absorbed through intestinal tract. Another example is antacids such as aluminum or magnesium hydroxide interacts with ciprofloxacin reducing its absorption by 85% due to chelate formation. Thus care must be taken to avoid administration of such substances together.

(d) Drug-induced mucosal damage: Anti-neoplastic agents such as Cyclophos-phamide, vincristine and procarbazine inhibit absorption of digoxin.

(e) Altered motility: An antiemetic drug metoclopramide increases stomach emptying time. This drug increases absorption of cyclosporine which may be toxic.

2. **Displaced protein binding**

Protein binding depends on the affinity of the drug to plasma protein. The most likely bound drugs are capable to displace other drugs. The amount of free drug is increased through its displacement by another drug with higher affinity. For example, Phenytoin is highly bound to plasma protein, tolbutamide and warfarin. Aspirin, sulfonamides and phenyl butazone drugs displaces phenytoin which remains as free form and is highly absorbed thus may exert toxic effects.

3. **Altered metabolism**

There are examples of drugs that effect metabolism of the other drugs changing its effectiveness. Although liver is the major site of drug metabolism, other organs WBC, skin, lung, and GIT can also contribute for the same.

(a) Enzyme induction: A drug may induce the enzyme that is responsible for the metabolism of another drug or even itself.
   (i)   Carbamazepine (an antiepileptic drug) increases its own metabolism.
   (ii) Phenytoin increases hepatic metabolism of theophylline leading to decrease in its level and reduces its action and vice-versa.

Enzyme induction involves protein synthesis therefore it needs around 3-week time to reach a maximal effect.

(b) Enzyme inhibition: Enzyme inhibition decreases rate of drug metabolism by another enzyme increasing the concentration of target drug leading to increased intoxicity. Inhibition of the enzyme may be due to the competition at binding sites, so the onset of action is short. For example, when carbamazepine (e.g. enzyme inducer) is administered with verapamil (an inhibitor) the effect of the inhibitor being predominant affects carbamazepine concentration and ultimately its effect. Some other examples of this type are inhibition of metabolism of astemazole and terfenadine by erythromycin. Increase in the serum concentration of the antihistaminic agents leads to increase in the life threatening cardiotoxicity. Omeprazole inhibits oxidative metabolism of diazepam.

(c) First-pass metabolism: Oral administration of drug increases the chance of its metabolism in liver and GIT leading to loss of some part of the drug dose that decreases its action. This effect is more prominent when such drug is an enzyme inducer or inhibitor. For example, Rifampin induces the hepatic metabolism of verapamil and thus lowers verapamil level in serum.

4. Altered renal execration

(a) Inhibition of renal tubular secretion: It occurs in the proximal renal tubules. The drug combines with a specific protein to pass through the proximal tubules. When a drug has a competitive reactivity to the protein (responsible for active transport of another drug) it reduces drug excretion and increases its concentration and hence its toxicity. For example, probenecid decreases tubular secretion of methotrexate.

(b) Alteration of urine flow and pH: Excretion and re-absorption of drugs occur in the tubules by passive diffusion which is regulated by concentration and lipid solubility. Ionized drugs are reabsorbed to lower level than non-ionized drugs. Thiazide diuretics indirectly increase proximal tubular re-absorption of Li^+ and can cause Li^+ toxicity in patients treated with lithium carbonate for mood disorders. The effect of urinary pH on the excretion of weak acids and bases is observed in patients under treatment of poisoning.

II. Pharmacodynamic Interactions

It means alteration of the drug action without change in its serum concentration.

1. Over doses

(a) Excessive single dose: Sometimes a single dose may become overdose depending on the health of the patient, e.g. a normal dose (taking body weight as 70 kg for an adult male) may be overdose for a under built person. However, it should not be more than 2 to 3 normal doses.

    (i)   A capsule containing atropine sulphate 6 mg and phenobarbital 360 mg to be taken three times a day before meals. The dose of both atropine sulphate and phenobarbital in this single capsule is 12 times the normal dose. The physician intends for 12 capsules to be dispensed but by mistake or may it be an incomplete prescription. Hence, before dispensing the pharmacist should consult the physician again and correct prescription as atropine sulphate 6 mg and phenobarbital 360 mg to be dispensed in total 12 capsules and label with direction as 'One capsule to be taken three times a day before meals'.

(ii) A capsule containing strychnine sulphate 20 mg and iron and ammonium citrate 500 mg. One capsule to be taken three times a day after meals. The dose of strychnine hydrochloride is 10 times overdose of than that of normal. The pharmacist should consult the physician and obtain the permission to change the dose. So, prescription needs to be corrected as strychnine sulphate 2 mg and iron and ammonium citrate 500 mg. One capsule to be taken three times a day after meals.

(b) **Excessive daily dose:** In this case, the daily dose of drug is exceeded. For example, a capsule containing codeine phosphate 15 mg and ammonium chloride 500 mg. Two capsules to be taken every hour for cough. The U.S.P. recommends that the prescribed dose should be taken after every four hours and not every hour. Hence the physician should be consulted.

(c) **Additive effect:** Additive effect occurs when two or more drugs having the same effect are combined and the result is the sum of the individual effects relative to the doses used. This additive effect may be beneficial or harmful to the client. There are certain drugs that possess similar pharmacological activity. In such case, advice of the physician is necessary. For example, a mixture containing amphetamine sulphate 20 mg and ephedrine sulphate 50 mg in syrup base to make 100 mL. The dose is 25 mL after every 4 hours. In this case, both drugs are sympathetic stimulants and are prescribed in their full dose. The formulation will produce additive overdose effect. Hence, the dose of individual drug should be reduced.

(d) **Synergistic effect:** Synergistic effect occurs when two or more drugs, with or without the same effect, are administered together to yield a combined effect that has an outcome greater than the sum of the single drugs active components alone. Propranolol with verapamil produces synergistic effect.

(e) **Potentiating effect:** Potentiating effect describes a particular type of synergistic effect of a drug interaction in which only one of two drugs exerts the action that is made greater by the presence of the second drug. For example, diuretics lower plasma potassium concentration and thereby enhance some actions of digoxin and predispose to glycoside toxicity.

(f) **Antagonistic effects:** Antagonistic effects are reactions with the opposite effect of synergism and result in a combined effect that is less than either active component alone. For example, protamine administered as an antidote to anticoagulant action of heparin. Another example is a β-adrenoceptor antagonist that diminishes the effectiveness of β-receptor agonists, such as salbutamol or terbutaline.

In a more simplified way, above mentioned effects of drugs when used together can be understood through following description.

Additive effect   = 1 + 1 = 2

Synergistic effect   = 1 + 1 = 3

Potentiating effect   = 1 + 0 = 2

Antagonistic effects = 1 + 1 = <1

2. Under dose

In this type of incompatibility, effect of one drug is reduced by the presence of another drug. The examples of this type of probable combination drugs are given below.

(i)   Stimulants like nux-vomica, strychnine sulphate, caffeine, etc. with sedatives like barbiturates, paraldehyde etc.

(ii)   Adrenergic drugs like ephedrine, nor-adrenaline with sympatholytic drugs like ergotamine.

(iii)   Sympathetic stimulants like methamphetamine with parasympathetic stimulants like pilocarpine.

(iv)   Purgatives like castor oil, liquid paraffin etc with anti-diarrheal agents like bismuth carbonates.

(v)   Acidifiers like dilute hydrochloric acid and alkalizing substances like sodium bicarbonate and magnesium carbonate.

For example, a capsule containing aspirin 300 mg and probenecid 500 mg. The dose prescribed is one capsule a day to treat gout. Aspirin is an Non-steroidal Anti-inflammatory Drug (NSAID) given to reduce the pain and swelling in case of gout attack. Probenecid blocks the active re-absorption of uric acid from the lumen of nephron, but aspirin blocks this action of probenecid. Hence, both of the drugs are antagonistic to each other, so its combination is therapeutically useless.

III. Improper consumption by the patient

In certain prescription, some special directions should be written. If the patients are not advised properly, the drugs may not produce the desired action due to low bioavailability. For example, a capsule contains tetracycline hydrochloride 250 mg. The usual dose is one capsule every six hour. Calcium present in milk inactivates the tetracycline; hence a patient may not get any therapeutic effect if he/she takes the capsule with milk. Thus, pharmacist should advise the patient to take the capsule with water and not with milk. In addition, the patient should not take antacid containing calcium salts.

IV. Contra-indicated drugs

Certain drugs should not be given in particular disease condition. For example:

(i)   Corticosteroids are contraindicated in patients with peptic ulcer.

(ii) Vasoconstrictors are contraindicated in hypertensive patients

(iii) Some drugs should not be given to asthmatic patients e.g. barbiturates, morphine, etc.

(iv) If a person is allergic to a drug such as penicillin injection, then it should not be given.

Certain combinations of drugs that are contraindicated include a capsule containing sulphadiazine 0.25 g, sulphamerazine 0.25 g and ammonium chloride 0.50 g. The direction is to 'Take two capsules after every six hours for cough'. In this prescription, ammonium chloride is a urinary acidifier and it could cause deposition of sulphonamide crystals in the kidney.

MODEL QUESTIONS

1. What is incompatibility? What are various reasons of incompatibilities?
2. Explain physical incompatibility with suitable examples.
3. List various remedies to avoid physical incompatibility.
4. Explain chemical incompatibility with suitable examples.
5. List various remedies to avoid chemical incompatibility.
6. Discuss reasons for therapeutic incompatibility.
7. Write a short note on:
   (i) Therapeutic incompatibility.
   (ii) Overdosing and under dosing.

■■■

Chapter **13**...

Semisolid Dosage Forms

LEARNING OBJECTIVES

Semisolid dosage forms are pharmaceutical formulations which contain one or more active ingredients dissolved or uniformly dispersed in a suitable base and any suitable excipients and are normally presented in the form of creams, gels, ointments, or pastes.

The objectives of this chapter includes

- To understand basic concept, need and advantages and disadvantages of semisolids.
- Recognize route of drug administration, mechanism and factors affecting drug dermal penetration and classification of semisolid pharmaceutical dosage forms.
- To know general various bases and other excipients used and formulation considerations of semisolid product development.
- To understand methods of manufacturing and various physical properties of semisolids.

13.1 INTRODUCTION

Semisolid dosage forms are pharmaceutical formulations which contain one or more active ingredients dissolved or uniformly dispersed in a suitable base and any suitable excipients and are normally presented in the form of creams, gels, ointments, or pastes. They are traditionally used for treating topical disorders. The majority of them are meant for skin applications. They are also used for treating ophthalmic, nasal, buccal, rectal, and vaginal ailments. Various categories of drugs such as antibacterials, antifungals, antivirals, antipruritics, local anesthetics, anti-inflammatories, analgesics, keratolytics, astringents, and mydriatic agents are incorporated into these products.

Drugs incorporated into semisolids either show their activity on the surface layers of tissues or penetrate into internal layers to reach the site of action. Systemic entry of drugs from these products is limited due to various physicochemical properties of dosage forms and biological factors. Systemic delivery of drugs from topical dosages is however feasible by suitable formulation modifications. Semisolid dosage forms are also used in non-therapeutic conditions for providing protective and lubricating functions.

Advantages:

(i)   Semisolid dosage forms can be used to avoid first pass metabolism of drugs.

(ii)   They have site specific action of drug on affected area.

(iii)   They are convenient to use by unconscious patients or patients having difficulty for oral drug administration.

(iv)   They are most suitable dosage form for bitter drugs.

(v)   They also are suitable for drugs that are degraded in stomach by acidic pH, intestine or metabolized by liver.

(vi)   Being applied externally there is no any interaction of drug with food, enzymes, drink and other GI flora maintaining drug integrity.

(vii)   Termination of therapy can be easily facilitated compared to other dosage forms.

(viii) They are more stable than liquid dosage forms.

Disadvantages

(i)   Semisolid dosage forms may cause skin staining.

(ii)   They are bulky to handle.

(iii)   Application of semisolid dosage forms with finger may cause contamination.

(iv)   They are physico-chemically less stable than solid dosage form.

(v)   They may cause irritation and may be allergic to some patients.

13.2 CLASSIFICATION

1. **Ointments:** Ointments are homogeneous, semi-solid preparations intended for external application to the skin or mucous membranes. They are used as emollients or for the application of active ingredients to the skin for protective, therapeutic, or prophylactic purposes and where a degree of occlusion is desired.

2. **Creams:** Creams are homogeneous, semi-solid preparations consisting of opaque emulsion systems. Their consistency and rheological properties depend on the type of emulsion, either water-in-oil (w/o) or oil-in-water (o/w), and on the nature of the solids in the internal phase.

3. **Pastes:** Pastes are homogeneous, semi-solid preparations containing high concentrations of insoluble powdered substances (usually not less than 20%) dispersed in a suitable base.

4. **Gels:** Gels are usually homogeneous, clear, semi-solid preparations consisting of a liquid phase within a three-dimensional polymeric matrix with physical or sometimes chemical cross-linkage by means of suitable gelling agents.

5. **Jellies:** Jellies are class of gels, which are semisolid systems that consist of suspensions made-up of either small inorganic particles or large organic molecules interpenetrated by a liquid in which the structural coherent matrix contains a high portion of liquid, usually water.

6. **Poultices:** Poultices are paste-like preparations used externally to reduce inflammation because they retain heat well. After heating, the preparation is spread thickly on a dressing and applied, as hot as the patient can bear it, to the affected area.

7. **Plaster:** Substance intended for external application made up of such materials and of such consistency as to adhere to the skin and attach to a dressing; plasters are intended to afford protection and support and/or to furnish an occlusion and macerating action and to bring medication into close contact with the skin.

Structure of skin

In order to understand mechanism of dermal penetration of drugs, one must know skin anatomy. The potential of using the intact skin as the port of drug administration to the human body has been recognized for several decades. However, the skin is a very difficult barrier to the ingress of materials allowing only small quantities of a drug to penetrate over a period of time.

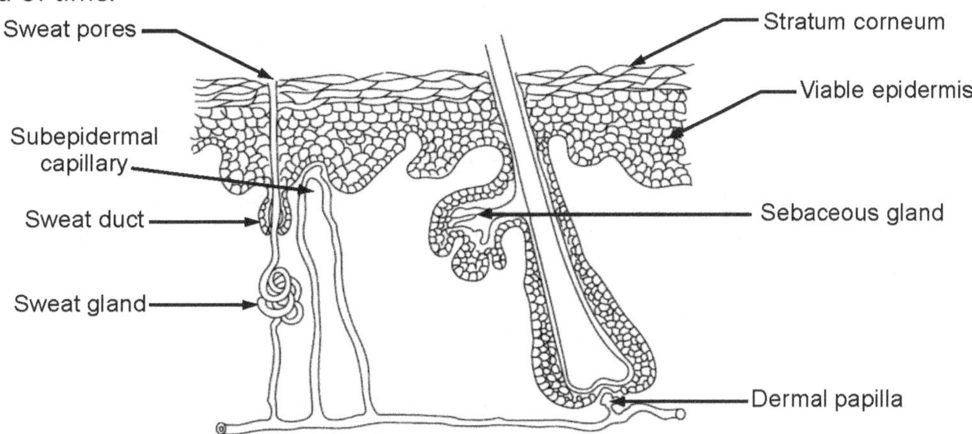

Fig. 13.1: Structure of Skin

Structure of the skin:

The human skin is the largest organ in our body with surface area of 1.8-2.0 m^2. It is composed of four main regions: the stratum corneum, the viable epidermis, dermis, and subcutaneous tissues. The skin is a well energized organ that protects the entire body against environmental factors and regulates heat and water loss from the body.

(i) **Stratum corneum:** This is the outermost layer of skin, also called horny layer. It is approximately 10 mm thick when dry but swells to several times this thickness when fully hydrated. It contains 10 to 25 layers of parallel to the skin surface, lying dead, keratinized cells, called corneocytes. It is flexible but relatively impermeable. The stratum corneum is the principal barrier for penetration.

(ii) **Viable epidermis:** This is situated beneath the stratum corneum and varies in thickness from 0.06 mm on the eyelids to 0.8 mm on the palms. Going inwards, it consists of various layers as stratum lucidum, stratum granulosum, stratum spinosum, and the stratum basal.

(iii) **Dermis:** Dermis is a 3 to 5 mm thick layer and is composed of a matrix of connective tissue which contains blood vessels, lymph vessels, and nerves. The continuous blood supply has essential function in regulation of body temperature. It also provides nutrients and oxygen to the skin while removing toxins and waste products.

(iv) **Subcutaneous tissues/Hypodermis:** The subcutaneous tissue or hypodermis consists of a layer of fat cells arranged as lobules with interconnecting collagen and elastin fibers. Its primary functions are heat insulation and protection against physical shock, while also providing energy storage that can be made available when required. Blood vessels and nerves connect to the skin via the hypodermis.

13.3 MECHANISM OF DERMAL PENETRATION OF DRUGS

Penetration of drug through the skin by various pathways is depending-up on physicochemical properties of the drug. Both lipophilic and hydrophilic drugs are absorbed from different routes. The upper stratum corneum of the skin opposes the absorption of drug but presence of various absorption routes facilitates the entry of drug and transport of drug to the systemic circulation.

The permeation of drugs through the skin involves the diffusion through the intact epidermis through the skin appendages (hair follicles and sweat glands). These skin appendages form shunt pathways through the intact epidermis, occupying only 0.1% of the total human skin. It is known that drug permeation through the skin is usually limited by the stratum corneum. Skin absorption pathways are divided into flowing transport mechanism:

1. **Epidermal route (across the intact SC)**

   (a) **Trans-cellular (intra-cellular) route:** Trans-cellular pathway means transport of molecules across epithelial cellular membrane. These include passive transport of small molecules, active transport of ionic and polar compounds, and endocytosis and transcytosis of macromolecules. Under normal conditions the transcellular route is not considered as the preferred way of dermal invasion the reason being the very low permeability through the corneocytes and the obligation to partition several times from the more hydrophilic corneocytes into the lipid intercellular layers in the stratum corneum and vice versa. The transcellular pathway can gain an importance when a penetration enhancer is used, for example, urea which increases the permeability of the corneocytes by altering the keratin structure.

   (b) **Para-cellular (inter-cellular) route:** In para-cellular route drug molecules transport around or between the cells. Tight junctions or similar situations exist between the cells. The principal pathway taken by a permeate is decided mainly by the partition coefficient (log k). Hydrophilic drugs partition preferentially into the intercellular domains, whereas lipophilic permeants (o/w log k >2) traverse the stratum corneum via the intracellular route. The intercellular route is considered to yield much faster absorption due to the high diffusion coefficient of most drugs within the lipid bilayer.

2. **Trans-follicular/shunt pathway (along the skin appendages)**

   Penetration of drug through skin appendageal route comprises transport via eccrine sweat glands, apocrine sweat glands and hair follicles with their associated sebaceous glands. These routes circumvent penetration through the stratum corneum and are therefore known as "shunt" routes. Trans-follicular route is considered to be of minor importance because of its relatively small area, approximately 0.1 % of the total skin area. In contrast, in the initial stages of a skin absorption process and in the case of large hydrophilic compounds and ions invasion through the appendages may play a considerable role.

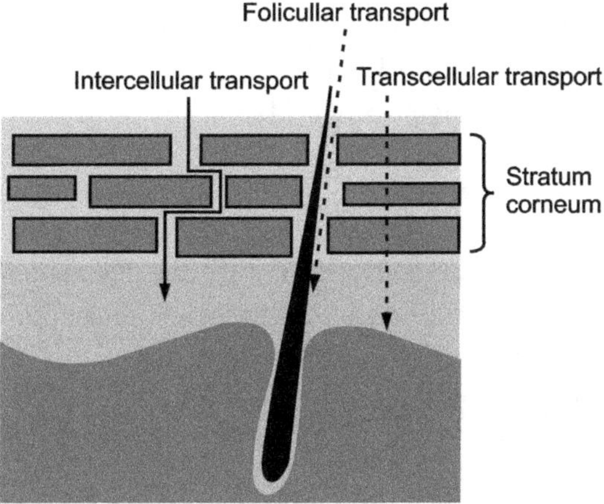

Fig. 13.2: Mechanism of Dermal Penetration of Drug

Skin absorption pathways

Drug penetration through skin may involve following steps:

(i)   Dissolution within and release from the formulation,

(ii)   Partitioning into the outermost layer of the skin, stratum corneum,

(iii)   Diffusion through the stratum corneum,

(iv)   Partitioning from the stratum corneum into the aqueous viable epidermis,

(v)   Diffusion through the viable epidermis and into the upper dermis,

(vi)   Uptake into the local capillary network and eventually the systemic circulation.

Diffusion of compounds across a membrane is described by Fick's first, which states that the flux (rate of transfer per unit area) of a compound (J, mass/cm^2 per second) at a given time and position is proportional to the differential concentration change dC over a differential distance dx (i.e. the concentration gradient dC/dx).

$$J = -D\frac{dC}{dx} \qquad \text{... (13.1)}$$

The negative sign indicates that the net flux is in the direction of decreasing thermodynamic activity which can often be represented by the concentration.

Fick's second law describing concentration within a membrane is derived by combining a differential mass balance in a membrane with Fick's first law and, when considering the skin, assuming that the compound does not bind, the compound is not metabolized, and its diffusion coefficient does not vary with position or composition.

$$\frac{dC}{dt} = \frac{Dd^2C}{dx^2} \qquad \text{... (13.2)}$$

Fick's first law can be applied to describe the diffusion processes in the individual layers of the skin, which are treated as pseudo-homogeneous membranes. For a membrane of thickness h, the flux at steady state (Jss) is given by:

$$Jss \ = \ \frac{D\ (C_1 - C_2)}{h} \qquad \qquad ... (13.3)$$

Where; C_1 and C_2 are the concentrations of the chemical in the membrane at the two faces (i.e. at x = 0 and x = h). When used to describe heterogeneous membranes like the stratum corneum, D is an effective diffusion coefficient.

13.4 FACTORS INFLUENCING DERMAL PENETRATION OF DRUGS

1. **Skin-Specific Factors**

    (a) **Site of Application:** Thickness of skin, nature of stratum corneum and density of appendages vary site to site. These factors affect significantly penetration. When semisolid formulation applied on various site of body, study reveals that, skin penetration, as indicated by the amount of chemical in the stratum corneum, was ranked as follows: arm ≤ abdomen ≤ postauricular ≤ forehead. It is noteworthy that whatever the compound applied, the forehead was about twice as permeable as the arm or the abdomen.

    (b) **Race:** Racial differences in skin function have been investigated. Study reported that, an increase in intracellular cohesion in black skin, while higher lipid content in black skin. Although relatively limited data are available on race, indications are that racial differences do exist among white and black skins, with regards to some anatomical and physiological functions of the skin, and that these differences could determine race related patterns in skin behaviour, namely the response to irritant chemicals and the penetration of topically applied drugs.

    (c) **Age of the Skin:** The young skin is more permeable than older. Children are more sensitive for skin absorption of toxins. Thus, skin age is one of the factors affecting penetration of drug from semisolid formulation. As the skin ages, some functional and structural changes take place that affect the transdermal absorption of molecules into it. Hydration plays an important role in transdermal absorption and decreases with age, as the skin loses its moisture content. The enzymatic activity in the skin also reduces with age, as well as the blood flow to the skin. A lower blood flow in older people suggests that the clearance of drugs in an older stratum corneum will be slower, which in turn would negatively impact on the drug flux gradient.

    (d) **Skin condition:** For most compounds, the rate of percutaneous absorption is limited by diffusion through the stratum corneum. However, the epidermal barrier may not be intact in diseased or damaged skin. Persons with diseased or damaged skin may be at special risk for the toxic effects of environmental pollutants as a result of increased percutaneous absorption. Damage to the skin may occur from mechanical injury (cuts, wounds, abrasions) or other insults such as sunburn. Any skin condition that compromises the capability of the stratum corneum to serve as a permeability barrier, including psoriasis, eczema, rashes, or dermatitis, may also result in increased percutaneous absorption in affected individuals.

(e) Hydration: In contact with water the permeability of skin increases significantly. Hydration is most important factor increasing the permeation of skin. So use of humectant is done in transdermal delivery. Skin occlusion with wraps or impermeable plastic films prevents the loss of surface water from the skin and this causes increased level of hydration in the SC thereby decreasing the protein network density and the diffusional path length. This increases skin penetration. Occlusion of the skin surface also increases skin temperature by 2-3°C resulting in increased molecular motion and skin penetration.

(f) Circulation to the Skin: Changes in peripheral circulation can affect penetration of drug. Prolonged skin exposure to organic solvents is known to result in vasodilation in areas that come into contact with these compounds. If the rate of chemical accumulation in the epidermis (via diffusion across the stratum corneum) is equal to or greater than the circulatory perfusion rate, then the rate-limiting step for skin permeation could become that of capillary transfer.

(g) Skin Temperature: Permeation of molecules across the skin is a passive process. An increase in temperature would thus result in an increase in kinetic energy of the drug molecules, which would therefore cause the molecules to move faster through the stratum corneum. An increasing temperature would also cause structural alterations in the stratum corneum and underlying tissue and result in a faster movement of the drug through the different skin layers.

(h) Skin metabolism: Skin metabolizes steroids, hormones, chemical carcinogens and some drugs. So skin metabolism determines efficacy of drug permeated through the skin

2. Compound/Drug-Specific Factors

(a) Solubility: Stratum corneum is a lipophilic membrane and the amount of a drug that accumulates in it bears some relationship to the solubility of that drug in some organic solvents, such as the highly lipophilic hexane. Saturated solutions better permeate through the stratum corneum, because they represent maximum thermodynamic activity. A very hydrophilic drug is unable to penetrate the skin, while a very lipophilic drug has the propensity to remain in the layers of the stratum corneum. While the stratum corneum is lipophilic in nature and favours the permeation of lipophilic drugs, the aqueous nature of the layers beneath the stratum corneum dictate that drugs should embody some hydrophilic properties to pass through them.

(b) Partition Coefficients: Penetration of the stratum corneum requires that a drug partitions into the membrane. Such partitioning is an important step in the penetration of the membrane. The optimal partition coefficient (K) is required for good action. Drugs with high partition coefficient are not ready to leave the lipid portion of skin. Also, drugs with low partition coefficient will not be permeated.

(c) Molecular weight: Drug penetration is inversely related to molecular weight; small molecules penetrate faster than large ones. Drug with molecular weight 500 Dalton are difficult to penetrate through stratum corneum.

(d) Ionization: The lipophilic nature of the stratum corneum had led to the belief that ionized drugs would be poor candidates for transdermal delivery. As a result of the complex structure of the skin, however, drugs can cross the skin via various pathways. The transcellular route is regarded as having intermediate properties, whereas the intracellular route is mainly regarded for allowing the delivery of lipophilic molecules. Ionized drugs hence cross the skin through the shunt route, but the amount of molecules that pass through that route is significantly less than unionized molecules that take the intracellular route.

(e) Hydrogen bonding: The varied skin components (lipids, proteins, aqueous regions, enzymes etc.) and possible drug penetrants (weak acids/bases, ionized/unionized species, neutral molecules etc.) suggest a multitude of potential interactions between drug substances and skin tissue. The formation of hydrogen bonds, or weak Van der Waals forces, would hence influence skin penetration of a permeating drug.

(f) Melting point: Generally, organic substances with high melting points and high enthalpy of melting have lower aqueous solubility properties, because solvents can't enter the crystalline structure of such molecules to dissolve them. An indirect relationship therefore exists between the melting point and the solubility of a drug. Lowering the melting point of a drug would hence cause an increase in its solubility in the stratum corneum and ultimately in its permeation across the skin.

(g) Compound/Drug concentration: A major determinant of the amount of a compound absorbed across the skin is the concentration or the amount of the compound at the skin surface. The flux is proportional to the concentration gradient across the barrier and concentration gradient will be higher if the concentration of drug will be more across the barrier.

13.5 EXCIPIENTS USED IN SEMI SOLID DOSAGE FORMS

1. Bases/Ointment base

The base is that substance or part of an ointment or other semisolid preparation which serves as carrier or vehicle for the medicament. Selection of an appropriate base for an ointment or cream formulation depends on the type of activity desired (for example, topical or percutaneous absorption), compatibility with other components, physicochemical and microbial stability of the product, ease of manufacture, pourability and spreadability of the formulation, duration of contact, chances of hypersensitivity reactions, and ease of washing from the site of application. In addition, bases that are used in ophthalmic preparations should be non-irritating and should soften at body temperatures.

The ideal base should possess the following characteristics**:**

(i)   They must possess affinity for skin and should be miscible with both aqueous and oily secretions of the skin.

(ii)   It should meet conditions of the skin particularly pH. Ideal pH should be 5-7.6.

(iii) It should be stable.

(iv)   It should be possessing property of permanency and smoothness.

(v)   It should be non-irritating and non-sensitizing properties.

(vi)   It must be inert to excipients that may be incorporated along with them.

(vii) It must be able to absorb water and solutions of chemicals.

(viii) It must be able to release easily its incorporated medicaments.

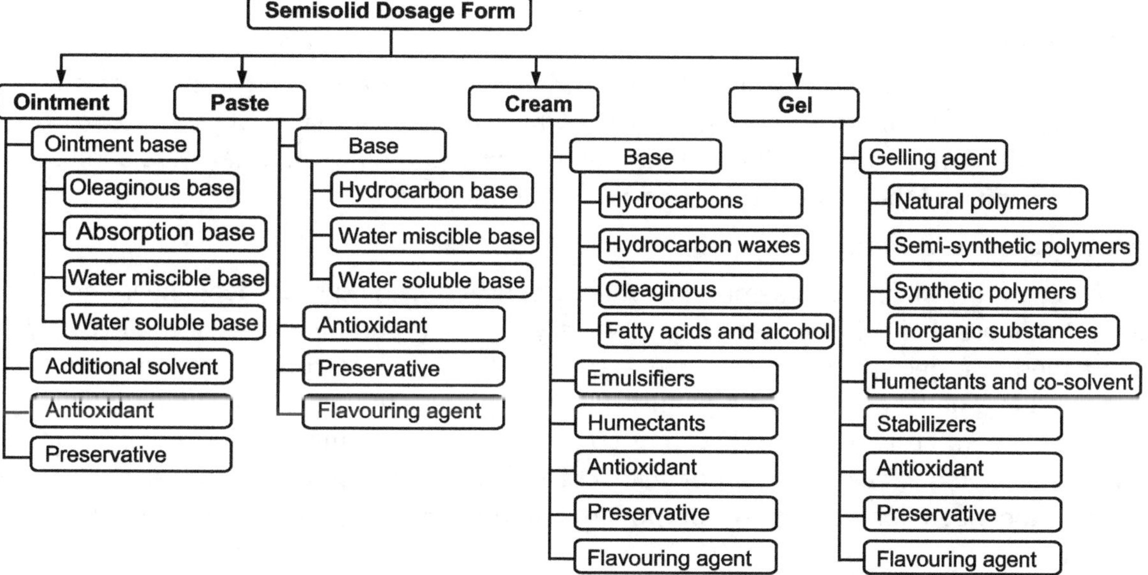

Fig. 13.3: Excipients used in Semisolid Dosage Forms

Important Constituents of Various Semisolid Dosage Forms

(Ointments, paste, creams and gel)

Classification of ointment base

Ointment bases are classified based on their composition and physical characteristics. The United States Pharmacopeia classifies ointment bases as**:**

(A) Oleaginous bases (Hydrocarbon bases)

(B) Absorption bases

(C) Water-miscible/removable bases

(D) Water - soluble bases

(A) Oleaginous bases (Hydrocarbon bases)

Oleaginous bases are non-aqueous formulations which provide emollient and protective properties and remain on the skin for prolonged periods. It is difficult to incorporate aqueous phases into hydrocarbon bases. However, powders can be incorporated into these bases with the aid of liquid petrolatum. Removal of hydrocarbon bases from the skin is difficult due to their oily nature. Hydrocarbon bases frequently contain the following components:

   (a) Hard paraffin

   (b) White/yellow soft paraffin

   (c) Liquid paraffin

   (d) Mineral oil

   (e) Microcrystalline wax.

Hard paraffin

It is a mixture of solid saturated hydrocarbons which are derived from petroleum or shale oil. Hard paraffin is a colorless or white wax-like material that is physically composed of a mixture of microcrystals. The melting point of hard paraffin is between $47°C$ and $65°C$. It is used to enhance the rheological properties of ointment bases.

White/yellow soft paraffin

It is a purified mixture of semisolid hydrocarbons (containing branched, linear and cyclic chains) that are derived from petroleum. White/yellow soft paraffin consists of microcrystals embedded in a gel composed of liquid and amorphous hydrocarbons that are themselves dispersed in a gel phase containing liquid and amorphous hydrocarbons. The melting range of the soft paraffin is between $38°C$ and $60°C$. White soft paraffin and yellow soft paraffin (the former being a bleached form of yellow soft paraffin) may be used as an ointment base without the need for additional components, although it may be combined with liquid paraffin.

Liquid paraffin (mineral oil)

This is a mixture of saturated aliphatic (C_{14}–C_{18}) and cyclic hydrocarbons that have been refined from petroleum. It is usually formulated with white/yellow soft paraffin to achieve the required viscosity for application to the required site. Formulations containing liquid paraffin require the incorporation of an antioxidant due to the ability of this material to undergo oxidation.

Microcrystalline wax

It is solid mixture of saturated alkanes (both linear and branched) with a defined range of carbon chain lengths (C_{41}–C_{57}). It is used to enhance the viscosity of ointments and creams. One of the advantages of microcrystalline wax is the greater physical stability provided to formulations containing liquid paraffin hence reduced bleeding of the liquid component.

Advantages of hydrocarbons bases

(i)   Emollient, thereby restricting water loss from the site of application due to the formation of an occlusive film that restricts the loss of moisture hence, keeps the skin soft.

(ii)   They are sticky hence ensures prolonged contact between skin and medicament.

(iii) They are almost inert. They consist largely of saturated hydrocarbons; therefore, very few incompatibilities and little tendency of rancidity are there.

(iv) They can withstand heat sterilization; hence, sterile ophthalmic ointments can be prepared with it.

(v)   They are readily available and cheap.

Disadvantages of hydrocarbon bases

(i)   It may lead to water logging followed by maceration of the skin if applied for a prolonged period.

(ii)   It retains body heat, which may produce an uncomfortable feeling of warmth.

(iii) Predominantly hydrophobic and therefore difficult to remove from the skin by washing and difficult to apply to (spread over) wet surfaces (for example, Mucous membranes, wet skin)

(iv) They are sticky, hence makes application unpleasant and leads to contamination of clothes.

(v)   Only a low concentration (< 5%) of water may be incorporated into hydrocarbon bases (with careful mixing).

(B) Absorption bases

Absorption bases contain small amounts of water. They provide relatively less emollient properties than hydrocarbon bases. Similar to hydrocarbon bases, absorption bases are also difficult to remove from the skin due to their hydrophobic nature. These may be either non-aqueous formulations to which an aqueous phase may be added to produce a water in oil (w/o) emulsion termed *non-emulsified bases* or water in oil emulsions that can facilitate the incorporation of an aqueous phase without phase inversion or cracking. The key properties of both non-emulsified bases and water in oil emulsions that are relevant to the formulation of ointments and pastes.

(i) Non-emulsified bases:

These are hydrophobic formulations to which water can be added. They assist oil soluble medicaments to penetrate the skin. Following application, a film is formed that offers occlusion and hence emollient properties; but these are less occlusive than hydrocarbon bases. They have more spreading properties than hydrocarbon bases. Non-emulsified bases are commonly composed of one or more paraffin and a sterol-based emulsifying agent. Examples of the types of emulsifying agents used in absorption bases include**:**

(a) Lanolin (wool fat)

(b) Hydrous lanolin

(c) Lanolin alcohols (wool alcohols)

(d) Beeswax (white or yellow).

Lanolin (wool fat)

Lanolin or wool fat is a refined, decolorized, and deodorized material obtained from sheep wool. It is available as a pale yellow, waxy material with a characteristic odour. Lanolin is typically mixed with vegetable oils or paraffin to produce an ointment base that can absorb approximately twice its own weight of water to produce water in oil emulsions. This property favors in preparing physically stable creams. Addition of soft paraffin or vegetable oil improves the emollient property of lanolin preparations. The usual concentrations of lanolin used in ointments (e.g. Simple Ointment BP) range from 5 to 10% w/w. Exposure of lanolin to higher temperature usually leads to discoloration and rancid like odor, and hence prolonged heating is avoided during the preparation and preservation of lanolin containing preparations. Gamma sterilization or filtration sterilization is usually employed for sterilizing ophthalmic ointments containing lanolin. Lanolin and some of its derivatives are reported to cause hypersensitivity reactions and therefore are avoided in patients with known hypersensitivity.

Hydrous Lanolin

Gradual addition of about 25 – 30% of water into molten lanolin with constant stirring gives hydrous lanolin. It is available as a pale yellow, oily material with a characteristic odor. The water uptake capacity of hydrous lanolin is higher than lanolin, and it is used for preparing topical hydrophobic ointments or water - in – oil creams with larger aqueous phase. Exposure of these preparations to higher temperatures results in separations of oily and aqueous layers. Hydrous lanolin that contains free fatty alcohols is avoided in hypersensitive patients.

Lanolin alcohols (wool alcohols)

Lanolin alcohol or wool alcohol is prepared from lanolin by the saponification process and is used as a hydrophobic vehicle in pharmaceutical ointments and creams. Wool alcohol is a crude mixture of sterols and triterpene alcohols and contains at least 30% cholesterol and 10–13% isocholesterol. It is available as a brittle solid material pale yellow in color with a faint characteristic odor. This is added to mixtures of paraffin (hard, so white/yellow soft or liquid) to produce the required consistency. The inclusion of wool alcohols (5% w/w) results in a 300% increase in the concentration of water that may be incorporated into paraffin bases. It is suitable for preparing dry - skin ointments, eye ointments, and water - in – oil creams. Creams containing lanolin alcohols do not show surface darkening and do not produce objectionable odor compared to lanolin - containing preparations.

Beeswax (white or yellow)

Beeswax is a wax that consists of esters of aliphatic alcohols (C_{24}–C_{36} even numbers) and linear aliphatic fatty acids (up to C_{36}, even numbers) that is combined with paraffin to produce non-emulsified bases.

- **Yellow beeswax:** It is obtained from honey combs. It contains about 70% esters of straight - chain monohydric alcohols, 15% free acids, 12% carbohydrates, and 1% free wax alcohols and stearic esters of fatty acids. It is available as non-crystalline pieces which are yellow in color and possesses a characteristic odor. It is practically insoluble in water and melts at 61–65°C. It is used in the preparation of hydrophobic ointments and water-in-oil creams because of its viscosity - enhancing properties. Concentrations up to 20% are used for producing ointments and creams.

- **White beeswax:** It is the bleached form of yellow beeswax hence is known as bleached wax or white bees wax. It contains about 70% esters of straight - chain monohydric alcohols, 15% free acids, 12% carbohydrates, and 1% free wax alcohols and stearic esters of fatty acids. It is available as granules or sheets which are white in color and possesses a characteristic odor. White wax is insoluble in water and melts between 61 and 65°C. It has stiffening and viscosity enhancing properties and therefore is used in hydrophobic ointments and oil-in-water creams. Although it is thermally stable, heating to above 150°C results in reduction of its acid value. White wax is incompatible with oxidizing agents. The presence of small quantities of impurities results in hypersensitivity reactions in rare cases.

(ii) Water in oil emulsions

It has property of absorbing greater concentration of water and can still provide similar performance to that provided by non-emulsified bases such as occlusion, spreading properties, etc. A common excipient that is employed in the formulation of this type of ointment base is 70-75% of hydrous lanolin and about 25–30% water. It is incorporated into paraffin and oils to produce a base that can incorporate the subsequent addition of an aqueous phase. The water content of bases that have been formulated using hydrous lanolin is significant, for example, Oily Cream BP is a water in oil emulsion ointment base that is composed of wool alcohols (50% w/w) and water (50% w/w).

Advantages of absorption bases:

(i)   They aid oil soluble medicaments to penetrate the skin.

(ii)   They are less occlusive but good emollient.

(iii) They are easier to spread.

(iv) They are compatible with majority of the medicaments.

(v) They are relatively heat stable.

(vi) They can absorb a large quantity of water or aqueous substances.

(vii) The base may be used in their anhydrous form or in emulsified form.

Disadvantages of absorption bases:

Absorption bases are difficult to wash; although they are hydrophilic in nature.

(C) Water-miscible/removable bases

Unlike hydrocarbon and absorption bases, a large proportion of aqueous phase can be incorporated into water - removable bases with the aid of suitable emulsifying agents. It is easy to remove these bases from the skin due to their hydrophilic nature. These are used to form oil in water emulsions for topical applications. British Pharmacopoeia describes three water-miscible/removable bases as Emulsifying ointment, Cetrimide emulsifying ointment and Cetomacrogol emulsifying ointment. Each of these contains 20% w/w liquid paraffin, 50% w/w white soft paraffin and 30% w/w anionic, cationic or non-ionic emulsifying wax.

(a) **Anionic emulsifying wax:** This is a waxy solid that, when incorporated into a paraffin base, may be used to produce an oil in water emulsion, for example, Aqueous Cream BP which contains 10% w/w anionic emulsifying wax. Anionic emulsifying wax: it is composed of 90 g cetostearyl alcohol, 10 g sodium lauryl sulphate and 1 mL purified water.

(b) **Non-ionic emulsifying wax:** This is also referred to as Cetomacrogol Emulsifying Wax BP and is composed of 800 g of cetostearyl alcohol and 200 g of cetomacrogol-1000.

(c) **Cationic emulsifying wax:** This is also referred to as Cetrimide Emulsifying Wax BP. Cationic Emulsifying Wax BP is composed of 900 g cetostearyl alcohol and 100 g of cetrimide.

Advantages of water miscible bases:

(i) They are able to accommodate large volumes of water, e.g. aqueous solutions of drug, excess moisture at the site of application.

(ii) They are not occlusive.

(iii) They may be easily washed from the skin and from clothing. Furthermore, they may be readily applied to (and removed from) hair.

(iv) Reduced interference with normal skin function.

(v) They are aesthetically pleasing.

(D) Water - soluble bases

Water-soluble bases are predominantly prepared using mixtures of different molecular weights of polyethylene glycol (macrogols) to produce the required ointment consistency. Polyethylene glycol (PEG) are mixture of polycondensation product of ethylene oxide and water. It has general formula:

$$CH_2OH \cdot (CH_2OCH_2)_n \cdot CH_2OH$$

Lower average molecular weights of this polymer (200, 400 and 600 g/mol) are liquids. As the average molecular weight increases, the consistency of this polymer changes from a liquid to a waxy solid ($\geq$1000 g/mol). It does not contain any oily or oleaginous phase. Solids can be easily incorporated into these bases. They may be completely removed from the skin due to their water solubility. Polyethylene glycol (PEG) ointment National Formulary (NF) is an example of water - soluble base.

Product with ointment like consistency can be obtained by mixing liquid and waxy form of PEG in suitable proportions. When 65 % of PEG 300 and 35 % of PEG 4000 mixed the product is suitable for ointment base (Macrogol ointment BPC).

Certain other substances that are used as water-soluble bases include tragacanth, gelatin, pectin, silica gel, sodium alginate, cellulose derivatives, magnesium-aluminum silicate and bentonite. In the true sense these substances are not water-soluble but they swell-up with the absorption of water.

Advantages of water soluble bases:

(i)   They are water soluble; hence, very easily removed from the skin and readily miscible with tissue exudates.

(ii)   They help in good absorption by the skin.

(iii)   They have good solvent properties. Some water-soluble dermatological drugs, such as salicylic acid, sulfonamides, sulfur etc. are soluble in this base.

(iv)   They are non-greasy.

(v)   They do not hydrolyze, rancidify or support microbial growth.

(vi)   They are compatible with many dermatological medicaments.

Disadvantages of water soluble bases:

(i)   **Limited uptake of water:** Macrogols dissolve when the proportion of water reaches about 5%.

(ii)   Less bland than paraffin due their hygroscopic nature.

(iii)   Reduction in activity of certain antibacterial agents, for example, phenols, hydroxybenzoates and quaternary compounds.

(iv)   Solvent action on polyethylene and bakelite containers and closures.

Additional/alternative solvents of ointment bases

These are hydrophobic liquid components that may be added to ointment bases predominantly hydrophobic or absorption bases are liquid silicone, vegetable oils, organic esters.

Liquid silicone

It is polydimethylsiloxane. This may be used in barrier ointments due to the water-repellent properties of this component.

Vegetable oils

Vegetable oils may be used either to replace mineral oils or, alternatively, may be added to hydrophobic or absorption bases to increase the emollient properties of the formulated product. Examples of oils that are used for this purpose are coconut oil and arachis oil.

Organic esters

These may be used partly to replace a mineral oil to enhance the spreadability and to enhance drug dissolution within the ointment base. One of the most commonly used example is isopropyl myristate.

Summary of Ointment Bases Properties

Property	Oleaginous Ointment Bases	Absorption Ointment Bases	Water/Oil Emulsion Ointment Bases	Oil/Water Emulsion Ointment Bases	Water-miscible Ointment Bases
Composition	Oleaginous compounds	Oleaginous base + w/o surfactant	Oleaginous base + water (< 45% w/w) + w/o surfactant (HLB $\leq$8)	Oleaginous base + water (> 45% w/w) + o/w surfactant (HLB $\geq$9)	Polyethylene Glycols (PEGs)
Water Content	Anhydrous	Anhydrous	Hydrous	Hydrous	Anhydrous, hydrous
Affinity for Water	Hydrophobic	Hydrophilic	Hydrophilic	Hydrophilic	Hydrophilic
Spreadability	Difficult	Difficult	Moderate to easy	Easy	Moderate to easy
Washability	Non-washable	Non-washable	Non- or poorly washable	Washable	Washable

contd. ...

Stability	Oils poor; hydrocarbons better	Oils poor; hydrocarbons better	Unstable, especially alkali soaps and natural colloids	Unstable, especially alkali soaps and natural colloids; non-ionics better	Stable
Drug Incorporation Potential	Solids (oil soluble only) or oils	Solids, oils, and aqueous solutions (small amounts)	Solids, oils, and aqueous solutions (small amounts)	Solid and aqueous solutions (small amounts)	Solid and aqueous solutions
Drug Release Potential	Poor	Poor, but > oleaginous	Fair to good	Fair to good	Good
Occlusiveness	Yes	Yes	Sometimes	No	No
Uses	Protectants, emollients (+/−), vehicles for hydrolyzable drugs	Protectants, emollients (+/−), vehicles for aqueous solutions, solids, and non-hydrolyzable drugs	Emollients, cleansing creams, vehicles for solid, liquid, or non-hydrolyzable drugs	Emollients, vehicles for solid, liquid, or non-hydrolyzable drugs	Drug vehicles
Examples	White Petrolatum, White Ointment	Hydrophilic Petrolatum, Anhydrous Lanolin, Aquabase™, Aquaphor®, Polysorb®	Cold Cream type, Hydrous Lanolin, Rose Water Ointment, Hydrocream™, Eucerin®, Nivea®	Hydrophilic Ointment, Dermabase™, Velvachol®, Unibase®	PEG Ointment, Polybase™

Source: The Pharmaceutics and Compounding Laboratory, UNC Eshelman School of Pharmacy.

2. Emulsifying agents

Emulsifying agents are also known as emulgent or emulsifier and are generally used in preparation of w/o or o/w type of creams and ointments. They reduce the interfacial tension between the two phases. i.e.; aqueous phase and oily phase thus make them miscible with each other and form a stable emulsion. No single emulsifying agents possesses all the properties required for the preparation of stable emulsion therefore sometimes it becomes necessary to use two or more than two emulsifying agents instead of one to get a product of desired qualities.

Examples:

(i)   Natural emulsifying agents: Acacia, tragacanth, agar, chondrus, pectin, wool fat, egg yolk etc.

(ii)   Semi-synthetic polysaccharides: Methyl cellulose, Sodium carboxyl methyl cellulose etc.

(iii) Synthetic emulsifying agents: *Anionic-* alkali soaps, metallic soaps, sulfated alcohols and sulphonates, *Cationic-* Benzalkonium chloride, benzethonium chloride etc., *Non-Ionic-* Glyceryl esters such as glyceryl monostearate, poly-oxyethylene glycol etc.

(iv)   Inorganic emulsifying agents: Several inorganic substances such as milk of magnesia, Mg oxide, Mg Tri-Silicate, Mg aluminum silicate etc. are used in the preparations of pharmaceutical emulsions. 5% suspension of bentonite is used as an emulsifying agent.

3. Gelling agent

Gelling agents are used to increase viscosity of dispersion in semisolid formulations. It acts as base for preparation of gel and as thickening agent for other semisolid formulations. A large number of gelling agents are commercially available for the preparation of pharmaceutical gels. In general, these materials are high molecular weight compounds obtained from either natural sources or synthetic pathways. They are water dispersible, possess swelling properties, and improve the viscosity of dispersions. An ideal gelling agent should not interact with other formulation components and should be free from microbial attack. Changes in the temperature and pH during preparation and preservation should not alter its rheological properties. In addition, it should be economic, readily available, form colorless gels, provide cooling sensation on the site of application, and possess a pleasant odor. Based on these factors, gelling agents are selected for different formulations.

Examples:

- **Natural polymers:** Natural polymers are those polymers which exist naturally and/or can be synthesized by living bodies, for example, Proteins like collagen, gelatine etc and polysaccharides like agar, tragacanth, pectin and gum etc.

- **Semi synthetic polymers:** These polymers are mostly derived from natural polymers by chemical modification, for example, cellulose derivatives like Carboxymethyl-cellulose (CMC), Methylcellulose (MC), Hydroxypropyl cellulose (HPC) and Hydroxyethyl cellulose (HEC).

- **Synthetic polymers:** The polymers which are prepared in laboratories are called synthetic polymers. These are also called man made polymers, for example, Carbomer carbopol 940, Carbopol 934, Poloxamer, Polyacrylamide, Polyvinyl alcohol and Polyethylene.

- **Inorganic substances:** Aluminium hydroxide and Bentonite.

4. Penetration enhancer

Penetration enhancers improve the solubility of the active drug in the stratum corneum and facilitate the diffusion of the drug through this barrier into the systemic circulation. An ideal penetration enhancer should reversibly reduce the barrier resistance of stratum corneum without damaging the skin cells. Ideal penetration enhancers should possess the following properties:

(i) It should be pharmacologically inert.

(ii) It should be non-toxic, non-irritating, and non-allergenic.

(iii) It should have rapid onset of action; predictable and suitable duration of action for the drug used.

(iv) It should be chemically and physically compatible with other ingredients.

(v) It should be readily incorporated into the delivery system.

(vi) It should be inexpensive and cosmetically acceptable.

Mechanism of chemical penetration enhancement

Penetration enhancers may act by one or more of three main mechanisms:

(i) Disruption of the highly ordered structure of stratum corneum lipid.

(ii) Interaction with intercellular protein.

(iii) Improved partition of the drug, co enhancer or solvent into the stratum corneum.

Examples: Commonly used penetration enhancers include DMSO (dimethyl sulfoxide), urea, and triethanolamine.

Other: *Alcohols-* methanol, ethanol, propanol, octanol, *Fatty Alcohols-* myristyl alcohol, cetyl alcohol, stearyl alcohol, *Fatty Acids-* myristic acid, stearic acid, oleic acid, *Fatty Acid Ester-* isopropyl myristate, isopropyl palmitate, *Polyols-* propylene glycol, polyethylene glycol, glycerol, *Anionic surfactants-* sodium lauryl sulfate, *Cationic surfactant-* benzalkonium chloride, cetylpyridinium chloride, *Amphoteric surfactants-* lecithins, Non-ionic surfactants- Spans®, Tweens®, poloxamers, Miglyol®, etc.

5. Buffers

The pH is important in drug formulations, especially because it affects drug solubility, activity, absorption, stability, sorption, and patient comfort. pH is related to certain physical characteristics, such as the viscosity of some polymers used as gel-forming agents. Buffer systems are sufficiently strong, however, to resist changes in pH under normal storage and use. Buffers (for example, phosphate, citrate) may be included in aqueous and hydro-alcoholic based gels to control the pH of the formulation.

Examples: Sodium acetate, sodium citrate, potassium metaphosphate.

6. Humectants

Humectants are agent which absorb moisture from surrounding and keep product wet. Loss of water can quickly lead to dry formulation in semisolids such as cream, gel and humectants   such as glycerol, propylene   glycol or   sorbitol   solution   may   be added to retain water.

7. Antioxidants

Antioxidants are added to minimize or retard oxidative processes that occur with some drugs or excipients on exposure to oxygen (air) or in the presence of free radicals. These processes can often be catalyzed by light, temperature, hydrogen ion concentration, presence of trace metals, or peroxides. Oxidation of a preparation may be manifested as an unpleasant odor or taste, discoloration or other change in appearance, precipitation, or even a slight loss of activity. The selection of an appropriate antioxidant is dependent on several factors, including solubility, location of the agent in the formulation (emulsions), chemical and physical stability over a wide pH range, compatibility, odor, discoloration, toxicity, irritation, potency, effectiveness in low concentrations, and freedom from toxicity, carcinogenicity, and sensitizing effects. The actual selection of an antioxidant depends on the type of product, route, dose, and frequency of administration, physical and chemical properties of the preservative used, presence of other components, and properties of the closure and container. Antioxidants are used in relatively low concentrations, usually from 0.001% to 0.2%.

In pharmaceutical ointments antioxidants are employed to prevent or reduce oxidation of either the non-aqueous components of the ointment base (for example, mineral/vegetable oils) and/or the therapeutic agent.

Examples: Lipophilic antioxidants (to be dissolved within the non-aqueous vehicle)-Butylated hydroxyanisole (BHA) 0.005–0.02%, butylated hydroxytoluene (BHT) 0.007–0.1%, propyl gallate ($\leq$ 1%), Hydrophilic antioxidants (to be dissolved in the aqueous phase)-Sodium metabisulphite 0.01–0.1%, sodium sulphite 0.1%.

8. Preservative

In semisolid formulations; some bases, although resist microbial attack but because of their high water content, it requires an antimicrobial preservative. Antimicrobial presservatives are used to prevent contamination, deterioration or spoilage of semisolid formulation by bacteria and fungi.

The first consideration in selection is the irritancy or toxicity of compound to the tissue to which the semisolid formulation is to be applied. For, instance methyl and propyl parabens are irritants to nasal passages. Boric acid may be toxic. Quaternary ammonium compounds or phenyl mercuric nitrates are better tolerated by nasal tissues. On occasions the plastic containers or rubber closures may take up some amount of preservatives thus reducing their availability for antimicrobial action. Sometimes the preservatives get complexed by other ingredients and are thus not available in sufficient concentration for microbial action. In presence of tween 80, methyl paraben, benzalkonium chlorie, benzoic acid, etc get inactivated to appreciable extents. The bacterial activity also depends upon the partition coefficient of antimicrobial compound between aqueous and oily phase. If both phases are to be protected additional amount may be needed.

Examples: Methyl hydroxybenzoate (Methyl paraben), Propyl-hydroxybenzoate (Propyl paraben), Chlorocresol, Benzoic acid, Phenyl mercuric nitrate, Phenols, Sorbic acid, Benzalkonium chloride, Chlorhexidine acetate, Benzyl alcohol and Quaternary ammonium salts etc.

9. Flavouring and Sweetening agents

Flavours and sweetening agents are only included in semisolid formulations that are designed for administration into the oral cavity, for example, for the treatment of infection, inflammation or ulceration. The choice of sweetener/flavouring agents is dependent on the required taste, the type and concentration selected to mask the taste of the drug substance efficiently.

10. Fragrances/Perfumes

These are added to semisolid formulations to mask unwanted odour of bases and other ingredients. The selection of perfume blend is a very tricky business and every manufacturer would like to give a distinctive odorific quality to this product.

Example: Lavender oil, rose oil, lemon oil, almond oil etc.

13.6 PREPARATION OF SEMISOLIDS

(A) Ointments

Ointments are homogeneous, semi-solid preparations intended for external application to the skin or mucous membranes. They are used as emollients or for the application of active ingredients to the skin for protective, therapeutic, or prophylactic purposes and where a degree of occlusion is desired. Ointments are formulated using hydrophobic, hydrophilic, or water-emulsifying bases to provide preparations that are immiscible, miscible, or emulsifiable with skin secretions. They can also be derived from hydrocarbon (fatty), absorption, water-miscible, or water-soluble bases.

Ideal properties of ointments are:

(i) It should be smooth and free from grittiness.

(ii) It should be chemically and physically stable.

(iii) It should melt or soften at body temperature and be easily applied.

(iv) The base should be non-irritant and should have no therapeutic action.

(v) The medicament should be finely divided and uniformLy distributed throughout the base.

Classification of Ointments:

Ointments are classified on the basis of penetration and their therapeutic use as follows:

(B) On the basis of penetration

 (a) Epidermic Ointments: These ointments are intended to produce their action on the surface of the skin and produce local effect. They are not absorbed. They act as protective, antiseptics and parasiticides.

 (b) Endodermic Ointments: These ointments are intended to release the medicaments that penetrate into the skin. They are partially absorbed and acts as emollients, stimulants and local irritants.

 (c) Diadermic Ointments: These ointments are intended to release the medicaments that pass through the skin and produce systemic effects.

(C) On the basis of therapeutic use

 (a) Antibiotic ointments: used to kill micro-organisms. Examples: bacitracin, chlortetracycline, neomycin etc.

 (b) Antifungal ointments: used to inhibit or kill fungi. Examples: benzoic acid, salicylic acid, nystatin etc.

 (c) Anti-inflammatory ointments: used to get relief from inflammatory, allergic and pruritic conditions. Examples: betamethasone valerate, fluocinolone acetonide, hydrocortisone and its acetate, triamcinolone acetonide etc.

 (d) Antipruritic ointments: used to relieve itching. Examples: benzocaine, coal tar etc.

 (e) Astringent ointments: used to cause skin cells or mucus membranes to contract or shrink, by precipitating proteins from their surface. When applied topically they dry, harden and protect the skin. They reduce bleeding from minor abrasions and are used to relieve skin irritations resulting from minor cuts, allergies, eczema, stretch marks, insect bites and so on. Examples: calamine, zinc oxide, acetic acid, tannic acid etc.

(f) Antieczematous ointments: used to prevent oozing and excretion from vesicles on the skin. Examples: hydrocortisone, ichthamol, salicylic acid, coal tar, sulphur etc.

(g) Kertolytic ointments: used to remove or soften the horny layer of skin. Examples: resorcinol, salicylic acid, sulphur etc.

(h) Counter-irritant ointments: applied locally to irritate the skin, thus reducing or relieving another irritation or deep cited pain. Examples: capsicum, methyl salicylate, iodine, oleoresin etc.

(i) Antidandruff ointments: used to treat dandruff. Examples: salicylic acid, cetrimide, etc.

(j) Ointment for psoriasis treatment: used to treat psoriasis. Examples: coal tar, corticosteroid, diathranol b, salicylic acid etc.

(k) Parasiticide ointments: used to destroy or inhibit living infestation like ticks and lice. Examples: benzyl benzoate, hexachloride, sulphur etc.

(l) Protectant ointments: used to protect skin from moisture, air, sunrays or other substances like soap and chemicals. Examples: calamine, zinc oxide, titanium dioxide, silicone etc.

Advantages of Ointments:

(i)   They avoid first pass metabolism of drug.

(ii) They provide means of site specific application of druq on affected area, which avoids unnecessary non-target exposure of drug thereby avoiding side effects.

(iii) They are suitable dosage forms for bitter taste drugs.

(iv) Convenient for unconscious patients having difficulty in oral administration.

(v)   Comparatively they are chemically more stable and easy to handle than liquid dosage forms.

Disadvantages of Ointments

(i)   These oily semisolid preparations are staining and cosmetically less aesthetic.

(ii) Application with fingertip may contaminate the formulation or cause irritation when applied.

(iii) As compared to solid dosage forms, ointments are bulky to handle.

(iv) Though semisolids allow more flexibility in dose, dose accuracy is determined by uniformity in the quantity to be applied.

(v)   Physico-chemically less stable than solid dosage forms.

Methods of preparation of ointments

Ointments are prepared by either incorporating the active ingredients into the selected base or by melting the base and active ingredient together.

1. Ointments prepared by Fusion method

When an ointment base contains a number of solid ingredients such as white beeswax, cetyl alcohol, stearyl alcohol, stearic acid, hard paraffin etc. as components of the base, it is required to melt them. The melting can be done in two methods:

Method-I: The components are melted in the decreasing order of their melting point i.e. the higher m.p. substance should be melted first, the substances with next melting point and so on. The medicament is added slowly in the melted ingredients and stirred thoroughly until the mass cools down and homogeneous product is formed. This will avoid over-heating of substances having low melting point.

Method-II: All the components are taken in subdivided state and melted together. The maximum temperature reached is lower than Method-I, and less time was taken possibly due to the solvent action of the lower melting point substances on the rest of the ingredients.

Precautions:

(i) Melting time is shortened by grating waxy components (i.e. beeswax, wool alcohols, hard-paraffin, higher fatty alcohols and emulsifying waxes) by stirring during melting and by lowering the dish as far as possible into the water bath so that the maximum surface area is heated.

(ii) The surface of some ingredients discolors due to oxidation for example, wool fats and wool alcohols and this discolored layers should be removed before use.

(iii) After melting, the ingredients should be stirred until the ointment is cool, taking care not to cause localized cooling, for example, by using a cold spatula or stirrer, placing the dish on a cold surface (for example, a plastic bench top) or transferring to a cold container before the ointment has fully set.

(iv) Vigorous-stirring, after the ointment has begun to thicken, causes excessive aeration and should be avoided.

(v) Because of their greasy nature, many constituents of ointment bases pick-up dirt during storage, which can be seen after melting. This is removed from the melt by allowing it to sediment and decanting the supernatant, or by passage through muslin supported by a warm strainer. In both instances the clarified liquid is collected in another hot basin.

(vi) If the product is granular after cooling, due to separation of high melting point constituents, it should be re-melted, using the minimum of heat, and again stirred and cooled.

Example: Simple Ointment BP

Wool fat	50 g
Hard paraffin	50 g
Cetostearyl alcohol	50 g
White soft paraffin	850 g

Method: Hard paraffin and cetostearyl alcohol on water-bath. Wool fat and white soft paraffin are mixed and stirred until all the ingredients are melted. If required decanted or strained and stirred until cold and packed in suitable container.

Uses: Unless otherwise directed, simple ointment prepared with white soft paraffin should be used as a base for white ointments and if it is prepared with yellow soft paraffin should be used as base in colored ointments. Wool-fat provides emollient action. By itself it is not readily absorbed but when mixed with soft paraffin or suitable vegetable oil it forms the cream which penetrate the skin and facilitates the absorption of therapeutically active ingredient. Hard paraffin works as stiffening agent. Cetostearyl alcohol improves the emollient properties of simple ointment.

Medicated ointment by fusion method: Completely or partially soluble solids should be added in fine powder to the molten base at very low temperature and the mixture stirred until cold. Liquids such as methyl salicylate and coal tar solutions and semi solids such as ichthamol should be added just as the base is thickening, at about 40°C. When a solid is soluble in liquid ingredient, (menthol in methyl salicylate), its more convenient to add it in solution. Insoluble solids (calamine, starch, zinc oxide) should be passed through a 180 um sieve and added in small amount while stirring to melted base, when it shows first sign of thickening. Sedimentation should be prevented. If the product has liquid paraffin or a fixed oil, small amount can be used to levigate powder before adding to base to produce a smoother product.

Example: Salicylic Acid Ointment BP

Salicylic acid	2% w/w
Wool alcohol ointment	q.s.

Wool Alcohol Ointment

Wool alcohol	60 g
Hard paraffin	240 g
White soft paraffin	100 g
Liquid paraffin	600 g

Method: Melt wool alcohol ointment BP which is used as base for this preparation and add salicylic acid in molten base with constant stirring until cold. In this preparation while preparing wool alcohol ointment; white soft paraffin is used as medicament is colorless.

Use: For the treatment of hyperkeratotic and scaling conditions such as psoriasis

Marketed products: Salicylic Acid Ointment 100 g (Gold cross), Salicylic Acid Ointment 450 g (Thornton and Ross Ltd.)

2. **Ointments prepared by Trituration method**

    This method is applicable in the base or a liquid present in small amount. Solids are finely powdered are passed through a sieve (# 250, # 180, #125). The powder is then taken on an ointment-slab and triturated with a small amount of the base (Levigation). A steel spatula with long, broad blade is used for this purpose. To this additional quantities of the base are incorporated and triturated until the medicament is mixed with the base. Finally, liquid ingredients are incorporated. To avoid loss from splashing, a small volume of liquid is poured into a depression in the ointment and thoroughly incorporated before more is added in the same way. Splashing is more easily controlled in a mortar than on a ointment slab.

    Examples: Whitfield ointment (Compound Benzoic Acid Ointment BPC)

Benzoic acid, in fine powder	6 g
Salicylic acid, in fine powder	3 g
Emulsifying ointment	91 g

Method: Benzoic acid and salicylic acid are sieved through No. 180 sieves. They are mixed on the ointment slab with small amount of base and levigated until smooth and dilute gradually.

Use: For treatment of fungal infection of the skin

Marketed products: Compound Benzoic Acid Ointment B.P. (Whitfield ointment) 500 g (Bell's Healthcare), Sibex® (Elixir Pharmaceuticals Ltd.), Benzalic® (Central Pharmaceuticals Ltd.), Fungalin® (Chemist Laboratories Ltd.), G-Benzosal® (Gonoshasthaya)

Example: Salicylic Acid Sulphur Ointment BPC

Salicylic acid BP	30 g
Precipitated sulphur BP	30 g
Oily cream BP	940 g

Method: Trituration method

Use: To treat acne and dandruff

Marketed products: SAStid®, Fostex®, Night CastR®

3. Ointments prepared by Chemical Reaction

Many ointment shows chemical reaction during its preparations.

(a) Ointment containing free iodine: Iodine is only slightly soluble in most fats and oils but very readily soluble in concentrated aqueous solution of potassium iodide due to formation of molecular complexes KI. I_2, $KI.2I_2$, $KI.3I_2$ etc. These solutions may be incorporated in absorption-type ointment bases.

Strong Iodine Ointment B.Vet.C (British Veterinary Pharmacopoeia) is used to treat ringworm in cattle. It contains free iodine. At one time this type of ointments was used as counter-irritants in the treatment of human rheumatic diseases but they were not popular because, they stain the skin a deep red color and due to improper storage the water dries up and the iodine crystals irritate the skin, hence glycerol was used some times to dissolve the iodine-potassium iodide complex instead of water.

Example: Strong Iodine Ointment B.Vet.C.

Iodine	4 g
Potassium iodide	4 g
Water	4 mL
Yellow soft paraffin	88 g

Method: Dissolve KI in water. Dissolve Iodine in it. Melt separately yellow soft paraffin on water bath. Melted mass is cooled to about 40°C. Then add iodine solution to melted mass in small quantities at a time with continuous stirring until a uniform mass is obtained. Cool to room temperature and pack.

Use: Ringworm in cattle.

(b) Ointment containing combined iodine: Fixed oils and many vegetable and animal fats absorb iodine which combines with the double bonds of the unsaturated constituents.

$$CH_3 \cdot (CH_2)_7 \cdot CH = CH.(CH_2)_7 \cdot COOH + I_2 = CH_3 \cdot (CH_2)_7 \cdot CHI \cdot CHI \cdot (CH_2)_7 \cdot COOH$$

Oleic acid   di-iodo stearic acid

Example: Non-staining Iodine Ointment BPC 1968

Iodine	5 g
Arachis oil	15 mL
Yellow soft paraffin...qs...	100 g

Method:

(i) Finely powder iodine in a glass mortar and add required amount to the oil in a glass-stoppered conical flask and stir it well.

(ii)   Heat oil at 50°C in a water-bath and stir continuously. Continue heating until the brown color is changed to greenish-black; this may take several hours.

(iii) Warm soft paraffin to 40°C. Add iodized oil and mix it well. Avoid further heating otherwise it will causes deposition of a resinous substance.

(iv)   Pack preparation in a warm, wide-mouthed, amber color, glass bottle. Allow it to cool without further stirring.

Use: Antiseptic and counter irritant

Marketed products: Iodex®, Iodoflex®, Iodosorb®

13.7 PASTES

Pastes are homogeneous, semi-solid preparations containing high concentrations of insoluble powdered substances (usually not less than 20%) dispersed in a suitable base. In short paste are ointments containing high proportion of powder dispersed in a fatty base. The pastes are usually less greasy, more absorptive, and stiffer in consistency than ointments because of the large quantity of powdered ingredients present. Some pastes consist of a single phase, such as hydrated pectin, and others consist of a thick, rigid material that does not flow at body temperature. The pastes should adhere well to the skin. In many cases they form a protective film that controls the evaporation of water.

Features of paste compared to ointments:

(i)   Pastes generally contain a large amount (50%) of finely powdered solids. So they are often stiffer than ointments.

(ii)   Because of the powder contents pastes are porous; hence, perspiration can escape. Since the powder absorbs exudates, pastes with hydrocarbon base are less macerating than ointments with a similar base.

(iii) When applied to the skin pastes adhere well, forming a thick coating protects and soothes inflamed and raw surfaces and minimizes the damage done by scratching in itchy conditions such as chronic eczema. it is comparatively easy to confine pastes to the diseased areas whereas ointments, which are usually less viscous, tend to spread on to healthy skin, and this may result in sensitivity reactions if the preparations contain a powerful medicament such as diathranol.

(iv)   Pastes are less greasy than ointments but since their efficacy depends on maintaining a thick surface layer they are far from attractive cosmetically.

(v)   Most of the pastes are unsuitable for treating scalp conditions because they are difficult to remove from the hair.

Preparation of Pastes

As like ointment base used for preparation of pastes are hydrocarbon base, water miscible base and water soluble bases. All other additives are same as like ointments. Pastes are also prepared by fusion and trituration method. Fusion method is used when the base is semisolid and/or solid in nature. Trituration method is used when the base is liquid or semisolid.

(a) Pastes prepared by fusion method

Example: Zinc and Coal tar Paste (White's Tar Paste)

Zinc oxide, finely sifted	60 g
Coal tar	60 g
Emulsifying wax	50 g
Starch	380 g
Yellow soft paraffin	450 g

Method-I: Melt emulsifying wax in petri dish at 70°C. Add weighed quantity of coal tar in melted wax. Melt separately yellow soft paraffin. Add half quantity of melted yellow soft paraffin to above mixture of coal tar and wax with continuous stirring. Add remaining quantity of melted yellow soft paraffin until homogeneous. Allow to cool at 30°C and add zinc oxide (which was previously passed through sieve no. 180) and starch with constant stirring. Continue stirring until cold.

Method-II: Melt emulsifying wax and yellow soft paraffin together; mix it well and stir until just setting. Mix zinc oxide powder with above melted wax on a slightly warm ointment slab by levigation and then incorporate coal tar. This method eliminates the risk of overheating.

Use: For treatment of psoriasis and eczema.

Marketed product: Elta Tar (Swiss-American Products, Inc)

(b) Pastes prepared by fusion and trituration method

Example: Compound Zinc Paste BP.

Zinc oxide, finely sifted	25 g
Starch, finely sifted	25 g
White soft paraffin	50 g

Method: Powder zinc oxide and starch and pass through sieve no. 180. Melt separately white soft paraffin on water bath. Take required quantity of powder in warm mortar and triturate well with melted white soft paraffin. Add rest of base gradually and mix it until cool.

Use: For the treatment of skin conditions including eczema and psoriasis. Can be used for sun protection.

Marketed products: Zinc Oxide Compound Paste 100 g (David Craig), Zinc Oxide Impression Paste (DE Healthcare).

13.8 CREAMS

Creams are homogeneous, semi-solid preparations consisting of opaque emulsion systems. Their consistency and rheological properties depend on the type of emulsion, either water-in-oil (w/o) or oil-in-water (o/w), and on the nature of the solids in the internal phase. Creams are intended for application to the skin or certain mucous membranes for protective, therapeutic, or prophylactic purposes, especially where an occlusive effect is not necessary. The term "cream" is most frequently used to describe soft, cosmetically acceptable types of preparations.

Method of preparation of creams

As creams are emulsions fatty bases, wax and different oils are used as oil phase and water as aqueous phase. Different emulsifiers are added to form emulsion or there is formation of soap by reaction between fatty acid and alkali during preparation of cream and this soap act as emulsifying agent (in-situ emulsification).

(i) **Preparation of oil phase:** Flake/powder ingredients, sometimes dry blended in advance, are dispersed into mineral oil or silicone oil. Heating may be required to melt some ingredients.

(ii) **Hydration of aqueous phase ingredients:** Emulsifiers, thickeners and stabilizers are dispersed into water in a separate vessel. Heating may be required to accelerate hydration.

(iii) **Forming the emulsion:** Both phases are mixed at same temperature under vigorous agitation to form the emulsion.

(iv) **Dispersion of the active ingredient:** The active ingredient often makes up only a small proportion of the formulation; this must be efficiently dispersed to maximize yield and product effectiveness. Generally, o/w creams are prepared at an elevated temperature and then cooled down to room temperature in order for the internal phase to solidify. The semi-solid form of a w/o cream is attributable to the character of the external phase.

(a) Oily creams (w/o)

These are hydrophobic creams and are usually anhydrous and absorb only small amounts of water. They contain w/o emulsifying agents such as wool fat, sorbitan esters, and monoglycerides.

Example: Oily cream /Hydrous ointment BP

Wool alcohols ointment	500 g
Phenoxyethanol	10 g
Dried magnesium sulphate	5 g
Purified water freshly boiled and cooled	485 g

Hydrous ointment is also known as oily cream. This is not an active ingredient as such, but works as a moisturizer by providing a layer of oil on the surface of the skin to prevent water evaporating from the skin surface. It is a very greasy moisturizer. It is made from a mixture of wool alcohols ointment and water, with Phenoxyethanol as an antimicrobial preservative.

Use: For all very dry skin conditions, particularly eczema and dermatitis.

Marketed products: Hydrous Ointment BP 500g (Pinewood Healthcare), AquaDerm® (Rxfarma)

(b) Aqueous creams (o/w)

These are hydrophilic creams contain bases that are miscible with water. They also contain o/w emulsifying agents such as sodium or triethanolamine soaps, sulfated fatty alcohols, and polysorbates combined, if necessary, with w/o emulsifying agents. These creams are essentially miscible with skin secretions.

Example: Aqueous cream, cetrimide cream, cetomacrogol cream.

Aqueous cream BP:

Emulsifying ointment	300 g
Phenoxyethanol	10 g
Purified water	690 g

Freshly boiled and cooled

Use: As an emollient for the symptomatic relief of dry skin conditions.

Marketed products: Aqueous Cream BP SLS Free (Zuche Pharmaceuticals Pvt. Ltd.), Aqueous Cream BP (Kingsley House Skincare).

(c) Cosmetic creams

These are both w/o and o/w types of creams used as cosmetic preparations.

Examples: All-purpose cream, baby cream, barrier cream, bleaching cream, cleansing cream, cold cream, hair cream, hand cream, vanishing cream.

Vanishing cream

Stearic acid XXX	24%
Potassium hydroxide	1%
Purified water	64%
Glycerin	10.5%
Perfume	0.5%

Use: Moisturizer and as foundation cream to hold face powder

Marketed products: Vanishing cream (LUSH), Afghan Snow (E. S. Patanwala Pvt. Ltd), Pond's

(d) Medicated creams

In this type of cream either w/o or o/w type of cream is used as base so as to carry medicaments.

Example: Hydrocortisone cream treat rashes like poison oak or poison ivy, psoriasis and eczema. Antibiotic creams are used to treat abrasions or small wounds and minor infections. Antifungal creams used in ringworm, *candida intertrigo* or *candida diaper* rash. Zinc oxide cream is used for sunblock activity and for infant diaper rash.

Terbinafine Hydrochloride 1% Cream

Terbinafine hydrochloride

Sodium hydroxide

Benzyl alcohol

Sorbitan stearate

Cetyl palmitate

Cetyl alcohol

Cetostearyl alcohol

Polysorbate 60

Isopropyl myristate

Purified water

Use: Antifungal cream

Marketed products: Lamisil[®] Cream (Novartis Pharmaceuticals UK Ltd.), Fungotek[®] Cream (FDC Ltd.), Exifine[®] Cream (Dr. Reddy's Lab), Terbicip[®] Cream (Cipla)

13.9 GELS

Gels are usually homogeneous, clear, semi-solid preparations consisting of a liquid phase within a three-dimensional polymeric matrix with physical or sometimes chemical cross-linkage by means of suitable gelling agents. Simply gels are semisolid preparations that contain small inorganic particles or large organic molecules interpenetrated by a liquid.

Gels are attractive delivery systems as they are simple to manufacture and suitable for administering drugs through skin, oral, buccal, ophthalmic, nasal, otic, and vaginal routes. They also provide intimate contact between the drug and the site of action or absorption. With the advancement in polymer science, gel – based systems that respond to specific biological or external stimuli like pH, temperature, ionic strength, enzymes, antigens, light, magnetic field, ultrasound, and electric current are being designed and evaluated as smart delivery systems for various applications.

Classification of Gels

(a) Hydrophilic gels: Hydrophilic gels are composed of the internal phase made of a polymer producing a coherent three-dimensional net-like structure, which fixes the liquid vehicle as the external phase. Intermolecular forces bind the molecules of the solvent to a polymeric net, thus decreasing the mobility of these molecules and producing a structured system with increased viscosity. Hydrophobic gel (oleogel) bases usually consist of liquid paraffin with polyethylene or fatty oils gelled with colloidal silica or aluminium or zinc soaps.

(b) Hydrophilic gels: Hydrophilic gel (hydrogel) bases usually consist of water, glycerol, or propylene glycol gelled with suitable agents such as tragacanth, starch, cellulose derivatives, carboxyvinyl polymers, and magnesium aluminium silicates.

(c) Non-Aqueous gels: Ethyl cellulose was successfully formulated as a nonaqueous gel with propylene glycol dicaprylate/dicaprate. The novel nonaqueous gel exhibited rheological profiles corresponding to a physically cross-linked three dimensional gel network, with suitable mechanical characteristics for use as a vehicle for topical drug delivery.

(d) Organogels: Sorbitan monostearate, a hydrophobic nonionic surfactant, and numbers of organic solvents such as hexadecane, isopropyl myristate, and a range of vegetable oils are present. Gelation is achieved by dissolving/dispersing the organogelator in hot solvent to produce an organic solution/dispersion, which, on cooling sets to the gel state.

(e) Controlled release gels: Drug delivery to nasal or ocular mucosa for either local or systemic action suffers from many obstacles. Gel formulations with suitable rheological and mucoadhesive properties increase the contact time at the site of absorption. However, drug release from the gel must be sustained if benefits are to be gained from the prolonged contact time. These gels are formed in simulated tear fluid at concentrations of polymer as low as 0.1%.

(f) Amphiphilic gels: Amphiphilic gels can be prepared by mixing the solid gelator like sorbitan monostearate or sorbitan monopalmitate and the liquid phase like liquid sorbitan esters or polysorbate and heating them at 60°C to form a clear isotropic sol phase, and cooling the sol phase to form an opaque semisolid at room temperature.

Amphiphilic gel microstructures consisted mainly of clusters of tubules of gelator molecules that had aggregated upon cooling of the sol phase, forming a 3D network throughout the continuous phase. The gels demonstrated thermoreversibility. Gelation temperature and viscosity increased with increasing gelator concentration, indicating a more robust gel network. At temperatures near the skin surface temperature, the gels softened considerably, this would allow topical application.

(g) Thermosensitive sol-gel reversible hydrogels: They are polymeric solutions which undergo reversible sol to gel transformation under the influence of environmental conditions like temperature and pH which results in in-situ hydrogel formation.

(h) Hydrogels: Hydrogels are gel systems in which water immobilized by insoluble polymer. The elements of hydrogels are water and a polymeric substance that is hydrophilic, but not water soluble. When exposed to water, the dry polymer swells and absorbs liquid. The polymer strands are cross-linked either chemically or by physical forces.

Formulation of gels

Gels are relatively easier to prepare compare to ointments and creams. Pharmaceutical gels primarily contain vehicle, gelling agents, buffers, preservatives, antioxidants, flavours/ sweetening agents and colours.

1. Vehicle

Purified water is the normal solvent/vehicle used in the formulation of pharmaceutical gels. However, co-solvents may be used, e.g. alcohol, propylene glycol, glycerol, polyethylene glycol (usually polyethylene glycol 400) to enhance the solubility of the therapeutic agent in the dosage form and/or (in the case of ethanol) to enhance drug permeation across the skin. If the drug has poor chemical stability and/or poor solubility in water or water-based vehicles, pharmaceutical gels may be formulated using polyhydroxy solvents, for example, propylene glycol, glycerol, polyethylene glycol 400 and polyacidic polymers, for example, poly (acrylic acid).

2. Gelling agents/ gel forming polymers

Polymer is simply a compound made-up of repeating units. Polymers are used to give the structural network which is essential for the preparation of gels. Gel forming bases or polymers is classified as follows:

(a) Natural polymers: Natural polymers are those polymers which exist naturally and can be synthesized by living bodies, for example, Proteins like collagen, gelatine etc and polysaccharides like agar, tragacanth, pectin and gum etc.

(b) Semi synthetic polymers: These polymers are mostly derived from natural polymers by chemical modification, for example, cellulose derivatives like carboxymethyl-cellulose, methylcellulose, hydroxypropyl cellulose and hydroxyethyle cellulose.

(c) Synthetic polymers: The polymers which are prepared in laboratories are called synthetic polymers. These are also called man made polymers, for example, Carbomer carbopol 940, carbopol 934, Poloxamer, Polyacrylamide, Polyvinyl alcohol and Polyethylene.

(d) Inorganic substances: Aluminium hydroxide and Bentonite.

(e) Surfactants: Sebrotearyle alcohol and Brij-96.

3. Buffers

As in other semisolid formulations, buffers (for example, phosphate, citrate) may be included in aqueous and hydro-alcoholic based gels to control the pH of the formulation.

4. Preservatives

Pharmaceutical gels require the inclusion of preservatives and, in general, the choice of preservatives is similar to that for ointments and pastes. Care should be taken while using certain preservatives, for example, parabens, phenolics, because they interact with the hydrophilic polymers used to prepare gels, thereby reducing the concentration of free (antimicrobially active) preservative in the formulation. Therefore, to compensate for this, the initial concentration of these preservatives should be increased.

5. Antioxidants

As in other semisolid formulations, antioxidants may be included in the formulation to increase the chemical stability of therapeutic agents that are prone to oxidative degradation. The choice of antioxidants is based on the nature of the vehicle used to prepare the pharmaceutical gel. Therefore, as the majority of pharmaceutical gels are aqueous-based, water-soluble antioxidants, for example, sodium metabisulphite, sodium formaldehyde sulphoxylate, are commonly used.

6. Flavouring/sweetening agents

Flavouring and sweetening agents are only included in pharmaceutical gels that are designed for administration into the oral cavity, for example, for the treatment of infection, inflammation or ulceration. Choice of sweetener/flavouring agents is dependent on the required taste, the type and concentration selected to mask the taste of the drug substance efficiently.

7. Coloring agents:

As per requirements FD&C certified colours can be used in pharmaceutical gels.

Methods of preparation of gels:

(a) **Fusion method:** In this method various waxy materials employed as gellant in non-polar media. Drug is added when waxy materials melted by fusion and stirred slowly until uniform gel formed.

(b) **Cold method:** Water is cooled to 4-10°C and placed it in mixing container. Gelling agent is slowly added and agitated until solution is complete. Temperature is maintained below 10°C. Drug is then added in solution form slowly with gentle mixing. Immediately transferred to container and allowed to warm to room temperature where liquid becomes clear gel.

(c) Dispersion method: Gelling agent is dispersed in water with stirring at 1200 r.p.m. for 30 min. Drug is dissolved in non-aqueous solvent with preservative. This solution is then added in above gel with continuous stirring.

Principles during gel formation

(a) Thermal changes: Solvated polymers (lipophilic colloids) when subjected to thermal changes causes gelatin. Many hydrogen formers are more soluble in hot than cold water. If the temperature is reducing, the degree of hydration is reduced and gelation occurs (Cooling of a concentrated hot solution will produce a gel), for example, Gelatin, agar sodium oleate, guar gum and cellulose derivatives etc. In contrast to this, some materials like cellulose ether have their water solubility to hydrogen bonding with the water. Raising the temperature of these solutions will disrupt the hydrogen bonding and reduced solubility, which will cause gelation.

(b) Flocculation: Here gelation is produced by adding just sufficient quantity of salt to precipitate to produce age state but insufficient to bring about complete precipitation. It is necessary to ensure rapid mixing to avoid local high concentration of precipitant, for example, solution of ethyl cellulose, polystyrene in benzene can be gelled by rapid mixing with suitable amounts of a non-solvent such as petroleum ether. The addition of salts to hydrophobic solution brings about coagulation and gelation is rarely observed. The gels formed by flocculation are thixotropic in behaviour. Hydrophilic colloids such as gelatin, proteins and acacia are only affected by high concentration of electrolytes, when the effect is to "salt out", the colloidal and gelation doesn't occur.

(c) Chemical reaction: In this principle gel is produced by chemical inter action between the solute and solvent, for example, aluminium hydroxide gel can be prepared by interaction in aqueous solution of an aluminium salt and sodium carbonate an increased concentration of reactants will produce a gel structure. Few other examples that involve chemical reaction between PVA, cyanoacrylates with Glycidol ether (Glycidol), toluene diisocyanates (TDI), methane diphenyl isocyanine (MDI) that cross-links the polymeric chain.

Examples:

Luxitop® Gel: Clindamycin phosphate-1.0 w/w (Luxica Pharma),

Clinderm Gel: Clindamycin-10 mg (Agio Pharmaceuticals Limited), used to treat acne. It helps to decrease the number of acne lesions.

Metrogyl V Gel: Metronidazole (Lekar Pharma), used to treat certain types of bacterial infections in the vagina (bacterial vaginosis)

Candid Gel: Clotrimazole (Glenmark Pharmaceuticals Ltd.), prevent fungal growth on skin.

Packaging and Storage

The packaging material, i.e., the container and closure system, should be compatible with the components of the formulation. Leaching from the container and closure system can increase the unknown degradable substances. Semisolid preparations are packaged either in large-mouth ointment jars or in metal or plastic collapsible tubes, tight containers, or other well-closed containers. Semisolid preparations must be stored in well-closed containers to protect against contamination and in a cool place to protect against product separation in heat. In some cases, special storage conditions are recommended: for example, protect from light, avoid exposure to excessive heat, avoid exposure to direct sunlight, avoid strong fluorescent lighting, do not refrigerate, and avoid prolonged exposure to temperatures exceeding 30°C. When required, light-sensitive preparations are packaged in opaque or light-resistant containers. In addition to the usual labeling requirements for pharmaceutical products, various pharmacopoeia directs the labeling for certain ointments and creams include the type of base used (for example, water soluble or water insoluble). The auxiliary label "For External Use Only" is required on all topical semisolid dosage forms.

Topical semi-solid dosage forms should be kept in well-closed containers. The preparation should maintain its pharmaceutical integrity throughout shelf-life when stored at the temperature indicated on the label; the temperature should normally not exceed 25°C. Special storage recommendations or limitations are indicated in individual monographs.

13.10 EVALUATION OF SEMI SOLID DOSAGE FORMS

Semisolid dosage forms are evaluated for various pharmacopeial and non-pharma-copeial tests to ascertain their physicochemical, microbial, *in-vitro*, and *in-vivo* characteristics. These tests help in retaining their quality and minimizing the batch-to-batch variations. Following are some common test performed for semisolid dosage forms:

(a) **Homogeneity and Surface Morphology:** The homogeneity of semisolid formulation is usually assessed by visual inspection and the surface morphology (of gel) by using scanning electron microscopy.

(b) **Minimum fill test:** This test is performed to compare the weight or volume of product filled into each container with their labelled weight or volume. It helps in assessing the content uniformity of product. A minimum - fill test is applied only to those containers that contain no more than 150 g or mL of preparation. It is performed in two steps. Initially, labels from the product containers are removed. After washing and drying the surface, their weights are recorded (W_1). In the second step, the entire product from each container is removed. After cleaning and drying, the weight of empty containers is recorded (W_2). The difference between total weight (W_1) and empty - container weight (W_2) gives the weight of product. The USP recommends that the average net content of 10 containers should not be less than the labeled amount. If the product weight is less than 60 g or mL, the net content of any single container should not be less than 90% of the labeled amount. If the product weight is between 60 and 150 g or mL, the net content of any single container should not be less than 95% of the labeled amount. If these limits are not met, the test is repeated with an additional 20 containers. All semisolid topical preparations should meet these specifications.

(c) Water Content: The presence of minor quantities of water may alter the microbial, physical, and chemical stability of ointments and creams. Titrimetric methods (Method-I) are usually performed for determining the water content in these preparations. These methods are based on the quantitative reaction between water and anhydrous solution of sulfur and iodine in the presence of a buffer that can react with hydrogen ions. Special titration setups and reagents (Karl Fischer, KF) are used in these determinations.

(d) pH: One gram of semisolid formulation is dissolved in 100 mL distilled water and stored for two hours. The pH is determined by using digital pH meter. In gel formulation many gelling agents show pH - dependent gelling behaviour. They show highest viscosity at their gel point. Determination of pH is therefore important to maintain consistent quality.

(e) Leakage Test: This test is mandatory for ophthalmic ointments, which evaluates the intactness of the ointment tube and its seal. Ten sealed containers are selected, and their exterior surfaces are cleaned. They are horizontally placed over absorbent blotting paper and maintained at 60 ± 3°C for 8 h. The test passes if leakage is not observed from any tube. If leakage is observed, the test is repeated with an additional 20 tubes. The test passes if not more than 1 tube shows leakage out of 30 tubes.

(f) Microbial Screening: Semisolid preparations are required to be free from any microbial contamination. Hence, most of the topical semisolid formulations are screened for the presence of *Staphylococcus aureus* and *Pseudomonas aeruginosa*. In some cases, screening for *Escherichia coli, Salmonella species*, and total aerobic microbial counts is recommended by the USP. In addition, preparations meant for rectal, vaginal, and urethral applications are tested for yeasts and molds. Suitable official microbiological methods are used to screen presence of micro-organism. The plate method or multiple - tube method is performed to estimate the total aerobic microbial counts.

(g) Drug content/Assay: The quantity of drug present in a unit weight or volume of semisolid dosage form is determined by various methods. Spectrophotometric, titrimetric, chromatographic, and in some cases microbial assays are performed. Selection of a particular method is based on the nature of drug, its concentration in the product, interference between the drug and other formulation components, and official requirements.

(h) Rheological Studies: Viscosity measurement for consistency determination is often the quickest, most accurate, reliable method to characterize semisolid formulations. It gives an idea about the ease with which formulation can be processed, handled, or used. Some of the commonly used tests for characterizing rheology of gels are yield stress, critical strain, and creep. Yield stress refers to the stress that must be exceeded to induce flow. This helps in characterizing the flow nature of non-Newtonian systems. Critical strain or gel strength refers to the minimum energy needed to disrupt the gel structure. Higher the critical strain, the better the physical integrity of gel systems. Creep or recovery helps in assessing the strength of bonds in a gel structure.

Based on the nature of the test material, different techniques are employed to measure the rheological parameters of semisolid formulations. Very sophisticated automatic equipment is commercially available for measurements. Cup - and - bob viscometers and cone - and - plate viscometers are widely used for viscous liquids and gels. Commercially available viscometers include Brookfield rotational viscometers, Haake rheometers, Schott viscoeasy rotational viscometers, Malvern viscometers, and Ferranti - Shirley cone - and - plate viscometers.

(i) Spread ability: One of the criteria for semisolid formulation to meet the ideal qualities is that it should possess good spreadability. It is the term expressed to denote the extent of area to which formulation readily spreads on application to skin or affected part. The therapeutic efficacy of a formulation also depends upon its spreading value.

About 500 mg of the test formulation is sandwiched between two slides, of 6×2 cm dimension each. The lower slide is fixed on the board of the apparatus and the upper slide is tied to a non-flexible string to which load (for example, 20 g) is applied with the help of a simple pulley. The time taken for the upper slide to travel the distance of 6 cm and separate from the lower slide under the influence of weight is noted.

Spreadability is calculated using following equation:

$$\text{Spread ability} = \frac{w.l}{t} \qquad \qquad \text{... (13.4)}$$

where, w is the weight tied to the upper slide (for example, 20 g), l is the length of the glass slide (6 cm) and t is the time in seconds.

(j) Extrudability: It is a usual empirical test to measure the force required to extrude the material from tube. The extrudability of the formulation is determined using extrudability apparatus in terms of mass in grams required to extrude 0.5 cm. ribbon of gel in 10 seconds.

(k) *In-vitro* drug release study: These studies are conducted to ascertain release of drug from the formulation matrix. Open - chamber diffusion cells such as Franz diffusion cells are used for performing in vitro studies. These cells consist of a donor side and a receiver side separated by a synthetic membrane such as cellulose acetate/nitrate mixed ester, polysulfone, or polytetrafluoroethylene. The membranes are usually pretreated with the receiver fluid to avoid any lag phase in drug release. The receiver side is filled with a known volume of release medium and is heated to $32 \pm 0.5°C$ by circulating warm water through an outer jacket. Aqueous buffers are used for water - soluble drugs. Phosphate buffer solution of pH 5.4 is considered most appropriate for dermatological products as it mimics the pH of skin. Hydro-alcoholic or other suitable medium may also be used for sparingly water soluble drugs. A known quantity of the test product is applied uniformly over the membrane on the donor side and samples are withdrawn from the receiver side at different time intervals. After each sampling, an equal volume of fresh medium is replaced to the receiver side. The receiver samples are analyzed by a suitable analytical method to quantify the amount of drug released from the formulation at different time intervals.

(l) *Ex-vivo* penetration study: *Ex-vivo* studies are carried out to examine the permeation of drug from semisolid through the skin or any other biological membrane. As with in vitro release studies, *ex-vivo* penetration is conducted using vertical diffusion cells or modified cells with flow - through design. In this case, the receiver side is filled with phosphate buffer solution of pH 7.4 to simulate the biological pH of human blood. Skin samples from different animal sources such as rats, rabbits, pigs, and human cadavers are used for screening dermatological products. The stratum corneum layer of the skin is separated from the dermis before mounting onto the diffusion cells. The epidermis is separated by immersing the skin sample in normal saline or purified water which is maintained at 60°C for 2 min followed by immersion into cold water for 30 sec. This layer is mounted between the donor and receiver sides and studies are conducted after application of test formulation over the surface of the stratum corneum in the donor side. Samples are withdrawn at different time intervals and analyzed for drug permeation by suitable analytical techniques.

(m) Skin Irritation and sensitivity study: In general, no semisolid formulation should possess irritant effect to eyes (in case of ophthalmic semisolid preparation) and on the skin or mucous membranes. The tests for irritancy can be carried out on the skin and eyes of rabbits or the skin in rats. Reactions are noted at intervals of 24, 48, 72 and 96 hours. Lesions on cornea, iris, conjunctiva are used for judging the irritancy to the eyes. Presence of patches on the skin within 2 weeks indicates irritancy to skin.

As various types of ingredients are used in semisolid formulation; there is a possibility of sensitization or photosensitization of the skin. Hence this sensitivity should be tested. This test is normally done by 'patch test'. The test sample is applied along with a standard market product at different places and effect is compared after a period of time.

(n) Stability studies: The stability studies of semisolid dosage forms are carried out as per ICH guideline. Preparations are placed at respective temperature and relative humidity as specified in guidelines and tested for various quality parameters after specified period of time.

MODEL QUESTIONS

1. Define semisolid dosage form. Give its advantages and disadvantages.
2. Classify and define various semisolid dosage forms.
3. Discuss mechanisms of dermal penetration of drug.
4. Discuss factors affecting dermal penetration of drug.
5. Classify various excipients used in semisolid dosage form.
6. Define and classify various types of ointments.
7. Classify and discuss various ointment bases.
8. Give advantages and disadvantages of ointment.
9. Comment on advantages and disadvantages of water soluble bases.
10. Comment on mechanism of penetration enhancers.
11. Discuss various methods of ointment preparation.
12. What are pastes? Give its silent features. Comment on preparation of paste.
13. What are creams. Classify them with suitable examples.

14. What are gels? What is principle behind gel formation?

15. Classify gels and enlist components used in preparation of gels.

16. Discuss in detail various tests used to evaluate semisolid dosage forms.

17. Write a short note on:

    (i)   Fusion method

    (ii) Trituration method

    (iii) Aqueous and oily creams

    (iv) Pastes

    (v)   Creams

    (vi) Gels

■■■

■■■